Health
Education

Health Education

A Process for Human Effectiveness

David A. Bedworth
State University College at Brockport

Albert E. Bedworth
New York State Education Department

Harper & Row, Publishers
NEW YORK, HAGERSTOWN, SAN FRANCISCO, LONDON

Sponsoring Editor: Jeffrey K. Smith
Project Editor: David Nickol
Designer: Katrine Stevens
Production Supervisor: Stefania J. Taflinska
Compositor: Maryland Linotype Composition Co., Inc.
Printer and binder: The Maple Press Company
Art Studio: Vantage Art Inc.

Health Education: A Process for Human Effectiveness

Library of Congress Cataloging in Publication Data

Bedworth, David A
  Health education.

  Includes bibliographical references and index.
  1. Health education. I. Bedworth, Albert E. joint author. II. Title.
RA440.B4   613'.07'1   77-21043
ISBN 0-06-040575-9

To Shirley and Susi,
for Their Love, Devotion,
Encouragement, and Patience.
To Jodi and Michael,
Who Represent the Future of Humanity

Contents

Part Three

The School/Community Health Education Program 185

Appendixes

Index   377

Preface

Health Education: A Process for Human Effectiveness was written because of the belief that there exists a critical need for a textbook that will bring into perspective current thinking about the philosophy and practice of health education. To accomplish this, the text emphasizes the psychological and sociological implications, rather than the biological and pathological foundations of health and education. Great emphasis is placed upon the complex processes necessary for the development of positive health behavior without ignoring the vital role that the acquisition of accurate health knowledge can and does have on establishing attitudes which ultimately direct this behavior. This book, therefore, provides the basic and essential understandings for health educators to develop and conduct health education programs that are health-oriented rather than disease-oriented.

Health Education: A Process for Human Effectiveness is a precursory effort which recognizes the scope of vital health issues, the potential for prevention, the role of education, and the need to deal with health problems within the context of the entire health care system. Both the philosophical basis and the practice of health education are described in terms of the needs and capabilities of people and the factors that influence their development and actualization. Emphasis is placed on the promotion of health and the prevention of disease, disability, and premature death. This is a distinct departure from some traditional philosophies of health education but consistent with national and international philosophies. Prevention through the promotion of health is the only viable solution to the costly (in terms of disability, death, and economics) therapeutic approaches that emphasize treatment. Methods by which the health educator can depart from these traditional practices are thoroughly discussed.

The fundamental philosophy underlying *Health Education: A Process for Human Effectiveness* is that health education consists of two major components which are inseparably interrelated. They are (1) the educational process, which is predicated upon the behavioral sciences, and (2) the health education content (information), which is predicated upon the findings of the health sciences. Their interrelatedness is given great emphasis throughout the text.

The book is intended as a basic text for the training of health educators regardless of what their primary interests may be—school health, community health, or clinical health. In this regard, the text is forward-looking, stressing the similarities of the three types of health educators as well as their distinct responsibilities; and stressing behavioral outcomes and experientially directed health learning related to the needs, goals, and characteristics of the learner. Since the health of people is determined by and dependent upon a variety of complex personal and social factors that are in constant interaction, this text brings them into proper perspective. It is this perspective that is essential if health education is to become stimulating, exciting, challenging, meaningful—a process for human effectiveness. Health problems can be solved only when educators, community leaders, and medical and other health professionals recognize the need to work together in a deliberate, concerted effort.

Since health education philosophy and practice are dynamic, changing as new discoveries become available, the book establishes a basis for a sound philosophy, but one that is adaptable to new conditions. Moreover, it is intended to stimulate thought and debate about what is presently known about health education and what future trends can be. The "Problems for Discussion" at the end of each chapter go beyond simple recall of information presented. They can provide the basis for health education students to begin to clarify their own understandings, provide greater insight into the whole complex area of health education, and help students begin to recognize that it is not, and should not be, a standardized course of study for all learners. In addition, each chapter is briefly summarized through the inclusion of a "Definitive Understandings" section. Its chief purpose is to provide the student with the major concepts discussed in the chapter and to clarify the ideas presented. In this regard, the book strives to provide a background for clarity of thought for personalizing the formulation of a philosophy of health education that is functional. The book is not intended to provide simple recipes to be followed by all health educators. To accomplish these complex goals, the book is organized into three major parts.

Part One, "Philosophical Foundations of Health Education," consists of four chapters that emphasize the necessity for the development of a philosophy of health education and discuss the various factors that influence health, the evolutionary patterns of health education, and the bases for health education. Chapter 1, "Why a Philosophy of Health Education?" not only answers the question, but explores many of the factors known to be the building blocks of effective health education programs. It emphasizes the necessity for students of health education to formulate their own philosophy as the guidepost for professional practice as health educators.

Since health itself is a complex concept, Chapter 2, "What Is Health?" describes in detail the factors affecting health, as well as the numerous ways in which it can be perceived and achieved. The student of health education will acquire a rather profound understanding of this elusive term and the most fundamental influence education has on the attainment of health.

Chapter 3, "Health Education in Transition," brings together the ecological forces affecting health education and describes a forward-looking model for a health care system with health education as its most basic element. In this regard, myths about health education are dispelled so that the reader can begin to develop a philosophy of health education based upon acceptable principles rather than on myths or obsolete notions.

The culminating chapter of Part One, "Bases for Health Education," provides a clear understanding of the chief elements that are recognized by health education authorities as those that constitute an effective program of health education. It describes the goals of health education, the importance of informational content, the scope and purpose of health education and introduces the importance and distinctions regarding learner and teacher objectives as the elements that direct the process of health learning.

Since current as well as future health education places great emphasis upon the importance of psychological and sociological influences, Part Two, "Psychological/Sociological Perspective of Health Education," consists of four chapters which stress the relation of human needs to health, how health contributes to human effectiveness, the principles of learning as a basis for health educational processes, and the role of human motivation.

Chapter 5, "Dimensions of Human Health Needs," directs attention to both the biological and psychosocial needs as powerful motivating forces that affect both health status and health learning. The chapter describes how needs and the means for satisfying them may be misinterpreted by the child or youth and become a vital factor in self-destructive behavior. In addition, concern is expressed about the need for health education programs to be based upon the recognition that learners must be helped to satisfy their needs in the most constructive way possible.

Chapter 6, "Health and Human Effectiveness," emphasizes the relationship of health and human effectiveness. A healthy person has the capacity for functioning effectively. Similarly, people with a handicap can function more effectively if appropriate changes in themselves or the environment are made. The chapter directs attention toward the holistic quality of people, the way they grow and develop, and the effects of health education on health and disease. In this regard, the similarities and differences of people are discussed as a basis for health education programs and methodologies to be used.

Since the educational process is concerned with learning, experiences provided the learner must be consistent with what is known about the psychology of learning. Chapter 7, "Principles of Learning Applied to Health Education," not only discusses how learning takes place, but describes how health education programs can be developed for maximum effectiveness along these lines.

One of the most perplexing problems that a health educator faces daily is how to motivate learning for all learners. Chapter 8, "Motivating for Health Learning," describes the basis for motivation and provides practical suggestions for applying strategies that will motivate learning.

Part Three, "The School/Community Health Education Program," directs attention to the practice of health education, building upon the philosophy and principles discussed in Parts One and Two. The practice of health education is predicated upon five interactional elements which compose a comprehensive health education program. These elements are discussed in the five chapters which constitute Part Three.

Chapter 9, "Professional Preparation of the Health Educator," discusses the importance of adequate training of the health educator, the need for establishing standards for developing competency, and how this can best be achieved. Attention is also given to the roles, both distinctive and common, of the school, public, and patient health educators as they function within their particular areas of responsibilities.

No health education program can survive long or be effective if it is not adequately organized and administered. Chapter 10, "Organizing for Health Education/Theory and Practice," describes the principles of organization, administration, and supervision of comprehensive health education programs and how these principles apply to school, public, and patient health education. Emphasis is again placed upon the need for the health administrator to be highly trained and skilled as an administrator as well as a health educator.

Chapter 11, "Curriculum Development in Health Education," describes the principles of curriculum development, the purpose and importance of written curriculum guidelines, and how to most effectively develop and implement these. The chapter presents several alternative designs and describes their advantages and disadvantages. No attempt is made to prescribe a particular design, since curriculum development is essentially a personal and individualized process.

The culmination of teacher preparation, organizing the program, and developing the curriculum is the application of these to the learning of children, youth, and adults. Chapter 12, "Health Education Methodology/Theory and Practice," discusses the varieties of methods that have been used and are still being used in health education programs throughout the country. It describes the basis for method selection, the advantages of some methods over others and relates these to the principles of learning and learner characteristics discussed earlier in the text, emphasizing strategies and techniques for motivating and individualizing health learning.

Chapter 13, "Evaluation in Health Education," emphasizes both the need for and the purpose of carefully planned and continuous evaluation of all aspects of the health education program. It describes the principles of evaluation and presents suggestions for the development of evaluative instruments. In addition, specific evaluative criteria are presented for adaptation in evaluating certain aspects of the health education program.

Each chapter contains illustrations of the relationships of the chief concepts being discussed. These illustrations are intended to add a visual dimension to understanding. They are included as a supplement for the reader and to ensure an understanding of the printed word. They are not intended for memorization, but rather for concept development.

Appendixes A and B consist of a glossary and resource list, respectively. The glossary is included for two purposes: (1) many terms used in health education are not included in the text but are important for a complete understanding of health education, and (2) the student of health education will find it valuable for quick reference and concise meanings of terms. The sources of health education resources is included to assist the health educator in locating learning aids that can be used by themselves or in conjunction with the teaching/learning process.

Appendixes C and D are provided for those readers who are interested in learning more details about the Health Systems Agency legislation and applying the principles and philosophy of health education presented in the position paper developed by the American Public Health Association.

It is important to state that the ideas presented in this book are those of the authors and in no way necessarily represent those policies of the State University of New York or of the New York State Education Department.

Finally, we would be remiss if we did not give recognition to the many people who provided us with guidance, suggestions, criticisms, and motivation, but most of all encouragement in writing this book. We gratefully acknowledge their assistance and extend our sincere thanks. We wish we could name them all, but we know they will understand. However, we would like to acknowledge Lucretia Dickson, who prepared the typed manuscript in its entirety and who sacrificed her personal time for this important endeavor.

The future does not belong to those who are content with today, apathetic toward common problems and their fellow man alike, timid and fearful in the face of new ideas and bold projects. Rather it will belong to those who can blend passion, reason, and courage in a personal commitment to the ideals and great enterprises of American society.

Robert F. Kennedy

A new era is about to dawn upon the health education profession. Never before has the profession provided such great potential for its success; and yet, never has the profession been confronted with such great obstacles that threaten its success.

AEB
DAB

Part One

Philosophical
Foundations
of Health
Education

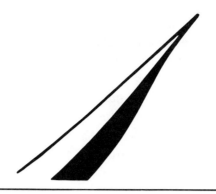

Why a
Philosophy
of Health
Education?

During the last few years a number of loosely related developments, both in and out of health education have converged, generated new social forces, a ferment of new ideas and new methods. All the signs are that once again health education is in a state of profound, even radical change.

Godfrey M. Hochbaum

The philosophy and practice of health education must take into account the multidimensional nature of people, their similarities and differences as determined by heredity and environment, and the cultural impact on health.

AEB
DAB

INTRODUCTION

Why health education?

On a very limited scale, scientists have succeeded in creating certain environments that are nearly perfect for human survival. One example is the interior of a space vehicle. It is relatively free of hazards, and the food for the astronaut is scientifically controlled. Astronauts receive training in which they learn precisely every move they must make and the exact times to make them if they are to survive their journey into space and return safely. Vital physiological signs are constantly monitored by precise scientific apparatus, which feed the data into computers to be sorted and interpreted. The slightest fluctuation of any kind or any indication of malfunctioning is immediately detected and diagnosed, and a treatment is prescribed if needed.

Not so in the real world. Not only is the environment not adequately controlled, but it is in a constant state of change, much of which is deterioration. Generally, people are left to their own devices to detect symptoms of physical or mental malfunctioning. Worst of all, medical personnel and other health personnel and facilities are often inadequate. *Consequently, we all must endeavor to learn what to do to stay healthy and what to do if there are signs that health is threatened.* We must also learn to distinguish between minor and serious health-threatening circumstances. In other words, people must learn to depend to a great extent upon themselves to maintain their health and to avoid hazardous situations. (This is discussed in more detail in Chapter 2.)

Therefore, it is the responsibility of social institutions to provide people with the opportunity to learn how to behave in order to preserve their health. This is unquestionably one of the most basic and vital functions of government. However, it is a responsibility that is too frequently preempted by other political priorities. Ironically, unless health is preserved and the environmental factors that threaten it are reduced or eliminated, society will not survive, for the adaptability of people, as with other forms of life, has limitations, and human extinction becomes a definite possibility.

Definitions

It is important to begin with a basic understanding of some of the terms associated with health education. Here we will define in simple terms *health, education,* and *health education* as a point of departure. In subsequent chapters these and other terms will be explored in some depth as they relate to specific elements of the educational program.

Health is usually defined as the quality of a person's physical, psychological, and sociological functioning that enables him or her to deal adequately with self and others in a variety of situations. *Education* is a complex process of experiences that influences a person's self-perception in relation to the social and physical environments. *Health education* incorporates both of these definitions in one educational discipline. All of those experiences—planned or unplanned, direct or indirect—affect the way learners think, feel, and act in regard to their own health as well as that of the community in which they live.

What is philosophy?

Historically, the beginnings of educational philosophy lie deep in the roots of primitive societies. Primitive people stressed education in those activities necessary to satisfy basic physical needs, religious training necessary to pacify the spirits, and training in tribal customs and taboos deemed important to observe if members were to live effectively together. This was their curriculum, and upon analysis, it is not radically different from current curricula. Their education, in short, consisted of the training judged to be vital for survival.

Simply speaking, philosophy is wisdom of the nature of things. It is a comprehension of the principles of reality, a body of knowledge that defines the perimeters of life and living. The philosophy of health education, therefore, includes the beliefs, concepts, attitudes, and theory of individual health educators and the profession in general. It sets the boundaries of practice, clarifying the areas of professional concentration; it is the cable that binds theory and practice.

PRINCIPLES OF HEALTH EDUCATION PHILOSOPHY

Philosophical dimensions

The health education profession consists of two fundamental dimensions: (1) its philosophical dimensions, and (2) its areas of practice. The philosophical dimensions are derived from the psychological, sociological, and biological sciences, which provide knowledge about the history, present research, and future expectations of the health of people. The principles governing the formulation of a philosophy are derived from both experiential and research data accumulated in the past, but especially from the knowledge and judgment of health authorities acquired in recent years. These principles emanate from (1) the present state of health affairs, (2) future health expectations, which become the forerunner for establishing purposes, goals, and practices, and (3) the efficacy of present practices, which provide the foundation and motivation for change. *In the final analysis, one's philosophy of health education is subjective, since it is based upon the way one perceives the factors surrounding it.* In developing a personal philosophy of health education, it is desirable to come to grips with what is, as well as with

The principles and philosophy of health education penetrate every aspect of the program and are the foundation for all practices that eventually ensue.

QUALITY OF THE HEALTH TEACHER AND ADMINISTRATOR PRE-EDUCATION AND POST-EDUCATION	QUALITY OF ORGANIZATION AND ADMINISTRATION OF THE HEALTH PROGRAM	QUALITY OF CURRICULUM DEVELOPMENT IN HEALTH EDUCATION	QUALITY OF TEACHING AND LEARNING METHODS, STRATEGIES, AND TECHNIQUES	QUALITY OF PROGRAM EVALUATION AND ADAPTATION

PHILOSOPHY AND PRINCIPLES OF HEALTH EDUCATION

what can be. Health professionals must recognize the constraints that exist, hoping to overcome them, but must also set their goals high, hoping to reach them. In this regard, a sound philosophy of health education should contain a high degree of pragmatism, seasoned generously with idealism.

Areas of practice

No philosophy of health education is of much value unless it results in practices that affect the health behavior of people and ultimately their health status. These practices are classified as (1) *professional preparation* of health educators, (2) *organization and administration* of the school/community health program, (3) *theory and application of curriculum development*, (4) *educational methodology and its application* to the health learning of people, and (5) *evaluation* of the effectiveness of the health program and its revisions for improvement. Although the philosophy of health education directly affects these areas of practice, it can in turn be affected by the differing interpretations that can and do change philosophy. This constitutes a cyclic phenomenon.

HISTORICAL BASIS

Primitive roots

What has history told us both from the viewpoint of health and the role education has played? Health education has always existed in one form or another from primitive times to the present and will always be needed as long as people exist. Certainly, the characteristics of today's health education have little in common with those of even a few decades ago; over the centuries, philosophy and practices have been quite different, but one aim has not changed markedly. Simply, this aim is to provide the essential knowledge necessary for survival. Today, we would expand that aim to include assisting individuals and society in living to full capacity by development of individual self-sufficiency.

Health movement

Health education has always been in a state of change. It has never "arrived," and it is likely that it never really will. This is basically because people and the way they live are constantly changing: new discoveries are being made about health; the health problems that confront us are changing, and it is even possible that we will, as we have in the past, create new and unheard-of health problems in the future.

It would serve little purpose to discuss in detail all of the events that have led to our present state of health education. However, a familiarity with some of the more significant health movements can result in a perspective that is important in understanding the various phases of development in school health that have occurred over the past century and a half. They will form a partial basis for the formulation of a personal philosophy of health education. Table 1–1 outlines these events.*

Historical developments in health and health education are frequently categorized according to certain historical periods. Anderson and Creswell[1] describe these periods as (1) *Egyptian* health practice from primitive peoples to 1000 B.C.; (2) *Hebrew* health code about 1500–500 B.C.; (3) *Greek* approach to health about 1000–200 B.C., (4) *Roman* health promotion about 100 B.C.–A.D. 500; (5) *Asceticism—Dark Ages—* 400–1000; (6) *Revival of concept of a sound body*, 1096–1248; (7) the premodern period of health—health from 1500 to 1800, and (8) *Modern era* of health—1850 to the present. The modern era is further divided into the miasma phase (1850–1880), the bacteriological phase (1880–1920), the positive health phase (1920–1960), and the social engineering phase (1960 to present). The characteristics of these periods were, respectively, (1) personal cleanliness, (2) formulation of a health code to include personal cleanliness and public health measures, (3) emphasis on a sound body, (4) sanitary engineering, (5) spiritual development, (6) sound body, (7) no unified health program, (8) odor-free environment, bacterial cause of disease, promotion of health, public health education, and other advancements in hygiene, and the health sciences.

Over the years, health education has undergone profound changes in its whole nature—philosophy, principles, purposes, and practices.

---

*For a more detailed discussion of these events, the reader is referred to Anderson, C. L., and William H. Creswell Jr., *School Health Practice*, the C. V. Mosby Company, Saint Louis, 1976, chapter 1; Jenne, Frank H., and Walter H. Greene, *Turner's School Health and Health Education*, the C. V. Mosby Company, Saint Louis, 1976, chapter 2; Means, Richard K., *Historical Perspectives on School Health*, Charles B. Slack, Inc., New Jersey, 1975.

TABLE 1–1 Significant Events Affecting Health Education

Date	Event
1842	Horace Mann advocated health instruction for school children.
1850	Report of the Sanitary Commission of Massachusetts by Lemuel Shattuck, advocating the teaching of physiology in all schools. This public health report recognized the value of health of the individual for adequate functioning.
1872	The first school medical inspector was employed by the Elmira (New York) Board of Education. The purpose was to deal with the smallpox crisis.
1875	The Women's Christian Temperance Union influenced legislation in 38 states requiring the teaching of the evils of alcohol, tobacco, and narcotics.
1880	The child health movement inaugurated the concept of child study as one basis for school activities.
1894	The first health examination in schools began in Boston. This concept spread to Chicago in 1895, New York in 1897, and Philadelphia in 1898. New York State passed legislation relative to alcohol education.
1899	Connecticut passed a law requiring the testing of vision of school children.
1903	The first school dentist was employed (Reading, Pennsylvania). Vermont required eye, ear, nose, and throat examination of *public* school children.
1904	The National Association for the Study and Prevention of Tuberculosis was founded.
1909	The American Association for the Study and Prevention of Infant Mortality was founded. Physical educators recognized that health was not synonymous with physical education.
1910	The First White House Conference on Child Health and Protection was held.
1914	A school health demonstration in Baltimore indicated that instruction in health could change a child's health behavior significantly.
1916	New York State passed legislation requiring physical education in the schools. The Child Health Organization of America was founded. It pioneered the acceptance of health education in the school curriculum.
1918	Health was established as the primary objective of education by the Commission on the Reorganization of Secondary Education. The Child's Health Organization was founded.
1922	The Massachusetts Institute of Technology conducted a two-year school health demonstration program in Malden,

TABLE 1–1 Significant Events Affecting Health Education (continued)

Date	Event
	Massachusetts, under the direction of Dr. C. E. Turner. The American Red Cross replicated this in Mansfield and Richland Counties in Ohio.
1923	The American Child Health Association was founded as a result of a merger between the Child Health Organization and the American Child Hygiene Association.
1930	The Second White House Conference on Child Health and Protection was held.
1935	Integration of all elements of the school health program was initiated. Health services, health instruction, and healthful living evolved.
1941	The Joint Committee on Health Problems in Education of the NEA and AMA published *Health Education*, a standard text for the profession today.
1942–1948	The W. K. Kellogg Foundation sponsored a school-community health project. It established the importance of cooperation between school and community health professionals.
1944	The American Council on Education recognized health objectives in its publication *A Design for General Education*.
1945	The charter *Suggested School Health Policies* was released by the National Committee on School Health Policies of the National Conference for Cooperation in Health Education.
1948, 1949, 1950, 1953, 1955	National Conferences on Professional Training in health education were held.
1950	The Mid-Century White House Conference on Children and Youth was held.
1971	Coalition of National Health Organizations was formed, made up of eight health organizations in the United States.
1973	The final report of the President's Committee on Health Education was released, calling for the establishment of a National Center for Health Education.
1974	The Bureau of Health Education was officially established as part of the Center for Disease Control under the authorization of the Secretary of HEW. The National Health Planning and Resources Development Act of 1974 was enacted.
1975	More than 60 bills with at least one health education component were before the Congress.
1976	The National Center for Health Education was established as a result of the recommendations of the President's Committee on Health Education.

Periods of drastic and significant advances brought about by social and political upheaval, new awareness of important health issues, and technological advances in the health and behavioral sciences have frequently occurred in the past. One such era, according to Hochbaum,[2] occurred about 1950, when new concepts of the nature and purpose of health education emerged. This resulted in the introduction of new approaches and new ways of preparing health professionals.

School health education study

A little more than a decade later (1961) the School Health Education Study (SHES) was conducted under the direction of Elena Sliepcevich. The results of this extensive research on the quality of health education practices revealed the need for new directions in curriculum design. A writing team of distinguished authorities was assembled and set out to study the literature on social changes, contemporary thought and practice, and what directions curriculum development was taking in other school disciplines. From this research emerged the "conceptual approach" to curriculum design. (Details of this approach are described in Chapter 11.)

Drug abuse crisis—1960s

Another example is the social upheaval that resulted from the massive drug abuse crisis of the late 1960s. Society's recognition of the extent of the drug problem affecting large numbers of young people in all walks of life resulted in a social and, in many instances, a political mandate to launch educational programs to reverse the trends of this critical health problem. Many states enacted legislation along these lines. However, since society's perception of the problem was tainted with misconceptions from the past, many actions were misdirected, being concerned primarily with treatment rather than causes and prevention.

New York State was one of the leaders in bringing about a new awareness of the urgent need to initiate educational programs that would concentrate efforts on the drug problem. Recognizing the need to keep this emphasis within the boundaries of a comprehensive health education program, New York enacted the landmark legislation Chapter 787 of the Education Laws of New York State. The late New York State Senator Edward Speno spearheaded the movement. Figure 1–2 provides the text of this law. It is important to mention that this law laid the foundation for, and stimulated enactment of, similar legislation in many other states. An analysis of this law reveals the extraordinary insight into the problem of combatting drug abuse.* In 1969, Senator Speno

---

* It's interesting to note that this law appropriated only $250,000 for five years to establish preventive education programs, while more than $51 million per year was appropriated for treatment and rehabilitation of drug addicts.

FIGURE 1–2   Education—Critical Health Problems—Five Year Program
CHAPTER 787
An Act directing the commissioner of education to establish a five year program
for critical health problems, and making an appropriation therefor.
Approved and effective May 2, 1967.

The People of the State of New York, represented in Senate and Assembly, do enact as follows:

Section 1. The legislature hereby finds and declares that the best interests of the citizens of the state of New York necessitate that the educational requirements regarding cigarette smoking, drugs and narcotics and excessive use of alcohol set forth in this act become the basis for broad, mandatory health curricula in all elementary and secondary schools. Such curricula shall include instruction appropriate for the various grade levels in nutrition, mental and emotional health, family living, disease prevention and control and accident prevention.

§ 2. The commissioner of education is hereby directed to establish a five year program for critical health problems designed to educate the citizens of this state with regard to the deleterious effects resulting from the use of cigarettes, drugs and narcotics and excessive use of alcohol with particular emphasis to be placed on the education of children attending schools in this state. Such program shall include, but shall not be limited to, the following:

(a) organization of a task force to conduct a series of conferences to which will be invited public, private and parochial school autorities, for the development of programs including:

(1) full descriptions of the stimulants, depressants and hallucinogenic drugs by competent authorities.

(2) presentation of experimental misuse of such drugs by representatives of the United States Food and Drug Administration.

(3) presentation of the narcotics problem, cigarette smoking and lung disease, and

(4) summaries by state health and state education department representatives.

(b) establishment of special training centers to provide health training for teachers;

(c) development of a state-wide in-training health program for teachers whereby school districts in the state may establish local health training programs for their teachers leading to certification by the department of education as health education teachers;

(d) development of cooperative health training programs between school districts and institutions of higher education whereby the qualified health personnel of such institutions would be available for local programs;

(e) utilization of the state bureau of radio and television to encourage participation in the program established by this act and to communicate to all the people of the state the objectives of such programs;

(f) establish new health curricula for use in the schools of this state including cigarettes, drugs and narcotics, alcohol, and such other health areas as shall be prescribed by the commissioner of education;

(g) contract with commercial agencies for the development of television tapes, kinescopes and films showing the evils involved in the use of cigarettes, drugs and narcotics;

(h) contract with the communications media of this state to show the above mentioned films during regular television hours;

(i) develop a state program to insure that the appropriate above mentioned films will be shown in all the elementary and secondary schools of this state;

(j) refine the health syllabus with the advice and counsel of the state department of health and other medical authorities.

§ 3. The commissioner of education is hereby designated to act as agent for the

FIGURE 1–2   (Continued)

state to receive any monies, in addition to the amount hereinafter appropriated, which may become available as a result of participation by the federal government, other states and/or public and private agencies in the health program established by this act.

§ 4. The sum of two hundred fifty thousand dollars ($250,000) or so much thereof as may be necessary, is hereby appropriated to the education department out of any moneys in the general fund of the state treasury to the credit of the state purposes fund not otherwise appropriated, to defray its expenses, including personal service and maintenance and operation, incurred in the development and initiation of the critical area health program established by this act. Such moneys shall be payable from the state treasury on the audit and warrant of the comptroller on vouchers certified or approved as prescribed by law.

§ 5. This act shall take effect immediately.

said, "When this social problem assumed alarming community-wide proportions, it became the obligation of the legislature to provide the laws and the finances to cope with it. The traditional niceties of non-involvement and separation of legislators from curriculum became a luxury."[3]

The New York State Education Department accepted the challenges of the new law by immediately implementing new health education programs in all of its elementary and secondary schools. The Regulations of the Commissioner of Education were revised accordingly; a team of experts was assembled under the leadership of John Sinacore, and a blueprint was developed. Briefly, this consisted of (1) developing a curriculum design that would be both practical and farsighted, (2) devising means for training teachers at both the preservice and in-service levels, (3) developing drug policy guidelines for use by school officials, (4) increasing the supervisory staff of the State Education Department, (5) developing learning resources for teachers, parents, and pupils, and (6) improving interaction with other state health-related agencies. Figures 1–3 and 1–4 provide, respectively, the text of the revised Regulations of the Commissioner of Education and the master plan for curriculum development.

Health education and optimal health

The Optimal Health Chart (Figure 1–4) is an overview of the health education program recommended by the New York State Education Department in 1970. It was designed to put into perspective the chief elements of a health education program—mission, goals, and content. To attain the mission of optimal health, health education programs should strive to provide the learner with education experiences directed toward achievement of the three goals: (1) the acquisition of relevant health knowledge, (2) the development or reinforcement of favorable health attitudes, and (3) the development or reinforcement of health behavior essential for effective living. The informational content is

FIGURE 1–3   Commissoner's Regulations
135.3   Health education.

(a) *Provision for health education.* It shall be the duty of the trustees and boards of education to provide a satisfactory program in health education in accordance with the needs of pupils in all grades.

(b) *Health education in the elementary schools.* The elementary school curriculum shall include health education for all pupils. In the kindergarten and primary grades, the health teaching shall be largely done by guiding the children in developing desirable health behavior, attitudes, and knowledge through their everyday experiences in a healthful environment. This guidance shall include systematic practice of health habits as needed. In addition to continued health guidance, provision shall be made in the school program of grades 4, 5, and 6 for planned units of teaching which shall include health instruction through which pupils may become increasingly self-reliant in solving their own health problems and those of the group. Health education in the elementary school grades shall be carried on by the regular classroom teachers.

(c) *Health education in the secondary schools.* The secondary school curriculum shall include health education as a constant for all pupils. In addition to continued health guidance in the junior high school grades, provision shall also be made for a separate one-half year course. In addition to continued health guidance in the senior high school, provision shall also be made for an approved one-half unit course. Health education shall be required for all pupils in the junior and senior high school grades and shall be taught by teachers holding a certificate to teach health. A member of each faculty with approved preparation shall be designated as health coordinator, in order that the entire faculty may cooperate in realizing the potential health-teaching values of the school program.

SOURCE: Rules of the Board of Regents and Regulations of the Commissioner of Education, New York State Education Department, Chap. II, Commissioner's Regulations, Subchapter G, Part 135, Section 135.3.

organized around five general "strands," which are further divided into topics that represented the chief health issues present in society at the time. (Optimal health is discussed in detail in Chapter 2).

HEALTH EDUCATION FOR THE 1980s

Health education/schoool health services/healthful school environment

Traditionally, the boundaries established for the school health program fall within three categories: (1) health education; (2) healthful school environment, and (3) school health services. Their functions were narrowly defined as follows: (1) school health services provided appraisals of pupils' health status, health counseling of pupils and parents, prevention of communicable disease, and emergency care for sick or injured pupils; (2) healthful school environment was concerned with the state of the physical environment of the school—ventilation, lighting, heating, and so on; and (3) health instruction focused chiefly on

FIGURE 1-4 Optimal Health Chart

The attainment of optimal health is related to the quality of one's health knowledge, attitudes, and behavior. These are influenced by the quality of health education one receives.

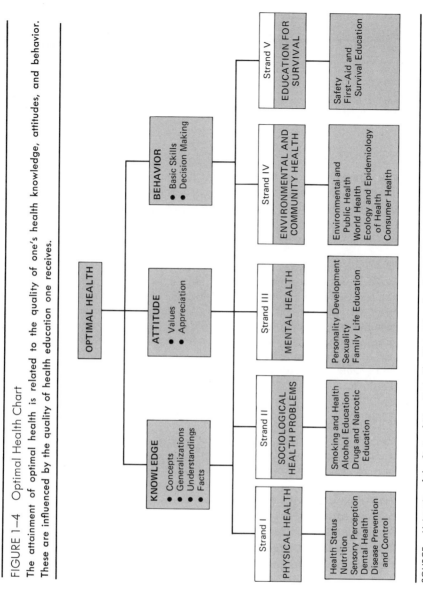

SOURCE: University of the State of New York, The State Education Department

teacher-centered approaches designed to indoctrinate pupils in certain aspects of health. As we will see, the perimeters of all of these areas have greatly expanded. Each of their roles in the school health program has necessarily altered considerably as more complex health problems have emerged and old ways of dealing with them were found to be no longer effective.

Looking toward the future

No one can tell for sure what the future holds for health education, but it will and must undergo many more changes in view of the technological advances being made in the health sciences and those changes taking place within the social and political spheres. Hochbaum recognized this in 1976 when he stated:

> We have little choice. If we wish to survive as an important and recognized professional entity, we must address ourselves to *all* the factors, *all* the forces, *all* the conditions that determine people's actions, not, as all too often we have done in the past, only to those that are responsive to direct communications and to other traditional educational interventions. In other words, our self-imposed new mission must be to *persuade* people to act wisely and change certain social conditions so as to remove barriers and *enable* people to take the very actions on which we have sold them. To do so, we will have to relinquish our comfortable role as "educators" and enter the struggle in the political, economic, social, and legal arenas on the local, state, and national levels. It is in these arenas where decisions are made, policies are shaped and resources allocated that will encourage or discourage, enable or disable, people to take the kinds of actions advocated by the health professions, and thus influence health behavior as well as or more than educational programs alone.[4]

Helen S. Ross pointed out in 1976 that as a result of the unprecedented national attention given to health education, the profession is challenged to reevaluate its practices and to begin to prepare for the future. She listed seven areas of urgent concern: (1) the dramatic changes in the organization and execution of health care delivery systems; (2) awareness that significant gains in the level of health will result only from major changes in the health behavior of people; (3) revenues for health education will increase when national health insurance and similar programs are operational; (4) the need for improving the quality of professional preparation of health educators; (5) the significant implications applying improved behavioral science research has for health education; (6) the increasing need for health educators to function at management and administrative levels requiring different knowledge than that of present training programs; and (7) the need for health educators to concern themselves with a body of ethics.[5]

What will health education for the 1980s be like? What influence will such factors as the development of telecommunications systems have on learning environments and communications approaches? What effect will political and social changes, new discoveries in the health sciences, advancements in space technology have on both the theory and practice of health education? Although we can not predict precisely what will take place or what impact these and many other developments will have on the health of people, we do know that leadership in any significant changes in health education must come from individuals within the profession. With the 1980's as our goal, we will explore in the following chapters the philosophy and practice of health education as it has been, as it is today, and as it must be for the future. Stop-gap measures are no solution; we must be concerned with the effects of today's theory and practice on the generations of tomorrow.

DEFINITIVE UNDERSTANDINGS

One of the most basic and vital functions of government is the provision of health education opportunities for all people. Each individual must learn ways to maintain health and to avoid situations that are hazardous. Society can not survive unless social and physical environments are improved and the health of people is preserved.

Philosophy is essentially wisdom regarding the principles of reality and of human nature. Philosophy of health education defines the boundaries of practice of the health educator and of the profession.

The two fundamental elements of health education are its philosophical dimensions and its areas of practice. The principles governing the formulation of a philosophy of health education are derived from knowledge gleaned from the experience and research of authorities. Health education philosophy should be both realistic and idealistic. It should result in practices that effect positively the health of the learner. These practices are professional preparation, organization and administration of the program, curriculum development, methodology, and evaluation.

Health education can be found in all societies from primitive times to the present. Health education today is quite different from that of even a few decades ago. Goals and approaches have changed but its primitive aim has remained essentially the same; to provide knowledge for survival. Today, we think also in terms of more than mere survival; we think in terms of fulfillment.

There are numerous historical movements that have been significant in the advancement of health education. Fairly recent examples include the School Health Education Study and the landmark legislation enacted in New York State. These and many other events have served to perpetuate and improve the health program. The health program consists of three interrelated elements: health services, healthful environment, and health education. Its goals are related to knowledge, attitudes and behavior.

The technological advances of the health sciences and the social changes taking place will significantly alter the philosophy and practice of health education in the future. The health profession must begin now to prepare for these changes.

PROBLEMS
FOR DISCUSSION

1. Explain why health education is vitally important in today's world.
2. Investigate the laws governing health education in your state. Analyze their provisions. Are they adequate? Do they require programs consistent with current health education philosophy?
3. Define philosophy.
4. What determines the principles upon which a philosophy of health education should be based?
5. It is stated that the principles of health education emanate from past, present and future health affairs and practices. Describe why this is true.
6. Describe why the formulation of a philosophy of health education is important.
7. Trace the historical development of health education over the past 50 years. What would you consider to be the three most significant events? Why?
8. Outline the essential areas to be considered in a philosophy of health education.
9. Formulate a philosophy of health education as you see it today. Keep it and make revisions as the course proceeds.

REFERENCES

1. Anderson, C. L., and William H. Creswell, Jr., *School Health Practice*, C. V. Mosby Company, Saint Louis, 1976, pp. 1–5.
2. Hochbaum, Godfrey M., "At the Threshold of a New Era," *Health Education*, 7 (4), American Alliance for Health, Physical Education and Recreation, 1976, p. 2.
3. Speno, Edward J., "Critical Health Legislation: A Blueprint for Action," *American Journal of Public Health*, American Public Health Association, New York, 59 (6), June 1969, p. 954.
4. Hochbaum, op. cit., p. 3.
5. Ross, Helen S., "Redefining the Future of Health Education", *Health Education*, 7 (4), American Alliance for Health, Physical Education and Recreation, 1976, p. 5.

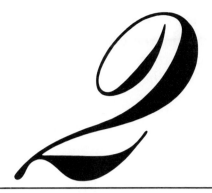

What Is
Health?

. . . one true measure of a nation is its success in fulfilling the promise of a better life for each of its members. Let this be the measure of our nation.

John F. Kennedy

Health education is fundamental for promoting individual and societal health, and the health needs of people determine its goals and actions.

AEB
DAB

INTRODUCTION

Approaches to health

It has been said that the American health system is not in business for people's health. Health and other social issues are simply given a low priority, being preempted by military and foreign policy commitments.[1] There are some evidences, however, that this situation will be rectified in the not-too-distant future. The spiralling costs of medical care alone have forced the American people to begin to ask questions and to demand answers. They are becoming less tolerant of exorbitant hospital bills, increasing cost and inadequacy of health insurance, and the prohibitive costs of essential prescription drugs and prosthetics. People are gradually becoming aware of what health educators have known for years: Health education and preventive health care are the most cost-effective approaches to our health care dilemma. We simply can not afford to get sick, at least not as much as we could in the past. The American economy can not continue to pour billions of dollars into treating afflictions while ignoring the fact that most of these can be prevented. What is needed is a health care system that directs its attention more to the promotion and maintenance of health than to the potential profits inherent in treating the sick. Also needed is a health education system that tells people that they don't have to get sick as often; that good health is an achievable condition for many people most of the time; that it is more efficient to *stay* well than to *become* well; that they don't have to tolerate exorbitant medical, hospital, and drug prices; and, above all, that they can do something to change the nation's priorities and attitudes towards health care.

The methods used to improve individual and societal health are *promotion, maintenance,* and *restoration,* and depend for their success upon the behavior of the individual. This is the common denominator illustrated in Figure 2–1. The fundamental factors that control how well one's health is promoted are (1) the quality of the individual's genetic potentials, and (2) the quality of the environment in which the individual lives. These two factors, heredity and environment, influence and are influenced by the life-style of the individual. Some hereditary potentials will develop more or less automatically, and can be positive, assisting in the promotion of health as they develop, or negative, resulting in a defect that may interfere with health promotion to varying degrees, depending upon the nature of the trait. (We will discuss the role of heredity in more detail later in this chapter.)

The quality of the environment is extremely important, for it can encourage the expression of desirable traits, and in many instances, discourage the expression of undesirable traits. Further, the behavior of the individual can have a direct bearing upon the degree to which

FIGURE 2–1   The Common Denominator for All Approaches to Health

Health education can affect significantly individual life-styles. It is the fundamental force necessary for health promotion, maintenance, and restoration.

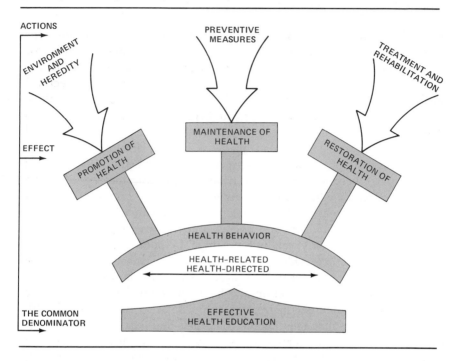

the environment can or will affect positive growth or the expression or development of an unhealthy condition. For example, all people inherit the potential to develop scurvy, but it can be prevented by the simple procedure of ingesting sufficient amounts of vitamin C daily.

The maintenance of health is very closely associated with health promotion, but there are some distinct differences. Health maintenance can be considered a sub-category of health promotion, for, obviously, if health *is* promoted—if one reaches a level of optimal functioning—a certain degree of health maintenance has been achieved. However, it is possible to achieve a level of optimal health but fail to sustain it. In this regard, health maintenance is defined as those measures one takes to insure that an optimal level of health continues. These measures can take the form of daily actions necessary to maintain health, such as adequate diet, physical activity, rest, recreation, freedom from undue emotional stress, or taking advantage of health technology—having periodic health checkups, receiving necessary immunizations, etc. The former activities are referred to as "health-related" behaviors and the latter are "health-directed" behaviors. Note that health maintenance is dependent entirely upon the behavior of the individual, while health promotion is significantly affected by genetic factors that may or may not be controllable.

Actions to restore health take place after attempts to promote and maintain health have failed. The success of health restoration measures is dependent upon (1) the quality of the individual's health knowledge and the motivation to act accordingly, (2) the quality and availability of appropriate health services, and (3) the individual's motivation to accept new behavior patterns necessary for recovery or rehabilitation and for preventing a relapse (health maintenance). For example, a person who has suffered a heart attack needs immediate medical attention. Availability of this attention is obviously extremely important for recovery. But in addition to this, the individual will have to learn to avoid those factors in the future that are associated with the onset of the heart attack. It might be necessary, for instance, to lose weight, stop smoking, change physical activities, or avoid emotional stresses. These latter activities, although a part of the rehabilitative process, are also examples of the kinds of health education that concern patient health educators. (Patient health education is discussed more fully in Chapter 9.)

In summary, education for health is an important influence on health behavior. Health behavior is associated with each person's style of living. One's style of living is the chief factor in the success of the three approaches to health—promotion, maintenance, and restoration. The urgency for directing our attention to the promotion of health and the prevention of disease is substantiated by the prohibitive costs of treating illness after it has occurred.

Current health education

Many of our current health problems are unnecessary, at least to the extent that they occur. It is unrealistic to think that we can eliminate all preventable health problems with existing resources, but it is realistic to assume that the majority could be. For this to happen, however, health educators, school and community agency administrators at all levels, and policy-making boards must recognize that it is essential for broad-based commitments to be made, directing attention toward the causative factors associated with these health problems and the means for preventing them. These factors include heredity, adverse environmental forces, individual emotional inadequacies, social impingements upon the individual's freedom to function adequately, the individual's acquisition of health misconceptions, and the individual's misperception of self, others, and the world in general.

Health education can play a significant role in alleviating many of the preventable health problems. It must, however, direct its energies and resources toward educational approaches that will result in each individual accomplishing the following objectives:

1. Developing basic decision-making skills necessary for dealing adequately with daily living problems.
2. Understanding the complex environmental forces that can interfere with normal growth and development and taking steps to avoid these when possible.
3. Developing a sense of self-sufficiency and recognizing that limitations are inevitable at times.
4. Acquiring insight into personal values and developing an appreciation for those of others.
5. Developing the skills necessary for changing or overcoming environmental hazards and social constraints on self-expression.
6. Understanding the nature of the health care system and developing the skills necessary to make the most effective use of it for personal growth and development and health maintenance.
7. Developing promotive health-related behavior or life-style.

Today's health education should be viewed as a pioneering effort that recognizes the scope of preventable health issues, the potential resources available, and the need to deal with the urgent health problems in the context of promotion and maintenance of health, prevention and treatment of disease, and rehabilitation of the disabled. The goals of health education must be based upon the needs and capabilities of individuals and the factors that influence their development. This is the only viable, logical, and economical solution to our present health care dilemma. It has become obvious that for positive change to take place, several things are necessary:

- Health education must become recognized as a fundamental and functional component of the health care system. It can no longer remain isolated from all health and medical activities.
- Health care must change from a disease orientation to prevention orientation. The medical profession, especially, must change from a chiefly pathologically-oriented profession to a preventive-oriented one.
- The training of health professionals must be improved by the establishment of health education centers.
- Health education must extend beyond the confines of the school and into the community and society. There must be a school/community interaction and coordination in all matters concerned with health. Health educators, medical providers and other health providers must begin to interact effectively.
- Individuals must be provided with learning experiences that are meaningful and pertinent to the issues they control. Their resulting behavior will contribute to a reduced incidence of disease.
- The massive quantity of health information must be organized in such a way that it is readily available to each individual, group, and educational or research institution.

Ways in which each of these goals can be achieved will be discussed in other chapters.

In conclusion, health education must be thought of as one of the chief means of influencing human effectiveness. It is imperative that people be provided with opportunities to acquire the accurate health information necessary for making intelligent choices about the behavior best suited for promoting health and preventing disease, disability and premature death. The most effective method for achieving this goal is through the establishment and implementation of comprehensive health education programs. These must be sequential and progressive; based upon the interests, needs and capabilities of the learner; taught by properly trained health educators; appropriately organized and administered; and suitable for both the health care system and the nature of the community in which the learner lives.

Modern health education
vs traditional approaches

America's health problems will be solved only when educators, community leaders, and medical and other health professionals recognize the need to work together in a deliberate, planned, and coordinated effort to promote and maintain the health of each individual. Traditional approaches to health education have emphasized disease rather than health, the teaching process rather than the learning process, teacher-centered rather than student-centered activities, passive rather than active learning, cognitive development rather than behavioral development, and symptoms of diseases rather than ways to control or prevent disease. In addition, health education has been confined to the classroom with little or no attention paid to the total community or the real health issues. For example, nearly every health curriculum guide and textbook devotes much of its content to discussing the characteristics of health problems that can *not* be prevented, controlled or even treated. Much space is frequently devoted to rare conditions that are unheard-of in America. Although some of these books may possess an element of interest for a small percentage of students, an in-depth study of them will do little to improve the health status of the learner.

More attention must be given to the health needs, interests, and capabilities of the learner and to the health issues over which the individual has some control. If this is not done, health curricula and textbooks will remain essentially irrelevant: The use of such materials will only cause intellectual boredom and a decrease in motivation. But more importantly, the preventable health problems will continue to plague, disable, and kill people unnecessarily.

FIGURE 2–2   Health is Relative to Conditions, Others, Self, and Achievement
Health status is associated with one's functioning ability at any given moment. It, in turn, is affected by the nature of disease or disability present and the means available to alleviate it.

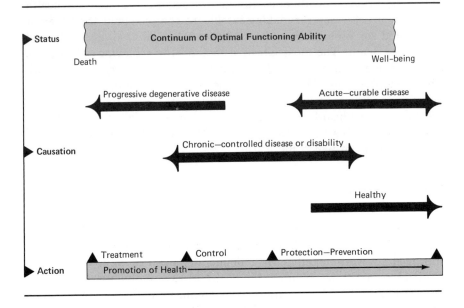

FACTORS AFFECTING HEALTH STATUS

What is health status?

If health status were to be placed on a continuum, as in Figure 2–2, we would find that functioning abilities would extend from near zero (death) to the opposite extreme of maximum output. For those with progressive degenerative diseases, the rate at which functioning becomes impaired can be decreased with proper treatment, especially if it is begun early enough. Most healthy people will from time to time contract conditions which are temporary or curable. Their ability to function may be hampered for a while, but with adequate treatment, health will return. Although many individuals may have a disability or disease which can not be cured, in most cases their ability to function can be improved through treatment and rehabilitation. Therefore, health status may be defined as *the level of functioning of the individual at any given moment.*

The World Health Organization's definition of health as a state of complete physical, emotional, and social well-being, not merely the absence of disease or infirmity, may be added to this concept as an ideal goal to be achieved. However, optimal health is more accurately described by the World Health Organization's objective as "the attainment by all people of the highest possible level of health."

Health education should direct its energies not only toward those who are well, but also toward those who are undergoing treatment for disease or disability, since they can learn to avoid in the future those factors which caused or contributed to their condition. Education is often essential in helping these individuals alter their life-style to accommodate the permanent disability they may have acquired as a result of the disease.

What factors influence one's health status?

Health status is determined by and dependent upon a variety of inter-related and interacting factors. These include, in addition to the multiple causations of ill health discussed earlier, the effectiveness and availability of the health care professionals, facilities, and programs. In addition, knowledge of the essential health information is necessary in order to behave appropriately during ordinary circumstances, as well as in times of crisis. Some authorities presume that health status can be improved mainly through periodic physical examinations, diagnosis and early treatment of disease. Sinacore points out, however, that "while we are to a greater extent looking outward to the community for means of attaining and maintaining health status, we have by no means outgrown our need for personal health responsibilities. Advances in the health sciences make it important for the individual to keep informed of these developments so that he may modify his behavior in accordance with their findings."[2]

Prevention vs treatment

As more and more people become unnecessarily ill and incapacitated by essentially preventable diseases, the demand for effective preventive measures will grow. Such health problems as cardiovascular diseases, lung cancer, drug abuse, alcoholism, and obesity, for example, are caused primarily by inappropriate individual behavior. The motivation for much of this behavior can be traced to the impact of social and physical environmental forces which initiate and perpetuate fallacies and misconceptions regarding a variety of health issues. These can be found, for example, in food, drug, and tobacco advertisements. Treatment approaches alone will not solve even our most basic health problems; they are expensive and time-consuming, but more importantly, they are failing to reduce the incidence, as well as the disabling effects, of these health problems. For example, the vast majority of lung cancer cases could be prevented if people would merely stop smoking cigarettes; many cardiovascular diseases could be prevented through a change in physical activity, dietary habits, and smoking behavior. These two diseases account for more than half a million deaths each year in the United States. The problem is compounded by the unknown amount of suffering and disability associated with the diseases.

Such health crises exemplify the failure of the therapeutic approach to solve many of our health problems. Society can not continue to build more hospitals without giving adequate attention to the causes of these critical health problems. For instance, by the time lung cancer can be diagnosed, it has progressed to the stage where treatment is generally ineffective in the vast majority of cases. As Rathbone and Rathbone have said: "Traditionally we have concerned ourselves with disease after it has developed. So much energy goes into plugging holes in the dike that no attention is given to building a better dike."[3]

Similarly, the educational community can not continue to stress academic achievement without giving equal emphasis to the basic health issues. A child withdrawing from heroin has little use for grammatical correctness; an adult cigarette smoker gasping for breath from emphysema will find little consolation in Shakespeare.

What is the role of the educational community?

The educational community must reevaluate its priorities and start emphasizing those fundamental issues which will be most valuable in teaching how to live in a society fraught with health hazards. This does not mean that other areas of the curriculum should be abandoned. It does mean that health education must be put in its proper place in the school curriculum so that today's children will be better prepared to avoid the vast numbers of preventable health problems prevalent today and predicted for the future. This is of equal importance for the health education of adults in the community.

We must begin to prepare people to assume more responsibility for their own health as well as for the health of others. Each individual needs to become aware of the technological factors that affect air and water pollution, the activities of industries that are more concerned with profit than with human health, and the activities (or inactivity) of government. Obviously, the real causes of our major health problems go deeper than individual health behavior; they lie in the numerous environmental obstacles preventing us from behaving healthfully or persuading us to behave in ways that contradict our intellect.

ATTAINING OPTIMAL HEALTH

What is optimal health?

Optimal health is attained when a person is functioning at the highest level possible under a given set of environmental circumstances. In this sense, optimal health will vary depending upon the complexity of the environmental constraints existing at the moment and the individual's capabilities for dealing with them. This can be as simple as the biological ability to resist disease or as complex as the ability to cope with psychological or sociological frustration, stress, and anxiety.

Although health can be improved at nearly any status level, the most logical point at which to promote optimal health is prior to the onset of disease and during the early formative years. The health education program should provide the basic health knowledge necessary to choose a life-style that can result in a better life and, ultimately, a better society. The sooner effective health education is begun, the more likely it is that individual attitudes and behavior will be positively affected. This will, in turn, result in a reduction of disease and disability and in an improvement in society's total health status. The enormity of the task confronting health educators is obvious.

How can optimal health be attained?

Our health affairs can best be dealt with by recognizing the interrelatedness of the physical, social, and psychological factors affecting health. Both personal and environmental factors must be given proper attention in any health education program, whether school or community based.

Life expectancy figures have for many years been recognized as valid, significant indicators of individual and societal health status. However, it is much more important to determine how well people function and how they contribute to society than to determine health in terms of longevity. Each individual needs to understand and apply the factors that aid functioning and avoid those that interfere with personal effectiveness.

For those who are essentially healthy the process is fundamentally one of learning how to live most effectively (health-related behavior). However, for those individuals who have a disease or disability, the process is much more complex. These individuals must acquire the knowledge necessary to understand their personal limitations and how best to develop their positive potentials. In addition, each person must learn when and where to seek competent health advice and care (health-directed behavior).

The role of heredity

It is vitally important to recognize that the horizons of human potentials extend beyond the imagination. Each person inherits certain biological traits which can continue to be developed or become dormant. Some of these traits contribute to the development of capacities to function effectively while others will interfere with it. For example, some genetic diseases can be detected in their early stages and prevented from progressing to the point of incapacitation. Phenylketonuria is a case in point. PKU is an inherited condition caused by the absence of the enzyme phenylalanine hydroxilase. This results in the inability of the infant to metabolize phenylalanine, an essential amino acid. Phenylketone bodies are then formed, damaging brain cells and causing mental retardation. This condition can be detected shortly after birth by the use of the Guthrie blood test and treated by altering the infant's diet to control the amount of phenylalanine consumed, thus preventing brain damage.

Similarly, desirable genetic potentials can be determined and provisions made to insure their development. These include the vast variety of abilities, both physical and mental, one possesses. As stated earlier, it is through this knowledge and the provision of an appropriate environment to enhance growth and development that the basis for the promotion of health is formed. Therefore, it is vital that the health sciences determine the real needs and capabilities of people and implement programs that will satisfy them.

The greatest need for all individuals is the ability to function adequately in a less than perfect environment. Health personnel and facilities must be made available to help everyone become a contributing, rather than dependent, member of society. Sinacore expresses great concern about the lack of health care facilities as well as the current misdirected efforts when he states: "While the health professionals are reorienting themselves from a disease and therapeutic orientation to one embracing the concepts of health and prevention, each individual needs to assess his own health values. He must do this, recognizing that if he makes mistakes there may be no one available who is capable of correcting them."[4]

The roles of the school and community

Figure 2–3 illustrates the role of the community and the school in helping people attain optimal health. Although many factors play important parts in this process, health education must be considered the most fundamental element.

Education for health can take place only to the extent that provision is made for opportunities to acquire basic health knowledge and effective learning experiences that influence health attitudes sufficiently to produce healthful behavior. The community must reinforce the school's efforts by providing an environment free of unnecessary hazards and conducive to health. Similarly, the school must reinforce the community. In addition, the community must provide health care by maintaining health through early detection and intervention programs and through appropriate treatment and rehabilitation procedures.

One of the most important factors associated with the attainment of optimal health is the need for positive interaction between the educational community and other social and health institutions. No institution can accomplish the task in isolation. Therefore, whether or not the initial steps are taken by the school, the health educator, or other health

FIGURE 2–3   Attaining Optimal Health

Emphases for achieving optimal health are inverted from school to community, but health education is necessary in both arenas.

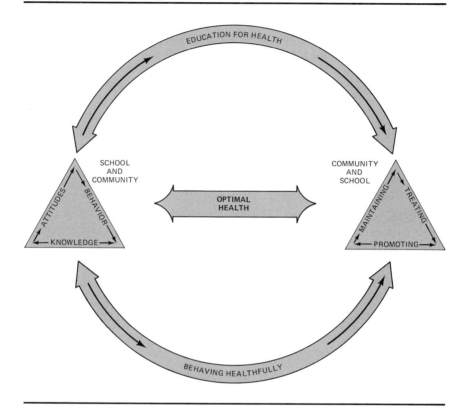

professionals, we must recognize the need to plan and implement programs in cooperation with all health-related agencies. Health will not just happen; conditions must be improved and individuals must learn to adapt to the nature of the community. If living conditions are improved significantly, however, one's health level can be raised since optimal health is defined in terms of both genetic potentials and environmental influences.

BECOMING HEALTHY(IER)

Improving individual and societal health

The President's Committee on Health Education emphasized the need to reevaluate our present approaches to solving health problems. We can no longer rely upon patient-doctor relationships alone. This is because the chief communicable diseases have been virtually conquered and are being replaced by diseases related to our social way of life. Their complexity requires attention beyond the expertise of the family physician, or, for that matter, the entire medical profession. The Committee states that "today, communicable disease has almost disappeared from the list of the most common causes of death. In its place, physicians and health educators are faced with new antagonists: diseases caused not by famine or contagion, but by aging, by our sedentary way of life, by nutritional excesses and dietary fads, by urbanization, by changes in the physical environment and by a mobile population whose movements have reduced traditional ties to the community and have compromised the traditional personal acquaintance between patient and physician."[5]

The chief cause of our major health problems

Changes have occurred, not only in the kinds of health problems, but also in the kinds and availability of health care. The once revered family physicians have all but vanished from the medical scene. In their place is the emergency room of a hospital or clinic. Home remedies have been replaced by thousands of sophisticated patent and prescription drugs. The cause of major health problems is no longer the microorganism but people themselves. Our most significant health problems, such as drug abuse, obesity, alcoholism, and lung cancer, are self-inflicted. Tragically, the way people live is all too frequently characterized by ignorance and misinformation regarding health matters; there is no valid excuse for this.

Fortunately, since life-styles are learned phenomena, the ones which result in self-inflicted diseases can be replaced by new and more beneficial ones. These conditions are essentially a manifestation of society's failure to come to grips with the health issues and to provide the necessary ingredients for promoting the development of individual potentials and establishing a health care system that works. The responsibility for rectifying this situation rests chiefly with the educational, medical, and political institutions. Leaders in these areas must recognize and understand what is needed, overcome apathy, and redirect society's resources accordingly. It is vital, therefore, that we no longer concentrate our health resources primarily on efforts to restore health while ignoring the fact that health can be better promoted, many diseases prevented, and health better maintained.

Health is relative

It has been said many times by many people that health is a relative thing. It is relative to (1) biomedical standards (the presence or absence of illness); (2) comparisons with others (statistical standards); (3) one's self (optimal health); (4) environmental circumstances which effect one's ability to function, and (5) a combination of these factors. Regardless of how health is described or what criteria are used, it is much more than a "state of well-being", as defined by the World Health Organization; it is an ever-changing and dynamic condition of the individual and should be measured in terms of effectiveness in achieving a particular task at a particular moment in time. Health and optimal functioning are interchangeable.

For example, one who is suffering from a disease may be very effective under certain conditions, while another person who is essentially healthy may fail in the same endeavor. You may recall that there is a relationship between personal potentials and environmental conditions. Under one set of criteria, the individual with the disease is considered unhealthy (even if functioning well) while the other person is considered healthy (even if unable to accomplish the task). Broadly speaking, one may be healthy in one situation and unhealthy in another. Health *is* relative, not only in regards to the status of others or to the presence or absence of disease, but in regards to emotional, social, and physical capabilities in achieving a particular goal under a given set of conditions.

What criteria should be used to ascertain one's health?

The "picture of health" will vary among individuals and from situation to situation. As Rathbone and Rathbone have put it, "An individual has a degree of health; he is more or less healthy. He is never healthy or unhealthy in an either-or sense."[6] At this point, it may be necessary to re-emphasize that each person must be provided with the basic ingredients necessary for self-development, and that all major aspects of society must be improved if health is to be promoted. This may require several things: the elimination of disease; a deeper insight into the self, the task to be achieved, the constraints to be overcome, and ways to achieve the goal; social, physical and psychological rehabilitation; or a change in the total physical environment. The criteria to be used to determine one's degree of health can be summed up in these questions:

- How well does one function in a variety of situations?
- Can the individual function better in a particular situation?
- Are there any significant handicaps?
- Is needless energy being expended?
- Is the task being accomplished efficiently?
- Does the individual possess a sense of self-worth?
- Does the individual have a social sensitivity?
- Is the individual free from diseases that interfere with functioning ability?

- Does the individual make judgments and choices based upon knowledge rather than feelings or emotions?
- Does the individual avoid self-destructive forms of behavior?

PROCESSES FOR PROMOTING HEALTH

Basis of health programs

Although each individual is similar in many respects to all others, each is also quite different. Consequently, society must provide opportunities for growth and development based upon these similarities *and* differences. A variety of programs are necessary to provide for these numerous variations. Our costly therapeutically oriented health care system is incapable of meeting the needs of the sick, to say nothing of health maintenance of the well. It is simply too narrow in its approach to meet the complex health needs of people.

The process for promoting health is, at best, extremely complex. There is no simple solution to our major health problems, but there is sufficient evidence to indicate that the route we have been pursuing is not likely to produce the desired results. Figure 2–4 illustrates a general approach by categorizing people into three broad levels of health status: (1) the *primary level*, (2) the *intermediate level*, and (3) the *secondary level*.

At the primary level, the chief action should be directed toward the provision of effective health education for those people who, for all practical purposes, are well. Such programs should emphasize the attainment of optimal health, the maintenance of health, and the prevention of disease and disability. This can best be achieved by establishing an informed public which can deal effectively with its own health affairs.

Although health education is important for those individuals at the intermediate level, a greater emphasis is placed upon treatment and restoration of health. Since most diseases afflicting people in this group respond to treatment, the individual's ability to function is usually only temporarily interrupted.

The secondary level group includes those individuals who have contracted conditions which, if left untreated, will result in disability or death. The primary goal is to halt the progress of the disease and to rehabilitate such people so that they can continue to function in spite of any incapacitation that may remain.

Determining program success

There are perhaps millions of people suffering needlessly whose health status is much lower than it should be simply because of a lack of basic health knowledge or inadequate health care facilities and personnel. John

FIGURE 2–4   A Process for the Promotion of Health

The approaches necessary for health promotion depend upon the level of health at which an individual is at any given moment in time.

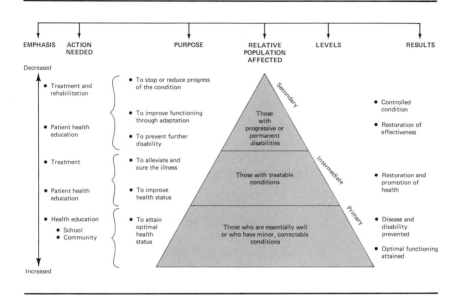

Stuart Mill expressed this concern when he stated that "preventable illness and disease caused mankind more suffering than all other causes put together. We have just begun to understand what public health services and the medical profession can do to lessen suffering, to increase the production of wealth, and to raise the intellectual and moral standards of mankind. We know that most of the painful and debilitating diseases . . . are no longer clinical problems, but problems only of adequate resources to wipe them out."[7]

As long as we continue to preoccupy ourselves with the sick at the expense of the well, to direct our resources toward building and staffing more hospitals and ignoring the urgency to build better and more healthful environments, and to wait for illness to occur instead of promoting health and preventing disease, we will continue to fail at eliminating needless human suffering. We still have a long way to go before we can reverse present attitudes about the best ways to deal with our health affairs. As Rathbone and Rathbone put it, "Promotion of health is still a frontier of public health work."[8] The following further illustrates the slowness of society to respond to the health needs of people, and is as true today as it was in 1932: "The problem of providing satisfying medical service to all the people of the U.S. at a cost which they can meet is a pressing one. At the present time, many persons do not receive service which is adequate, and the costs of service are inequitably distributed. The result is a tremendous amount of preventable physical pain and mental anguish, and social waste. Furthermore, these conditions are . . . largely unnecessary. The U.S. has the economic resources, the organizing ability, and the technical experience to solve this problem."*

PEOPLE, PURPOSES, AND ACTION

What determines the health action needed?

A well-planned health care system directed toward specific goals and related to the needs of people can result in improved individual health behavior. However, if the actions of health professionals are inappropriate, the results may be frustration, misunderstanding, and a deterioration of personal health behavior. Each element of the health care system, especially health education, must function in cooperation with other elements in order to be successful in keeping healthy people healthy and restoring health to those with disease or disability. The major goal should be to facilitate individual adaptability to internal and external influences. To achieve this, the following factors must be determined:

- What is the existing health status of the community?
- What kinds of health problems exist? How prevalent are they?
- How preventable are present or impending health problems and issues?
- What is the quality of existing health care in terms of facilities and personnel?
- What is the availability of health care to all people?
- What is the level of understanding that people have about what the health care system can do for them?
- What is the degree of motivation each person has for taking advantage of the health care that is available?
- How urgent is the demand for new programs to meet health needs?

The foundational elements of a health care system

Figure 2–5 diagrams the necessity for turning our attention to a health care system whose programs are directed toward satisfying the health needs of the people. This is related to the specific needs of individuals and groups. When actions are directed positively toward the satisfaction of these needs, they are more likely to result in the achievement of the desired goals. On the other hand, programs that are sporadic and primarily disease-oriented, are more likely to result in failure to solve the health problems. As we will see later, the foundations for a success-

---

* N.Y. Penn News, Nov., 1975. "These opinions were contained in the final report of the Committee on the Costs of Medical Care, published on Oct. 31, 1932."

FIGURE 2–5   People, Purposes, and Actions
The needs of all people determine the health goals to be achieved which, in turn, determine the kinds of actions necessary to achieve these goals. The results of the actions taken
will influence need satisfaction, and the cycle begins again.

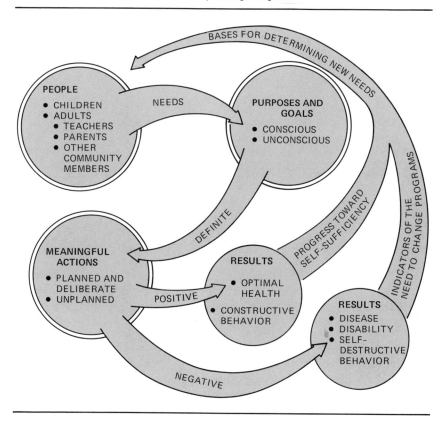

ful health care system must be within the context of a comprehensive, positive health education program for all people, but especially for the new generation.

AND SO . . . HEALTH EDUCATION

Life-styles and health education

The high incidence of many of today's major health problems represents the failure of past health education efforts. A noteworthy example is the high incidence of lung cancer. Approximately 90 percent of lung cancer occurs among cigarette smokers. There are an estimated 91,000 new cases and 81,000 deaths each year from this essentially preventable disease. Health educators have failed to convince young people that cigarette smoking is lethal and that advertisers are concerned with sales increases, not the detrimental effects of smoking on people. The federal government, contributes to this problem by continuing to allocate millions of dollars each year to subsidize the tobacco industry.

It is obvious that health education programs that place emphasis on not beginning the cigarette habit and on overcoming the insidious persuasion of advertisements will contribute to the elimination of lung cancer as a significant health problem. The President's Committee on Health Education emphasized the importance of health education when it pointed out that "while health education is not a panacea that will solve all health problems, it is undeniably a fundamental part of any logical attack on the problems."[9]

It is important to stress that community health resources should and must continue to be directed toward the restoration of health for those who have contracted temporary and treatable diseases, and for those who have disabilities which can not be cured, but which can be treated. Adequate and timely health education must be the foundation for any successful health care system. Although one's own health is ultimately a personal responsibility, one must depend to some extent upon others for a healthful environment and the maintenance of health. The awesome responsibility for making this possible rests with the educational community and society.

The major components of health education

Today's health education programs consist of two major components: (1) the *educational process*, and (2) the *informational content*. The educational process is predicated upon the findings and principles of the behavioral sciences. It should concentrate on those principles concerned with human motivation, the developmental process, the nature of learning, individual potentials and expectations, and social health needs. Each of these will be discussed in detail and perspective in subsequent chapters.

The informational content is based upon the research findings of the various health sciences. The health content should provide each individual with accurate health information regarding those health problems that can be prevented, controlled and/or treated. The information should assist the individual to make beneficial health decisions. This includes both health-related and health-directed behaviors.

The emphasis of today's health education program

The emphasis of any health education program must be placed upon the psychological and sociological implications (including causation) of today's critical health problems, rather than only upon the physiological or pathological ramifications. Extensive discussion of the pathological nature of disease is not consistent with current health education philos-

FIGURE 2–6   The Chief Components of Health Education

The principles and practices of health education programs are derived from the behavioral *and* health sciences which determine both the process and content. Selection of process and content are derived from learner characteristics.

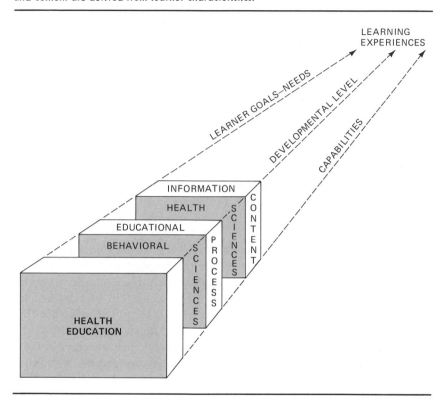

ophy and practice. This is especially true if it is substituted for more positive health matters or in place of health issues related to adverse effects on the ability to realize one's potentials.

Health educators must recognize that each person has needs and desires which must be fulfilled to assure the continuance of humanity and society and progress toward a better life for future generations. This becomes the basis for the development of any viable health education program since what society's institutions do today for the betterment of people will determine the kind of society that will exist in the future. Undoubtedly, one of the most important and influential social institutions is the educational community. Its design and effectiveness will be a chief factor in determining the quality of life for those who will follow, the children of today. Therefore, current goals of health education should be based upon the kind of society hoped for tomorrow. This is what health education is all about.

DEFINITIVE UNDERSTANDINGS

Health is a dynamic and relative state of functioning. The more effective you are, the more healthy you are said to be. Health can be interpreted in terms of good (healthy) or bad (unhealthy). Health can be promoted and, frequently, restored. Many diseases can be prevented.

Health status is also dynamic rather than static and refers to one's total physical, mental, emotional, and social functioning ability at any given moment.

Optimal health is the point at which one functions at the highest level possible in terms of individual potential and the existing environmental conditions. Optimal health is one way of expressing an individual's health status. Other ways include comparisons with others and the presence or absence of disease.

The promotion of health is the process of advancing one's physical or mental condition to a more productive level of functioning, that is, toward the attainment of optimal health. It includes the provision of an environment that will allow for full growth and development of the individual.

Both heredity and the environment influence the incidence of disease and disability, as well as the state of health. People inherit certain basic potentials that are influenced by the environment. Human potentials are latent physical and intellectual characteristics which can be classified in terms of abilities (athletic, musical, intellectual, etc.). The role that the social and physical environments play is to provide opportunities for these abilities to develop, or, conversely, to prevent their development.

The prevention of disease and disability is any process that precludes the onset of a condition that interferes with normal functioning. It may occur medically, by means of improved environment, or behaviorally, through improved life-styles. Many diseases can also be prevented from progressing by providing adequate and timely treatment. In this way, disease can be controlled.

A disability is any physical or mental condition which results in infirmity. A disease is any condition which results in decreased functioning ability and which is disabling to a lesser or greater extent depending upon a variety of circumstances. A disease such as polio may result in a permanent disability. Not all diseases are disabling to the same extent; relatively few result in permanent disability.

Health education is one of several processes for improving human effectiveness. It is much more than the acquisition of health knowledge: Health education results in a deep personal insight which affects health attitudes and behavior as well as health knowledge. Health education consists of two major components referred to as the educational process and the informational content.

The goals of the health care system, including health education, should be determined by the health needs of people. Action programs must be developed and implemented in accordance with achievement of these goals. This is the only way health will be improved and the incidence of disease and disability reduced.

PROBLEMS
FOR DISCUSSION

1. Identify several factors supporting the concept that effective health education is the key to our health care crisis.
2. Discuss the advantages and disadvantages of a health care system that is prevention-oriented.
3. What role does modern health education play in the health care system?
4. List five reasons why health education programs of the past were ineffective.
5. List six changes that must occur before health education can become an effective process for the promotion of health and the prevention of disease, disability, and premature death.
6. Discuss the ways in which genetics, experience, environment, and self-understanding affect one's attainment of full actualization.
7. List five of the major health problems in the United States and indicate the cause of each. What can be done by society and individuals to reduce their incidence?
8. Define health.
   a. Compare your definition with that of the World Health Organization's.
   b. What is the chief factor that differentiates today's concept of health with that of the recent past?
   c. Is your definition a functional one? Explain.
9. What is meant by the statement "Health is relative"?
10. Explain why health status is never static.
11. What factors affect one's health status? Are they the same for all people?
12. Explain why a therapeutically oriented health care system can not solve today's major health problems.
13. Define optimal health.
14. How can optimal health be achieved for each individual?
   a. Is optimal health a static or dynamic state? Explain.
   b. What criteria are used to determine whether or not one is healthy?
15. Differentiate between the following:
   a. health status
   b. optimal health
   c. promotion of health
   d. prevention of disease
   e. maintenance of health
16. Discuss the process of promoting health in relation to the three levels of health status.
   a. How do the actions taken for each level contribute to improved health?
   b. Why should there be increased emphasis placed on the primary and intermediate levels?
   c. In your opinion, should more resources be directed toward treatment than toward prevention? Explain.
17. Give several reasons why the action of health agencies and professionals should be determined by the actual health needs of the community.

18. List the two major components of the health education program and discuss how they are related.
19. In general, what should the outcomes of a health education program be? What should determine these outcomes?

REFERENCES

1. Ehrenreich, Barbara, and John Ehrenreich, *The American Health Empire*, Vintage Books, New York, 1970 (Preface).
2. Sinacore, John S., *Health: A Quality of Life*, Macmillan Publishing Co., New York, 1974, p. 7.
3. Rathbone, Frank S. Jr., and Estelle T. Rathbone, *Health and the Nature of Man*, McGraw-Hill Book Company, New York, 1971, p. 10.
4. Sinacore, op. cit., p. 10.
5. U.S., Department of Health, Education and Welfare, *The Report of the President's Committee on Health Education*, 1973, p. 15.
6. Rathbone, op. cit., p. 14.
7. Baker, Noel, "Human Rights in 1968," *World Health: The Magazine of the World Health Organization*, Oct.–Nov., 1968, p. 5.
8. Rathbone, op. cit., p. 10.
9. U.S., Department of Health, Education and Welfare, op. cit., p. 17.

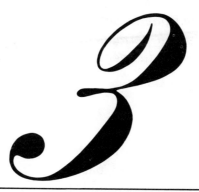

Health
Education
in Transition

No social unit, even one as small as the family, can live on permanent change, innovation, and experiment.

Barbara Ward and Rene Dubos

The present generation has inherited the mistakes and successes of past generations. The unborn will inherit those of this generation. What will we leave for the future of humanity?

AEB
DAB

MORE ON HEALTH EDUCATION—
FACTS AND MYTHS

Introduction

Unlike most areas of the school curriculum, health education is a relatively new discipline. This is especially true as far as the educational community's recognition of the potentials of *effective* health education for preventing many of our major health problems, as well as the ways in which it can contribute to the promotion of individual and societal health. Marked changes in the philosophy of health education have occurred in recent years. Health authorities generally agree that health education is, and should be, concerned with much more than merely the acquisition of health facts or the development of health concepts. These concepts must be applicable to the individual and to society.

The establishment of health education as a viable and integral part of the total educational program has been, and continues to be, a painfully slow process. One of the chief reasons for this is the lack of understanding and agreement among educators, especially school administrators, about what health education is, or is not, and what it can contribute to the educational program. This issue will be clarified in the following discussion.

What really is health education?

Health has been defined as many things: "dynamic and relative state of functioning," the ability to achieve a task under certain environmental circumstances, a "quality of life," as Sinacore stated, a state of well-being, the freedom from disease. If it is all these things and more, then health education must be defined in terms of the ways it contributes to the promotion and maintenance of health and the prevention of disease.

Kilander has defined health education as "the sum of all experiences that favorably influence knowledge, attitudes, and practices relating to individual and community health."[1] Willgoose, on the other hand, states that, "health education is an applied science concerned with relating research findings in health to the lives of people."[2] And Grout says "health education is the translation of what is known about health into desirable individual and community behavior patterns by means of the educational process."[3]

It is evident that health education is a *process* in which behavior is modified so that it reinforces tendencies concerned with integration and health. Each person strives to protect the self and to develop innate potentials. How people go about doing this is the result of interpreting the relevant factors in the environment and of the skills acquired. This behavior is the application of health knowledge to life and living and the development of decision-making skills. The recognition of health education as a process is reflected in a statement of purpose in the Comprehensive School Health Education Act introduced in Congress: "It is the purpose of this act to encourage the provision of comprehensive programs in elementary schools with respect to health education and health problems by establishing a system of grants for teacher training, pilot and demonstration projects, and the development of comprehensive health education programs."*

A careful analysis of the above definitions indicates that health education is concerned with two major elements: (1) the body of *health information*, and (2) the *processes* for making what is known about health a dynamic part of people's lives. That is, health education should positively affect the way individuals think, feel, and act regarding personal, as well as societal, health.

Obviously, health education can be defined in a variety of ways. The significant factor is that no matter how it is defined, certain basic concepts always appear: learning experiences, accurate and timely health information, improvement of health behavior, and the application of learning to society. In general terms, health education is *one* of several processes for improving health effectiveness. In this context, it is important to consider those educational elements which determine what the process will be. Specifically, they include the following:

- *The nature of the learner.* Learners may be students in elementary or secondary school or in college; teachers and other school personnel; patients recovering from illness, or the general public.
- *The quality of the teacher.* Most elementary school teachers have had little or no training in health education. Tragically, many are required to teach the health concepts. Most states that mandate health education in secondary schools require teachers to have certain minimum training in this important area of the curriculum. However, many states still do not recognize health education as a fundamental part of the total school curriculum. The quality of health education will be determined, in the end, by the qualifications of the teacher.
- *The quality of the learning environment.* Health education requires that the classroom environment be stimulating, as well as healthful. The school can be a very specialized environment for health learning. It should provide learners with experiences they can not get in other situations and/or reinforcement of non-school health learning experiences. Health education should not be confined to the walls of a classroom; it should extend beyond the school grounds. It is vital that health learning take place as a part of the total school/community environment.
- *The quality and availability of learning resources, both material and human.* In recent years, multimedia resources have become abundantly

---

* Senate Bill S. 3074, introduced by Senator Richard Clark, February 27, 1974. This bill never reached the floor of the Senate or House.

available in nearly all segments of health education. Although some cost a significant amount, many are free, or relatively inexpensive.* Teachers need to become familiar with the sources and select those which provide students with the best learning experiences possible. In addition, many health professionals have recognized the contributions that they can make to the health education program—school and community based. These resources should be utilized when appropriate.

- *School and community support.* One of the chief reasons health education has been slow in achieving the recognition and status it deserves is the lack of support from school administrators and community. This has resulted mainly from a lack of understanding as well as from widespread misconceptions about what health education is and what it can contribute to the total education of people. Health educators, generally, have failed to communicate this message adequately to decision-makers in the community and school.
- *The educational organizational structure.* It has been only in very recent years, and unfortunately only infrequently, that health education has become an important part of the organizational structure of the school.
- *The approaches selected for providing learning experiences.* Health education does not lend itself to indoctrination, lecture approaches, recitation, or to many of the traditional forms used in most other disciplines. Methodology in health education is discussed in detail in Chapter 12. Suffice it to say here that health education must be stimulating and relevant to the developmental levels of all pupils. Approaches can take the form of direct, correlated, integrated, or incidental learning experiences, or a combination of two or more of these. The important point is that at some point the student must be exposed to deliberate and direct health education under the guidance of a highly trained health educator.
- *The evaluation of learner progress.* Evaluation in health education is affected by a number of elements involved in the learning progress of the student. These include effectiveness of the teacher, selection of curriculum and its design, the methods used, the learning aids used— the total impact of the learning experiences on individuals. In essence, the key to evaluation lies in the answer to the question, "What positive effects result from the collective impact of all facets of the health education curriculum?"

Myths about health education

There are many misconceptions about the purpose, process, and content of health education. Some noteworthy examples are:

---

* See Appendix B for the addresses of sources of health education materials. See also Chapter 13, which describes selection criteria and ways these materials can be evaluated.

- *Health education is primarily a program of instruction.* Although the literature is rich in statements associating health education with programs of instruction nothing could be further from the truth. Except in very limited health areas, people can not be "instructed into" healthful behavior. Furthermore, today's health affairs require attention by those who are educated in making logical decisions about a variety of very complex health issues. Therefore, "health instruction" is an antiquated term which implies simply the impartation of health facts, the development of simple physical habits, and a process of indoctrination. In reality, health education is one of the most complex disciplines in the school's educational program.

- *Health education is concerned with disease entities.* In-depth discussions of pathology are appropriate in medical training, but not in health education of elementary and secondary school students. Health educators are concerned with promoting and maintaining health, not curing disease.

- *Health education is primarily a study of human anatomy and physiology.* Although some knowledge of the structure and function of the human body may be important in understanding some health issues, it does not necessarily help people appreciate or understand themselves better. Certainly, such information is not required to make intelligent health decisions. A study of anatomy and physiology should be undertaken only when it is related directly to solving a particular health problem or understanding more thoroughly an important health issue. It should never become a central part of the health education course of study in and of itself.

- *It is important for learners to memorize a body of health facts if they are to become healthier.* Health facts are essential only to the extent that they are relevant in helping people understand themselves and arrive at positive health decisions. Health facts should be acquired as a result of inductive learning experiences rather than as a result of deductive learning. (This concept is discussed in detail in Chapter 12.)

- *Health education is an opportunity for the teacher to tell students how to live healthfully.* Lectures and sermons on health issues have been shown to be ineffectual in altering the health behavior of individuals. As a matter of fact, such approaches are more likely to result in diminishing returns. Students learn best through involvement and personal discovery.

What is the nomenclature of health education?

One of the most fundamental factors influencing the quality of a philosophy of health education is a complete understanding of the meaning and implications of the terminology of education for health. Meanings may change with the acquisition of new information, or as a result of research findings in the health sciences. In this regard, the health educator must remain ever alert to the changes in society and alter philosophy accordingly. One of the most recent definitions of health education which reflects some of these changes has been developed by the Joint Committee on Health Education Terminology.[4] In 1973, the committee stated that health education is "a process with intellectual, psychological, and social dimensions relating to activities which increase the abilities of people to make informed decisions affecting their personal, family, and community well-being." This definition recognizes the wholeness and interrlatedness of individuals, society, and its institutions. The committee goes on to state that "this process, based on scientific principles, facilitates learning and behavioral change in both health personnel and consumers, including children and youth." Thus, health education has finally become a *recognized* component of the total health care system. The next step is to make it a *functional* component, and this is the responsibility of the health educator.

Steps in this direction are being made, but it has yet to become widespread. The establishment of health maintenance organizations illustrates this awareness. The medical profession as a group needs to be enlightened about the essential contributions that health education can make to the health care system. The burden of this task rests upon the shoulders of the health educators.

Once health educators have an understanding of the latest approaches to defining health education, it is important that a working knowledge of other terms related to the subject be acquired. Educators must become familiar with terms and concepts such as these:

- The components of a total health program
- The community health program
- The school health program
- Health education: community, school, and patient
- Health instruction
- Health education resources: material and human
- Health care system
- Community health organizations
- Administration of the school health program
- Administration of the health program
- Health educator: school, public, and patient
- Health services: school and community
- The health environment: school and general
- Health behavior: practices and habits
- Health knowledge (understandings)
- Health attitudes (feelings, beliefs)
- Health guidance and counseling
- School nurse-teacher
- School nurse
- School physician
- School dentist

- Dental hygiene teacher
- Direct health experiences (education)
- Integrated health experiences
- Correlated health experiences
- Incidental health experiences
- Health sciences
- Health curriculum
- Health education methodology
- Health goals and objectives
- Behavioral objectives
- Cognitive domain
- Affective domain
- Psychomotor domain
- Voluntary and official governmental health agencies
- Health professions*

These concepts will be discussed later on in their appropriate context. It is sufficient here to recognize the fact that knowledge of the terminology of the philosophy of health education is essential if health professionals are to communicate with each other.

As a result of research and experience, the meaning of many health terms has changed markedly, and their application to the health learning process has undergone similar alteration. The application of these terms is included in the discussion of health education practices in Part III.

Evaluation of health education

In addition to the changes in the language of health, there have occurred over the years important insights into the *foundational principles* upon which effective health education is based. Modern health education finds its roots in the activities of the voluntary health agencies during the nineteenth century. These health workers recognized the need to educate the public about communicable diseases. It is significant that this occurred at a time when no emphasis was placed on the promotion of health. In fact, the promotion of health is a concept which has appeared only in very recent years. There were, however, some attempts to prevent communicable disease from spreading. During the nineteenth and early twentieth centuries, health education was thought of merely as the transmission of health information. The emphasis at that time was on providing facts about diseases, rather than improving health. This disease orientation persists today, but a transition is underway and is rapidly acquiring momentum.

Until a decade or so ago, nearly all health education programs focused attention on discussions of the human anatomy and physiology

---

* The reader is referred to Appendix A for a concise definition of these terms.

and on pathology. Today, the focus is on the sociological, psychological, and physiological implications of all health issues. The goal today is the promotion of health and the prevention of disease and disability. Wilner, Walker, and Goerke point out that today "health education is the process through which individuals, social groups, and communities attend to and assimilate information about health and disease, and mobilize appropriate behavior for health-promotive ends."[5]

Thus a new era has been launched with the development of foundational principles of health education based upon the research findings of the behavioral sciences and the health sciences. These principles provide the framework for a modern and dynamic philosophy of health education and dictate what its functional components will be. The School Health Section of the American Public Health Association stated in their position paper released in 1974 that "health education should be a continuing process, from conception to death, and that such education must be comprehensive, coordinated, and integrated in *all* community planning for health." (See Appendix E for the complete text.)

Today's health education programs are organized around the purposes, goals and objectives of health education; the curriculum and its design; methodology, procedures, strategies, and techniques of health education; the informational content; the organizational structure, and the techniques for evaluating the effectiveness of the programs. Wilner and his collaborators acknowledged the need for this new emphasis when they stated: "A new focus, not by any means yet fully realized for many practical reasons, is to view health education as a form of *planned intervention.* In this sense there is an effort to influence largely unplanned, natural processes in such a way as to bring about improved health status. Health education thus [has come] to abandon primary preoccupation with pamphlets and lectures and rather to rely increasingly on the theory and methodology of the behavioral sciences."[6]

The principles of health education that are derived from the behavioral sciences include such broad categories as the principles governing education and learning, human growth and development, human needs and motivation, and maturation and personality development. These, and others, are discussed in Part II.

Further evidence of the realization that health education must establish itself as a method for insuring people's health is furnished in the introductory statements of legislation introduced in Congress in 1974:

SEC. 2. (a) The Congress finds that—

(1) Health education in the schools has the potential for enhancing the quality of life, raising the level of health for the student's lifetime by significantly reducing those health problems susceptible to educational intervention, and favorably influencing the learning process;

(2) the provisions of a comprehensive program with respect to health education and health problems for children and youth of the Nation should be given high priority; and

(3) most children and youth of the Nation now do not have an opportunity to participate in comprehensive health education programs, since health education in many schools either is nonexistent or is provided on a fragmented and inadequate basis.[7]

Thus, health education is slowly transcending the obsolete notions of the past and the societal and political obstacles which have existed too long. If we and all social institutions are sincerely concerned with the health of people, this movement forward must not be impeded. The responsibility for continued progress in health education rests with those members of all of the health professions, whether their primary concern is treatment, rehabilitation, or prevention.

ECOLOGICAL CONSIDERATIONS

What factors have influenced the progress of health education?

Many factors have played important roles in the progress of health education over the past century. Particularly noteworthy are those related to a more profound understanding of the nature of people and the influence of the total environment (physical and social) on overall health. Tosteson makes this revealing statement about the personal aspect involved in the improvement of health education: "It is important to recognize that the public is not a monolithic entity but rather consists of distinct and different persons. Although we may consider policies of health education for the entire group, the actual process of educating about health is, like all other forms of education, a highly individual matter."[8]

Teachers must always be aware of the fact that the younger children are, the less likely it is that they will understand a health fact or concept or correctly interpret a learning experience. The child's perception of self and environment at this point in life is apt to be quite different from what it will be in a few years. Therefore, extreme care must be taken by the teacher in selecting learning activities and in evaluating their effectiveness. Otherwise, misconceptions about health could be easily, often unconsciously, acquired by the learner. Such misconceptions could be detrimental to the child's future health behavior and might be extremely difficult to change later in life.

The personal and environmental factors affecting the development of health education are interrelated. As more information regarding health and disease becomes available, we must acknowledge this interrelatedness. The sooner this becomes universally recognized, the sooner health education will make the complete transition from the "dark ages" approach of the past to the "renaissance" of the future. This, of course, necessitates that health educators make provisions for a variety of rich and meaningful learning environments and experiences that will accommodate the similarities and differences of the learner. It was Aristotle who said that "true equality consists in treating unequal talents unequally." This concept can be applied to the health education of children: health experiences which will favorably affect one individual may not be appropriate for the talents of another. Since individual and societal needs vary, learning environments must be adjusted accordingly. Schools have never been more capable of making these adjustments than today, yet all too few have done so.

Prior to the turn of the century, there were practically no efforts, nor recognition for the need, to provide programs of health education in schools. What little recognition there may have been centered largely around rather feeble attempts to control communicable diseases (which were, admittedly, significant health problems at the time). We also find references to rather unorganized and haphazard instruction in physiology and hygiene. Additionally, during the late nineteenth century, most states required instruction in the ill effects of alcohol and narcotics.

Progress in the recognition of the importance of implementing effective health education programs in schools has been chiefly influenced by two factors: (1) massive health crises, and (2) the work of prestigious and influential educational and health groups. For example, as a result of the large numbers of young men rejected for military service during World Wars I and II because of preventable physical and emotional diseases, the educational community was motivated to accept some responsibility for providing health education programs for elementary and secondary school pupils. Some states went so far as to mandate such programs.

A more recent example of a health crisis precipitating more effective health education in schools is the drug abuse crisis of the late 1960s and early 1970s. Even more recent is the recognition of the alcohol abuse crisis that began in the early 1970s. Unfortunately, the educational community's response to these and other health crises is generally slow and often inadequately funded. Too often it is directed toward relieving the symptoms rather than the causes. Nevertheless, with each crisis, health education moves slowly forward. In the meantime, the slowness of society to respond results in thousands of people dying or becoming sick or disabled unnecessarily.

What distinguishes modern from past health education?

Since health problems have changed considerably in the past five decades, today's health education should bear little or no resemblance to that of even a few decades ago. Current health learning environments should manifest progress in the following ways:

- use of a variety of learning resources covering every preventable health issue appropriate for the developmental levels and capabilities of the learner.
- inclusion of laboratory experiences to solve health problems
- provision for both small and large group discussions
- provision of field experiences outside the confines of the school
- use of team teaching and team learning
- encouragement of cooperative learning rather than competitive learning
- use of a variety of sensory stimuli
- increased specialization to challenge learner curiosity and interest and develop special talents
- provision for individualized learning
- use of available learning media
- use of available community resources.

Health education today should be so unlike the health (or hygiene) teachings of just two decades ago that the past will remain merely an historical memory. Above all, learning environments should be flexible so that immediate adjustments for learning can be made as new health information becomes available.

Unfortunately, the focus of health education in many schools and communities is still on the disease entity. However, more and more educational leaders are recognizing the need to give greater attention to the ways educational approaches can contribute to promoting and maintaining the health of children. There is evidence that health educators and medical professionals are beginning to cooperate in this movement. In this regard, health education is becoming increasingly concerned with the factors that influence health and with how education can best utilize individual potential and environmental influence to promote health.

For too long health educators have overdignified cognitive development while ignoring the value of affective development. Each individual has personal qualities which can be classified as physical (biological), psychological (mental and emotional), and sociological (inter- and intra-personal). Genetics play a major role in determining these potential qualities, but equally important is the impact of environment and experience. The richness of learning experiences, therefore, has the greatest significance for affective development. Cognition is vital for planned, conscious behavior, but in the long run, the quality of one's life is determined by: (1) retention and application of health concepts, (2) establishment of feelings toward the experience, (3) clarification of personal values, (4) development of health attitudes, and (5) motivation toward creative health behavior (self-actualization). New York State Commissioner of Education Ewald Nyquist, in a commencement address, offered an explanation of the purpose of education: "Education is learning how to make a living, but it is also learning how to live a life—a sensitive, creative, humane life. The purpose of education is not really how to earn your bread; rather it is to make each mouthful sweeter."* This definition is valid, but it can not, in itself, be the panacea for all the ills of humanity. It is, however, the adhesive force which holds together the numerous partial solutions that were discussed in Chapter 2. Without it, the only recourse that remains is a return to the appeasement of the "evil spirits," since the other "solutions" will remain in an isolated vacuum with limited availability and application to people's lives.

As we begin to identify the ecological factors associated with programs of action for improving people's health three fundamental factors must be considered. These factors are the cause of both good health and ill health, and, as such, they become the most fundamental elements upon which a health system is constructed. They are (1) genetic defects and how we can detect them, prevent them, and treat or control them; (2) the environment itself, which includes both the physical and social aspects, and how health is affected by it; and (3) the positive potentials of people and how they are associated with human productivity.

Genetic influences on health

People can and do inherit certain diseases. Over 2000 genetic diseases have been identified. Genetic disorders are found in all ethnic groups. There is evidence that each individual possesses more than six defective genes that could, under proper circumstances, result in serious or even fatal illnesses in future generations. Genetic disorders fall into three categories: (1) those caused by a single, faulty gene, (2) those resulting from faulty chromosomal combinations, and (3) those resulting from the collaboration of genetic and environmental factors known as polygenic or multifactorial factors. Recent advances in the genetic sciences makes it imperative that health educators become familiar with this area and what the future may hold for genetic health. Below is a list of some of the varieties of genetic disorders that fall into these categories.

- *Down's syndrome* (mongolism) is a common form of mental retardation caused by faulty chromosomal formation. It occurs most frequently in infants born to women over 40 years old; a 1 in 70 chance, as compared with women under thirty, who have a 1 in 1500 chance. Overall, approximately 1 out of every 600 births is affected by Down's syndrome. It can be predicted by amniocentesis. Interestingly, mongoloids are highly susceptible to developing leukemia.
- *Tay-Sachs disease* is a nervous system degeneration resulting in death by the age of four. Tay-Sachs disease is most common in children of Jewish parents of Eastern European origin. Blood tests can determine whether or not potential parents are carriers of the disease.
- *Thalassemia* (Cooley's anemia) is most common in children of parents

---

* 125th Commencement of Geneva College, Beaver Falls, Pa., May 6, 1975.

of Italian or Greek origin. It is a form of anemia characterized by the production of abnormally thin red blood cells.

- *Phenylketonuria* (PKU) is most prevalent in infants born to parents of Irish or North European origin. It is a form of mental retardation caused by the inability to metabolize an essential amino acid known as phenylalanine. This inability exists because the person does not possess the enzyme phenylalanine hydroxilase necessary for this metabolism.
- *Sickle-cell anemia,* most prevalent in blacks, is due to an abnormality of the hemoglobin in the blood. The red blood cells become twisted (sickled) and are easily destroyed. Sickle-cell anemia is quite easily diagnosed by microscopic examination of the blood (Sickledex Test).
- *Cystic fibrosis* is one of the leading causes of death among white children. It is characterized by the secretion of thick, sticky mucus from mucus glands, interfering with normal functions of the organs in the digestive and respiratory systems.
- *Genetic cataract* is characterized by an enzyme (galactolinase) deficiency. Galactolinase is essential for metabolizing galactose, a sugar found largely in milk. If this enzyme is absent or insufficient, galactose builds up in the lens of the eye, causing cataract.
- *Fabry's disease* affects males only. It is a sex-linked disorder characterized by a deficiency of an enzyme necessary for the breakdown of glycolipids in the body. As glycolipids pile up, severe pain, rash, and fatal kidney disorders are produced. Although still in the experimental stages, enzyme replacement therapy holds great hope for treating Fabry's disease.
- *Porphyria* is an inherited defect in the body's ability to produce heme, the oxygen-carrying component of hemoglobin. It is characterized by an abnormal production of porphyrins (a type of pigment), resulting in severe abdominal pain, neurologic dysfunction, and psychiatric disturbances. Symptoms may be precipitated by the use of barbiturates, estrogens, sulfa drugs, and possibly alcohol.
- *Huntington's chorea* is a genetic degenerative brain disorder which manifests itself in middle age.

It is clear that genetic disorders are among the most critical health problems affecting humanity. According to the National Genetics Foundation, approximately 44 percent of all heart attacks in males 45 years of age and younger are due to genetically related defects; 1 out of every 3 pediatric hospital admissions is for gene-dependent illnesses; 40 percent of infant mortalities are due to genetic causes, and 25 percent of all institutionalized handicapped people have genetic-related diseases. In all, it is estimated that some 15 million Americans suffer from some form of genetic-related defect. This does not include those who are born dead or die shortly after birth.

Although cures for most genetic diseases await future research, many of them can be detected, predicted, and treated to some degree.

Through genetic screening, carriers can frequently be identified. Over 50 of the approximately 2000 genetic-related disorders can be diagnosed by the process of amniocentesis. Genetic counseling has become an important form of health education and must be included in any program of health education. Through genetic counseling, prospective parents can make better decisions about (1) having children, when a genetic defect may be transmitted, (2) monitoring the development of the fetus during pregnancy through amniocentesis (and other techniques), and (3) therapeutic abortion, if the results of amniocentesis indicate abnormal development of the fetus. Thus, genetic health can be promoted and some genetic diseases prevented.

Overcoming environmental influences

A second element associated with the development of a model for health and health education is the concern for the numerous health hazards resulting from the environment, both natural and artificial. These include a wide variety of communicable and noncommunicable diseases, many of which can be prevented, eliminated, or alleviated by (1) massive improvements in the environment, and (2) changes in the way individuals react to their environment. Some diseases, for example, are the result of infectious agents (natural environment), but many can be prevented through immunity programs, improved sanitary measures, etc.; and, as emphasized earlier, some diseases are self-inflicted (artificial environment) by the individual's inappropriate behavior.

Positive health potentials

A third element which must be considered as we begin to develop our model is related to the positive attributes of people. As has been emphasized earlier, each person inherits certain positive potentials. These are responsible for providing people with (1) the capacity for a broad range of adaptations; (2) the ability to learn and to alter behavior accordingly, and, finally, (3) the ability to change both their natural and artificial environments to make adaptation easier and living more healthful and productive. In this sense, our model must emphasize (1) the varieties of people and their potentials, (2) positive, as well as negative, health, (3) environments as they exist and what they can become, (4) goals which must be achieved (the end result) and the time factors involved, and (5) the approaches necessary to achieve the goals most economically and expeditiously. Figure 3–1 illustrates the relationships between the actions and the elements needed for establishing a model for health *and* health education.

The comprehensive health program: a model

In developing a workable model for health and health education it is important to give proper consideration to the ways in which all com-

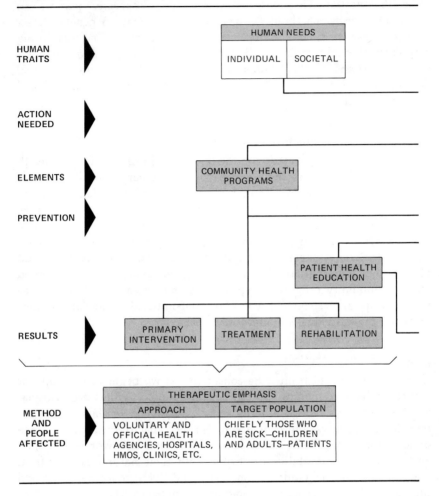

FIGURE 3–1 A Model for Health and Health Education

A Comprehensive health program in any community must be based upon known human traits, emphasizing health promotion and prevention, but not ignoring the therapeutic and rehabilitation needs of people.

ponents are interrelated, interactional, and interdependent. The comprehensive health program must be based upon those human traits which contribute to the attainment of health. Essentially, they include *individual and societal needs*, the *dimensions of health* (physical, mental, emotional, and social), and *genetic and environmental influences*.

Basic human needs are directly related to the dimensions of health, and are fully discussed in Chapter 5. The four dimensions of health may be described briefly as follows:

• The *physical dimension* is the most concrete and observable. As a result, it frequently receives the greatest attention. The physical

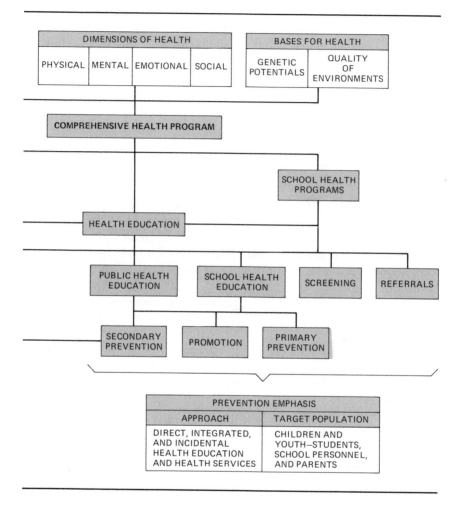

DIMENSIONS OF HEALTH				BASES FOR HEALTH	
PHYSICAL	MENTAL	EMOTIONAL	SOCIAL	GENETIC POTENTIALS	QUALITY OF ENVIRONMENTS

COMPREHENSIVE HEALTH PROGRAM

SCHOOL HEALTH PROGRAMS

HEALTH EDUCATION

PUBLIC HEALTH EDUCATION	SCHOOL HEALTH EDUCATION	SCREENING	REFERRALS

SECONDARY PREVENTION	PROMOTION	PRIMARY PREVENTION

PREVENTION EMPHASIS	
APPROACH	TARGET POPULATION
DIRECT, INTEGRATED, AND INCIDENTAL HEALTH EDUCATION AND HEALTH SERVICES	CHILDREN AND YOUTH—STUDENTS, SCHOOL PERSONNEL, AND PARENTS

dimension is associated with the biological aspects (structure and functions) of the individual.

- The *emotional dimension* of health refers to the ability to express feelings adequately and in appropriate ways. It has to do with values, appreciations, and the like, as they contribute to worthwhile achievements.
- The *mental dimension* of health is related to the individual's ability to learn and to behave accordingly. It is associated with rationality, logic, decision-making, etc.
- The *social dimension* of health is associated with interpersonal rela-

tions. One's social health depends upon the ability to deal effectively with the social environment.

The dimensions of health are interactional: the state of one dimension affects the state of all others. The School Health Education Study puts it this way: "Health is a quality of life involving dynamic interaction and interdependence among the individual's physical well-being, his mental and emotional reactions, and the social complex in which he exists."[9]

ELEMENTS OF THE HEALTH PROGRAM

Environment/Education/Services— the three elements

The primary elements of the comprehensive health program fall into two broad areas: (1) the *community health program*, which consists of public and patient health education, primary intervention, treatment, rehabilitation, and research; and (2) the *school health program*, which consists of health education of pupils, teachers, and parents, and health screening, counseling and referrals, and primary intervention. It will be noted that health education is a fundamental component of both the community and school health programs and is essential for the success of both.

The majority of activities in the community health program revolve around therapy as the means for improving the health of people. However, health education plays an integral part in the promotion of health and primary prevention of disease through the efforts of the public health educator. In addition, the clinical (patient) health educator helps individuals recovering from an illness understand the nature of their condition and the actions they may take to prevent further occurrences (secondary prevention). (The kinds of health educators and their functions will be discussed in detail in Chapter 9.)

The comprehensive health program is concerned with all human health affairs. It must be a school *and* community health program. The school health component consists of all of the health activities that are initiated by the educational community, but it does not limit itself only to the school, nor should it. From either the viewpoint of the school or of the community, the *three chief elements* of the health program can be summarized as follows:

- Provision for a healthful school/community *environment*.
- Provision for a comprehensive school/community *health education* program.
- Provision for an adequate school/community *health services* program.

FIGURE 3–2   The Components of the School/Community Health Program

All efforts of the school or community must be coordinated and interactional, resulting in consistency and reinforcement. Efforts are related to environments, services, and education.

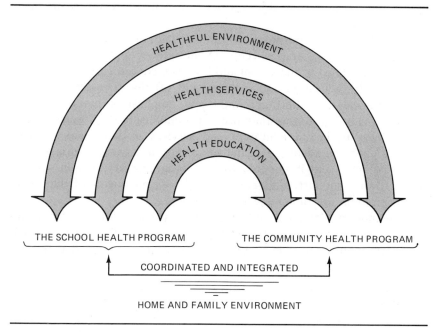

THE SCHOOL HEALTH PROGRAM   THE COMMUNITY HEALTH PROGRAM

COORDINATED AND INTEGRATED

HOME AND FAMILY ENVIRONMENT

All three of these elements must be adequately coordinated, since each contributes to the effectiveness of the others. For example, an individual needs to understand what health services are available and when to seek appropriate medical attention. In the same way, health services personnel have many opportunities to educate patients regarding their particular health problems. The need for this coordination effort is illustrated in *Figure 3–2*.

Finally, the promotion of health and prevention and alleviation of today's health problems require both a prevention and therapeutic emphasis. Solutions to our health problems will result only through the implementation of health programs at both the general community level (local, state, and national), and the school level (for all pupils, teachers, and parents). It is not a question of either-or; it is both.

Intra-school and extra-school aspects of the school health program

The school health program is concerned chiefly with promotion of health and prevention orientation. Its elements consist of the school health education program and the school health services program. The school health program directs its attention mainly toward pupils who are well; although concerted efforts are also made to identify, through health screening and counseling, those pupils with health problems. Appropriate referrals to community health agencies or private practitioners are made when necessary.

For all practical purposes, it can be said that the school health program has two general aspects: (1) the *intra-school* aspect, which is essentially confined to the school and is chiefly concerned with pupil and teacher health education and services, and (2) the *extra-school* aspect, which extends into the community and emphasizes parental health education as well as appropriate use of community health resources. The effectiveness of health education and services is dependent in large measure upon the adequacy of the *supporting influences.* These are the factors which make it possible for the programs to function—funds, administrative support, motivation, etc. These components of the school health program are illustrated in Figure 3–3.

The most fundamental unit of society is the individual. Each person is subject to constant, persistent change as a result of the normal growth and maturation process. In addition, children are confronted with arti-

FIGURE 3–3   Elements of the School Health Program

The school health program should extend into the community (extra-school). The success of school health efforts will depend upon the quality of health education and services available *and* the quality of the supporting influences.

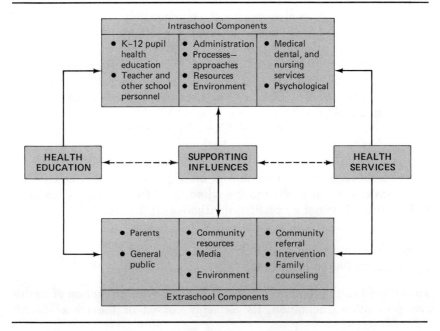

TABLE 3-1   Contributions of Each of the Elements of the School/Community Health Programs

	Health Education	Health Services	Supporting Influences
CONTRIBUTIONS:	Provides health learning experiences for all pupils, teachers, school administrators, other school personnel, and parents.	Provides health services and counseling for pupils, teachers, and school administrators. Provides health liaison with parents.	Provides the means by which the total health program can become effective: motivation for health learning, organization and administration, and community acceptance.
PROCESS:	1. Planned, comprehensive health education program in grades K–12. 2. Teacher in-service health education programs. 3. Planned educational programs in cooperation with community health agencies. 4. Formal and informal parent health education in cooperation with the continuing education departments. 5. Establishment of learning resource centers.	1. Establishes a health services program staffed by trained medical and dental personnel: school physician, school nurse-teachers, dental supervisor, and dental hygiene teachers. 2. Maintains a close working relationship with the school psychological services: school social worker, psychologist, and guidance counselor. 3. Maintains a close working relationship with community health agencies; makes referrals. 4. Makes health screenings as appropriate. 5. Works closely with the custodial staff in the maintenance of a healthful school environment.	1. Administrators support the total program by insuring adequate organization, facilities, learning environments, and budgetary allocations. 2. Provides opportunities for the implementation of effective learning experiences, such as student-centered classes, student involvement, teacher-student planning, and relevant health information. 3. Maintenance of community and government awareness and support through school-community communications.

ficial changes resulting from what is commonly referred to as "progress." This progress is also responsible for drastic change in the second fundamental unit of society, the family. These two factors of change, social progress and maturation, along with the multitude of experiences from other sources (television, for example), present today's youth with continuous change, exposure to both accurate and inaccurate health information and to a variety of social and emotional situations with which to cope. The educational community must provide the essential stabilizing intellectual, social, and emotional influence. It must further provide the means by which each individual can accurately interpret both personal growth and social progress. We are surrounded with motivations for health learning; health educators must recognize their existence and harness them for use by young people. This is the most important challenge confronting the health professions today.

DEFINITIVE UNDERSTANDINGS

Generally, health educators have failed to convey to the general public, politicians, and school administrators what health education is, what it is not, and what it can contribute to the improvement of the health of society. As a result, many misconceptions continue to exist among both school officials and the general public, and in many cases, among the health professionals themselves.

Essentially, health education is concerned with both the informational content and the processes needed for affecting the way individuals think, feel, and act. There are eight specific factors that influence the success of the process of health education: the nature of the learner, the quality of the teacher, the quality of the learning environment, the quality of learning resources, school and community support, the way in which health education programs are organized and administered, the quality of the learning experiences, and the validity and application of evaluation.

Health education is no longer concerned primarily with such factors as indoctrination, disease as such, human anatomy and physiology, the memorization of health facts, and teacher dominated classes.

Health education is a fundamental component of the health care system. It is gradually undergoing changes which will, in time, become a true health care system rather than a disease care system. The health educator has a direct responsibility for assuring that this change continues and becomes a reality. As with all disciplines, health education has a unique vocabulary. This is necessary to assure that health professionals communicate accurate meanings when dealing with matters concerned with health and health education. The formulation of a functional philosophy of health education is based upon accurate understanding of what it is and what it is not, what it can or can not accomplish, and the processes available for these accomplishments. Consequently, there are foundational principles upon which one must base a philosophy of health education. Broadly speaking, these emanate from the research findings of the health and behavioral sciences. On the one hand, we are talking about health information, while on the other hand, we are concerned with the processes which will affect positively the health behavior of people.

Health education must take into account personal as well as environmental variables that effect the health of people. The health educator needs to recognize the similarities and differences of individuals and apply this knowledge to the educational process and adjust the learning environment accordingly.

Health education programs have improved considerably during the past few decades, but they still lag behind what they should be. Strides forward have been motivated chiefly by social health crises and the dedicated, persistent work of health professionals and agencies. However, we must be reminded that health education in itself can not be the cure for all the ills of humanity; expectations must be kept within proper perspective.

An awareness of the part that genetics play in the establishment of the health of individuals is critical to finding solutions to health problems. Genetic disorders themselves must be considered one of our most pressing health problems. Health counseling for individuals at high risk is an important activity for preventing some genetic disorders. It is, however, limited. Early detection of some genetic-related disorders can result in a prevention of the consequences of the disease. Therapeutic abortion may be deemed necessary by some individuals. Amniocentesis is one technique used to discover abnormal development of the fetus. It is usually performed about the fifteenth week of pregnancy.

Essentially, our health care system is therapeutically oriented. Much more money (and other resources) is allocated and spent for the treatment of disease and rehabilitation programs than for the promotion and maintenance of health. According to the United States Department of Health, Education and Welfare, more than $116 billion are spent annually on health care. Only about four percent of this goes for prevention and health education. This scale needs to be brought more into balance before we will see a realistic health care system.

Therefore, any model for health must take into account both the therapeutic and the prevention aspects of health. In this regard, plans for the health care system must be ever mindful of its purposes—the improvement, maintenance, and restoration of health of all people. Consequently, a comprehensive health program should be predicated upon (1) human health needs, (2) the dimensions of health, and (3) genetic and environmental influences.

The comprehensive health program consists of the community-based component and the school-based component. The community component emphasizes a therapeutic approach while the school component emphasizes a health promotion and disease prevention approach. On the one hand, we are dealing chiefly with well people, while on the other hand we are dealing chiefly with sick people. Regardless of where the program is "housed" there are three fundamental elements which are common: a healthful environment, health education, and health services. The quality of the school health program is influenced by the intra-school aspects, the extra-school aspects, and the supporting factors.

PROBLEMS
FOR DISCUSSION

1. Identify the factors which contribute to the health of an individual; to the health of society. How do they differ?
2. Develop criteria to be used to distinguish a healthy person from an unhealthy person.
3. What is health education?
4. How can health, disease, and education be conceptualized into a philosophy of health education?
5. Should a philosophy of health education be founded upon a pragmatic or idealistic viewpoint? Support your contention.
6. Discuss the ways in which health behavior affects the (1) promotion of individual health, (2) maintenance of individual health, and (3) restoration of individual health.
7. Identify some factors to support the contention that the quality of the teacher will determine the quality of health education. Is this also true regarding the other health professions?
8. Explain why the examples given in the text regarding what health education is not are valid in view of current thinking.
9. Describe what constitutes the foundation principles of health education. How do these differ from two or three decades ago?
10. Analyze how learner similarities and differences are likely to affect the kind and quality of health education programs.
11. Compare current learning environments in the school with those of twenty years ago. How are they alike? Different?
12. Basically, what stimulates progress in program development in health education? Why?
13. By diagram or explanation, show how the dimensions of health, domains of objectives, and goals of health education are interrelated.
14. Describe why this statement is valid: "Genetic disorders must be perceived as among the most critical health problems affecting humanity."
15. List and describe the functions of the elements which constitute a comprehensive health program. How does this differ from a comprehensive health education program?
16. Compare the community health program with the school health program. How are they similar? How do they differ?
17. Distinguish between the intra-school and extra-school components that influence the school health program.

REFERENCES

1. Kilander, H. Frederick, *School Health Education*, Macmillan Publishing Co., New York, 2d ed., 1968, p. 9.
2. Willgoose, Carl E., *Health Education in the Elementary School*, 3d ed., W. B. Saunders Co., Philadelphia, 1969, p. 30.
3. Grout, Ruth E., *Health Teaching in Schools*, W. B. Saunders Co., Philadelphia, 4th ed., 1963, p. 2.
4. Joint Committee on Health Education Terminology, *Health Education Monographs* no. 33, SOPHE, Inc., San Francisco, 1973, pp. 65–66.
5. Wilner, Daniel M., Rosabelle Price Walker, and Lenor S. Goerke, *Introduction to Public Health*, 6th ed., Macmillan Publishing Co., New York, 1973, p. 437.
6. Ibid.
7. U.S., Congress, *Comprehensive School Health Education Act*, S. 3074 and H.R. 13084, 93d Congress, Feb. 27, 1974.
8. Tosteson, Daniel C., M.D., "The Right to Know: Public Education About Health," *Journal of Medical Education*, Feb. 1975.
9. School Health Education Study, *Health Education: A Conceptual Approach to Curriculum Design*, 3M Education Press, St. Paul, 1967, p. 10.

The real solution to health care cost does not lie in the health field at all, as we know it today. It lies in reducing the need and demand for health care. And that means somehow influencing people to accept responsibility for their own health, reducing their dependence on the health care system.

Bernard R. Tresnowski

The bases for health education are predicated upon the goals and processes that in some way influence the favorable development of children as they progress toward maturity; toward self-actualization; toward the attainment of self-sufficiency; toward the development of capabilities for improving and enhancing their lives and the lives of others. Adequate development of the intellect, decision-making skills, wisdom about living, compassion for others, clarification of values, maintenance of physical, psychological, and social health—these form the bases for health education and a social mandate that can not be ignored.

AEB
DAB

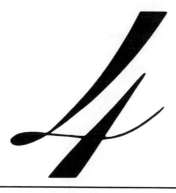

Bases
for Health
Education

INTRODUCTION

The need for health education

To a great extent, the American people are misinformed or simply lack basic information regarding health matters. This was revealed by the School Health Education Study conducted in the early 1960s, the results of which were released in 1963, and by the National Health Test conducted by CBS on national television in 1966. Both of these studies revealed that the majority of American people lacked even the most elementary knowledge about their health and that many people possessed a variety of misconceptions about many aspects of personal health.

More specifically, a vast majority of our major killing and crippling diseases need not be serious health problems. Some examples have been cited earlier. Further examples include the following:

- Glaucoma, a leading cause of blindness in the United States, which can be controlled. Blindness can be prevented through early detection and competent treatment. There are two types of glaucoma: (1) acute glaucoma, which appears suddenly and is manifested by extreme pain in the eyes when they lose their plasticity and become hardened. Immediate and proper medical attention is imperative. Surgery is indicated; and (2) the chronic form of glaucoma (the most common), which can be detected and diagnosed early and treated with drugs or surgery. In both types, there is increased pressure within the eyeball that causes damage to the retina. Early treatment is essential to halt progress and to prevent further and permanent retinal damage. Glaucoma occurs most frequently in people over 50 years of age. Periodic eye examination and prompt treatment where indicated can prevent most cases of blindness due to glaucoma.
- Skin cancer. Approximately 300,000 cases are diagnosed each year in the United States. About 5000 people die each year as a result of untreated skin cancer or prolonged delay in seeking treatment. The incidence of skin cancer could be greatly reduced by the elimination of the misconception that suntans are healthful. Most skin cancer results from an overexposure to the sun's rays.
- Breast cancer. Approximately 89,000 new cases of breast cancer are diagnosed each year. Most of these can be detected early through breast self-examination, mammography, thermography, xerography, and periodic physical examination by a physician. If women would examine their breasts each month and report any change to their physician, most of the 33,000 deaths each year from breast cancer could be prevented.
- Uterine or cervical cancer. There are about 46,000 new cases of uterine or cervical cancer diagnosed each year. Uterine cancer can be detected

in the early stages of development, even before a problem arises, through the use of the Pap test. Every woman who has had sexual intercourse should have a yearly Pap test. Through this early detection technique, nearly all of the 11,000 deaths each year from uterine cancer could be prevented.

These examples along with others cited elsewhere in this book should provide us with sufficient evidence of the need for effective health education programs in each community setting. The economics of prevention alone dictate that our society can not afford to ignore these numerous, preventable health issues. Medical, paramedical, health insurance, and hospital costs demand that the American people not remain ignorant about basic health matters. Health is a fundamental right of each individual. It is obvious that education about health is a vital weapon against disability, premature death, and exorbitant medical costs. Health education, therefore, becomes a fundamental right of each individual, and each individual should demand that this right not be preempted by other, less important, social projects.

The breadth of health education

As emphasized earlier, the health education program is directed toward all individuals: pupils from kindergarten through college; parents and teachers; school administrators; and the general public. Since the specific needs of each of these groups will be different, approaches to health learning will necessarily vary. Some health education programs will be initiated and implemented by the school while others will be initiated and implemented by community health-related agencies. But health education programs regardless of their origin or setting should never be isolated from each other.

There are no limits to the breadth of health education. There are, however, priorities. Directors of health education programs must be instrumental in determining these priorities, but the one basic criterion should be, "How important is the health issue to causing disease, disability, and premature death and can it be prevented?" The health issues may include such areas as dental health problems, communicable and degenerative diseases, complex social and emotional disturbances, nutritional deficiencies and excesses, genetic disorders, disturbances related to growth and development, environmental health problems, and health economics, to cite a few.

The breadth of health education programs also includes the numerous varieties of processes, techniques, and environmental conditions which affect or cause learning in people. It also includes the ways programs are established, organized, administered, staffed, financed, evaluated, and revised for greater effectiveness for the target population. Essentially, health education is concerned with all the factors that influence human effectiveness; it is concerned with finding better ways of favorably influencing human behavior through the educational process; it is concerned with developing a health educated society.

GOALS OF HEALTH EDUCATION

What is a health goal?

A goal is defined as the end toward which a particular process is intended to progress. A health goal may be distinguished from an aim in that an aim is the mission of the accumulated learning experiences, while the goal or goals are the intermediary guideposts which direct the individual toward the achievement of the mission. The mission of health education is to provide the individual with the ingredients necessary for more effective living. Health goals are related to these ingredients. A health goal, therefore, is the predetermined purpose of the health learning experiences. It has been generally agreed by health education authorities that the chief goals of health education are threefold: (1) the acquisition of health knowledge, (2) the improvement or reinforcement of health attitudes, and (3) the improvement or reinforcement of health behavior.

Health goals may be defined further as terminal or enabling goals. A *terminal goal* is the ultimate end result of the learning experience or experiences. It describes the conditions under which the learner's need is satisfied and learning motivation is complete. The *enabling goal* is defined as achievements necessary for the learner to satisfy the terminal goal. It provides the teacher and learner with the direction needed and the process to be used in pursuing the terminal goal. Some authorities refer to these as enabling or terminal *objectives*. Figure 4–1 illustrates how the health education program is composed of the relationships between the health goals, learner, and process. Figure 4–2 shows how the foundational principles of health education are related to the achievement of the terminal goals and the aim of the program.

Below is a list of criteria that should be used by the teacher when planning the health education program, establishing goals, and selecting methodologies.

- How will the learner's health knowledge, attitudes, and behavior be different as a result of the program experiences?
- Are program experiences selected with favorable change in mind?
- What health information is most important in influencing the learner's intellectual development?
- What kinds of learning experiences will influence positively the learner's health attitudes?
- To what extent will the learning process affect positively the learner's health behavior?

FIGURE 4-1   The Relation of Learner to Goals and Process

The health education program, conceived in terms of the learner, should establish aims, goals necessary to accomplish the aims, and the learning process most likely to achieve the goals.

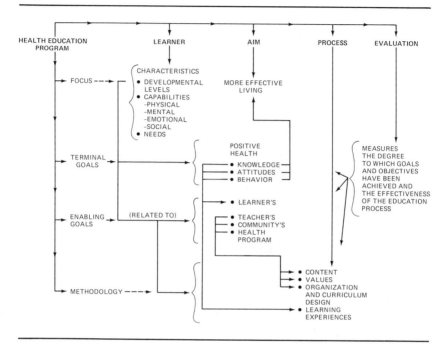

- At what developmental level are particular learning experiences most appropriate to achieve the goals?
- What enabling goals should be used as aids for the achievement of the terminal goals?
- Are goals and approaches sufficient for completing the health education mission?
- Are the goals of health education oriented toward the learner or toward the teacher, curriculum, or program?

Health knowledge, attitudes, and behavior

The acquisition of health information and the development of health knowledge are frequently interpreted as being one and the same. Health information should be viewed as unorganized or unrelated health facts. Health information becomes more usable when the learner understands not only what the facts are, but why they are significant and how they relate to other information that has already been acquired. The acquisition of health information is an illustration of the process of assimilation described by Piaget and discussed in Chapter 6. Not until the health

FIGURE 4–2 The Foundations of Health Education

The foundational elements of the health education program dictate *how* the goals shall be achieved.

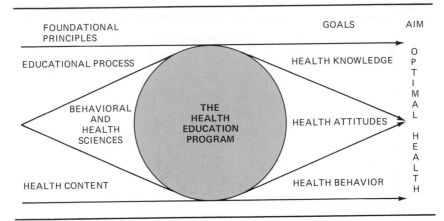

information becomes a predisposition (creates a readiness to respond) can it be properly described as health knowledge. Health knowledge implies comprehension, and comprehension implies the ability to behave according to the individual's perception of the usability of the information. It now becomes the basis for health decision-making. In other words, once the health information influences the individual's adaptability, accommodation has taken place.

Health knowledge can be either factual or fallacious. It can be perceived accurately or inaccurately; acquired through direct and conscious learning experiences or through indirect and subliminal learning experiences; immediately or potentially usable. Health knowledge may be found in a variety of forms characterized by simple familiarity, comprehension, insight, and wisdom. Although health knowledge can frequently be inferred from healthy behavior, the possession of such knowledge does not guarantee health-promoting actions. For example, if we observe a child brushing his or her teeth correctly, we can conclude that the child knows how to brush the teeth; but a youngster who knows how to may not always do it correctly. Therefore, health knowledge is essentially potential in the sense that it *can* direct the individual's behavior accordingly, but it may not since there are a number of other factors besides knowledge that direct behavior.

Finally, health knowledge can be viewed as having three levels of application. It may manifest itself through observable adaptation as illustrated in the above example; through unobservable behavior as a feeling or belief; or as potential usable knowledge. Observable manifestations, for example, may be the simple recall of facts or events or the application of knowledge for solving complex personal and social

FIGURE 4–3   Levels of Application of Health Knowledge

The application of acquired health knowledge is motivated by the kind of predisposition it establishes and may be manifested as observable or nonobservable behavior or as potentially usable behavior for future actions.

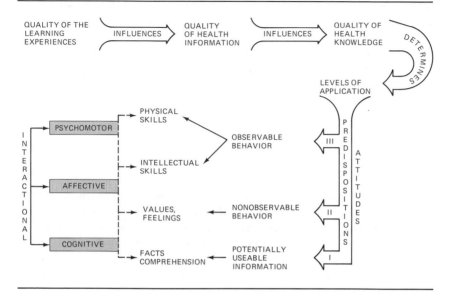

health problems. Figure 4–3 illustrates the possible levels of application of health knowledge.

Health attitudes are learned. They are predispositions to respond to environmental stimuli. Generally, attitudes begin to develop during the early childhood years. They are influenced chiefly by learning experiences associated with the social environment, especially through social contacts with parents and peers. Although attitudes can be changed, it is extremely difficult once they are established. First and early impressions can be lasting. However, it is important to recognize that the ways in which individuals express their attitudes can be influenced through the acquisition of new knowledge and greater insight into self, others, and the situation that exists. As was stated earlier, assimilated health knowledge determines the level of predisposition to respond. Therefore, health knowledge and health attitudes are inseparably intertwined, and as we will see, the quality of health behavior is dependent upon these two factors.

Health behavior is any isloated reaction to social or physical environmental stimuli; it is organized, purposeful reactions, or goal-directed actions, all of which can be observed. In addition, health behavior includes the variety of internal thoughts and feelings experienced by the individual and may be inferred from the external behavior. In essence, health behavior is the interpersonal, intrapersonal relations one possesses or expresses; personal values and philosophy; the totality of one's internal and external actions or reactions that are associated with all facets of health functioning. Generally, behavior can be viewed as any activity of the organism from the simplest reflex to the expression of complex physical and intellectual skills. Except for innate reflex actions, all human behavior is learned. As stated earlier, health behavior can be either health-related or health-directed. Some authorities believe that all behavior is health-related but only special kinds are health-directed.

CONTENT OF HEALTH EDUCATION

Major categories

The content of the health education program should be much more than merely factual health information. It should also include the learning experiences, the use of resource materials and people, the many evaluative techniques being used: all of the factors that affect the health learning of each individual. In other words, the health education content is the curriculum, and the curriculum is the total design for health learning and its application to the learner.

The informational content of health education programs should be identified on the basis of the three dimensions of health: physical, psychological, and sociological. Specific health areas and issues can be organized within these categories. The informational content areas are identified for convenience in planning the health education program since, as we will see, there is an interrelationship between both the categories and the topics.

To adequately discuss the factors which influence one's social health, for example, we must also consider the psychological impact of cultural influences upon one's personal values, self-concept, etc. One's interpersonal relations are, in turn, dependent to a great extent upon how well one views the self, especially in regards to others. The impact of a specific physical health problem upon the three dimensions of health can be seen in the case of a coronary thrombosis or heart attack. Coronary thrombosis is basically a physical health problem: It is caused by a blood clot present in a coronary artery and is characterized by physical pain in the chest which may extend to other proximal parts of the body, the arms and neck, for instance. Since most people experiencing a heart attack survive, there will necessarily be a change in their life-style to decrease the possibility of a recurrence. These changes may include changes in attitudes toward self, others, job, etc.; changes in physical activities, such as recreational participation and the kinds and frequency of social functions. In this example, we observe effects upon the social and psychological, as well as physical health of the individual, exemplifying the holistic interrelationship of the three dimensions of health.

Health facts should be stressed only when they are essential for the learner to achieve the health objectives. Basically, the acquisition of health information should *result from* the learning experience, rather than *being* the learning experience. For instance, it may be necessary to concentrate on health facts when such information is needed to solve the health problem. However, as health educators, we should avoid the pitfall of merely presenting health facts for memorization, recall, and recognition. This process of learning about health usually results in minimal and short-lived retention with little or no application by the learner for improving health behavior. Health facts become important when they are internalized by learners; when they have an influence upon how they think, feel, or act. One of the most effective ways to avoid teacher-dominated presentations is through the use of the inductive learning process rather than the deductive learning process.

Physical health

Physical health topics consist of areas that deal with the individual's biological well-being. They include areas that relate to personal health, factors which can be controlled to some extent, or which affect tissues, organs or systems of the body favorably or adversely. Physical health topics are associated with anatomy and physiology; however, they are not a study of human anatomy and physiology. They are a study of the internal and external environmental conditions which play an important role in the health of the anatomy and its ability to function in accordance with its intended purposes. The following list describes some of the chief physical health topic areas.

- *Foods and nutrition* affect the individual's growth, development, and functioning ability. Nutritional abuses can result in inadequate growth, emotional problems, and some disease conditions. Proper nutrition can enhance growth and development and, along with other factors, prevent the onset of some diseases. Some genetic disorders are closely associated with nutritional behavior, as well as other health topic areas included in this list.
- *Sensory perception and sensory health* are concerned chiefly with the five senses, but especially hearing and vision. Perception is an intellectual process characterized by an awareness of, and interpretation of, environmental stimuli. The health of the sense organs will determine the intensity and accuracy of the stimuli received by the brain, and this, in turn, will determine the quality of perception and ultimate behavior of the individual.
- *Disease prevention and control* implies the multitude of personal, social, epidemiological, medical, and other actions or procedures employed to decrease the likelihood of a pathological condition occurring

or interfering with normal functioning. Disease is essentially any of a number of physical, social, or psychological pathological conditions. Disease prevention occurs when the individual behaves appropriately, society provides a healthful environment, or the health sciences, especially the medical profession, provide essential immunizing agents. Disease control takes place when known methods to prevent the condition from expressing itself are employed. For example, scurvy, basically an inherited predisposition to a disease state, can be *prevented* from expression through the ingestion of adequate amounts of vitamin C. Diabetes mellitus can be *controlled* by the artificial administration of insulin.

- *Dental health* is more appropriately labeled *oral health* since it includes the maintenance of health of all of the oral structures: teeth, gums, tongue, etc. Proper nutrition, oral hygiene, the avoidance of such irritants as tobacco and tobacco smoke, and excessive use of alcohol, along with measures to prevent infections of the oral structures are important for oral health.
- *Genetic health* is described here as a physical health topic because it is related to the biological determiners of human potentials even though the manifestation of genetic ill-health may be psychological in some instances.
- *Personal safety* results when individuals avoid injury or take steps to eliminate or reduce hazardous environmental conditions. It is a physical health topic that is closely associated with both the psychological and social health topic categories, since many unsafe conditions are created by society and some individuals appear to be more accident-prone than others. Proneness to accident has been suggested to be allied with unconscious mental factors which place people in situations that are more likely to result in personal injury than for others who do not possess this proneness. On the other hand, accident proneness may be simply a manifestation of carelessness due to a lack of safety knowledge, poor perception of the situation, or a preoccupation with an unrelated event.

Psychological health

This category includes health topic areas that are concerned with the intellectual and emotional development and behavior of the individual. Health education programs should address the overall factors that influence the individual's total personality development, self-concept, mental and emotional health, thinking and reasoning, as well as the factors that influence interpersonal relations. Emotions may act as powerful motivators. They are complex and intense feelings which involve both internal, physiological responses and overt, observable reactions to environmental stimuli. Emotions can influence the individual's quality of reasoning and decision-making either positively or adversely. In like manner, the intellect can influence the quality of emotional expressions. Health education is, therefore, directed toward providing people with an understanding of their feelings so that expressions can be directed intelligently toward constructive forms of behavior. The psychological health topic areas are described as follows.

- *Human needs,* the satisfaction or deprivation of which, act as motivators of human behavior. Learning experiences in this topic area should center around an understanding of the nature of basic needs, how they influence behavior, and how they can best be satisfied and used to achieve desirable personal and social goals.
- *Human emotions* can be either positive or negative forces. Love, for example, may provide one with the motivation to succeed, enhance the quality of life, and is often accompanied by pleasant sensations. Conversely, love may elicit unpleasant sensations and actually interfere with the ability to function. Love is an emotion associated with the desire to possess, a desire that can be expressed in terms of selfish or shared behavior. Other emotions may also elicit desirable or undesirable reactions. Learning about the various facets of emotion is important in using them as mechanisms for achieving desirable ends.
- *Values clarification* is a topic area that has only recently acquired popularity among health educators. It is described as a health methodology in Chapter 12. Essentially, it is a complex series of processes designed to help learners examine and understand their own value system. It is presumed that such insight will result in the ability to deal objectively with such significant influences as social mores and the varieties of personal moral issues and beliefs.
- *Personality development* is an extremely broad and complex topic encompassing all of the topics mentioned in this list. Learning experiences related to this topic should emphasize chiefly the genetic and environmental factors that affect the growth and development of people. Personality is defined as the total organized characteristics of the individual including external appearance and behavior and self-awareness. These characteristics distinguish us from all others and determine how others will respond to us (social stimulus value). The components of one's personality are quite permanent and are generally, acquired early in life. Experiences and interpretations during the first few years of life are important in forming personality.
- *Coping mechanisms* are also called defensive mechanisms or ego defense mechanisms. Coping mechanisms are unconscious reactions employed by the individual and designed to maintain a feeling of adequacy and to seek relief from emotional conflict and anxiety.
- *Psychophysiologic health* is synonymous with psychosomatic health. Generally, the literature refers to this area only in terms of disorders. We prefer to emphasize the health aspect of this topic rather than the pathological aspects. Viewing this area positively exemplifies the close relationship between the mental health of an individual and some aspects of physical health. Emotional stresses can affect organs,

usually under the control of the autonomic nervous system, which results in physical dysfunction and often actual tissue damage. Disorders whose etiology is at least partially emotional are called psychosomatic or psychophysiological disorders. Maintenance of emotional health is a chief preventive for this class of diseases.

- *Neurotic and psychotic behavior* are two rather extreme groups of manifestations that indicate that mental health has failed. Neurotic reactions (psychoneuroses) are characterized by mild personality disorders: emotional maladaptation associated with anxiety, resulting from unresolved, unconscious conflicts. Psychoses are a group of disorders characterized by gross personality disorganization and distortion or misinterpretation of reality. Psychoses may manifest themselves as mild or severe, temporary or permanent. The etiology of psychoses may be emotional or organic. The organic etiology can be associated with nervous tissue damage from chemicals, mechanical injury, or infection.
- *Mental health maintenance* is a general topic area that should be given priority for all developmental learning levels. It should direct its attention toward providing the learners with insight into their whole behavioral make-up: self-concept, self-worth, personal capabilities, and ways of dealing with emotions, stresses, conflicts, anxieties, and frustrations. It includes the factors affecting mental health, the influence of the social environment, social expectations, and reactions needed to function effectively. Finally, mental health maintenance is concerned with the people and agencies available to provide assistance when needed, their purposes, and how to make use of them most effectively.
- *Human motivation* is basic to effective functioning. An understanding of the factors that motivate an individual is important for sustaining psychological health.
- *Human sexuality* is an important topic area that receives unwarranted, adverse, and controversial attention. Although everyone at sometime in life learns that there are essentially two sexes whose life's roles are, in some respects, similar, and in other respects quite different, and that human sexuality refers to this total social role of sexes alone or together, there is a tendency for some people to become obsessed with the morality of heterosexual, homosexual, or bisexual intercourse. Human sexuality is concerned with much more than this expression of people for people. It is rather concerned with the totality of human beings functioning in a variety of social settings. In this regard, human sexuality might better be categorized as sociological health rather than psychological health. But the basic health dimension which has the greatest impact on this area is the psychological dimension. However, it can not be separated from the social dimension any more than the social dimension can be separated from the psychological dimension.
- *Grief education* is more popularly called death or dying education.

It is a sensitive area with a variety of psychological and social ramifications. The health educator must be specially prepared to adequately implement programs designed to assist the learner to cope with situations that result in extreme grief.

Sociological health

The social and physical environments affect the physical and psychological development and functioning of the individual and the group. They play the most important role in affecting the quality of human behavior. This is especially true in regards to the ways people are expected to react to their "significant others". As illustrated in Figure 4-4, some significant others are in almost continuous contact with us as we proceed through the growing years. Other aspects of the social environment that are also important influencers of sociological health include the particular social institutions, community agencies, media, and formal and informal social groups. These components tend to be less direct and more sporadic than the direct relations one has with the significant others. Sociological health addresses such issues as family living, cultural influences, changing social mores, and interpersonal relations. The general topic areas of sociological health are listed below.

- *Public and community health* includes the psychological and physical environments in which we must live. It is concerned with the health problems and issues whose solutions rest with organized, coordinated mass procedures directed toward the prevention of disease, promotion of health, and prolongation of life. Today, we must think in terms much broader than a single community setting; public health must encompass the whole of all societies on a world-wide scale.
- *Consumer health* views all individuals as users of health products (drugs, devices, etc.) and health services (medical, nonmedical, paramedical, hospitals, etc.). In addition, all individuals are purchasers of these through direct or indirect payment procedures. These include the cost of health and accident insurance, whether through private or governmental sources. Furthermore, consumer health is concerned with the purchase and/or use of products and services that have been proven ineffective or not beneficial (quackery, nostrums, etc.).
- *Epidemiology* is, according to Mausner and Bahn, "the study of the distribution and determinants of diseases and injuries in human populations." They go on to say that "epidemiology is concerned with the *extent* and types of illnesses and injuries in *groups* of people and with the *factors* which influence their distribution."[1] In health education we are concerned with more than what epidemiology is; we are concerned with its methods as well. The epidemiologist applies the methods of inductive investigation for understanding health and disease. These principles are applicable to the health education methodology.

FIGURE 4-4   Significant Others
Some social forces are indirect and sporadic. The significant forces are direct and continuous. They consist chiefly of peers, siblings, parents, and teachers.

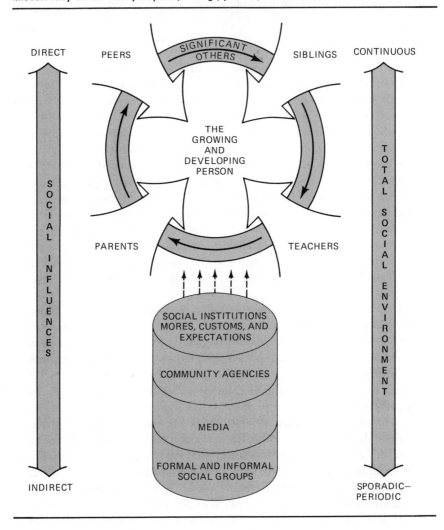

- *Marriage and family health* have undergone significant changes in the past few decades. The roles of individuals have also undergone changes. Since the family is the second basic unit of our society (the individual being the most basic), its health may very well be the only important indicator of the health of society. New standards governing marriage and family structure have been introduced. Society must evaluate these and make judgments about whether or not they tend to strengthen the family unit and are consistent with the goals of American society.
- *Safety and first aid* are frequently considered to be a single topic area

since first aid is usually performed following a careless act which results in injury or accidental poisoning. In this context, we are considering this topic area as a sociological health problem because safe behavior protects more than just the individual (as in automobile safety, for example). First aid usually involves two or more people.

- *Drug education* is concerned with legal drugs such as prescription and over-the-counter drugs, and their use and abuse (alcohol and tobacco, for example) as well as illicit drugs (marijuana, cocaine, heroin, etc.). The drug problem is an extremely complex one which aroused the curiosity, interest, political activity, and greed of thousands of people in less than ten years. It has been dealt with by many sources, but chiefly through law enforcement and treatment and rehabilitation of the drug dependent. Although billions of dollars have been channeled through these sources, little, if any, progress has been made in reducing the incidence of drug abuse or reducing the number of drug addicts. The remaining approaches—research into causes, education, prevention, and improved environments and living conditions—have been virtually ignored as possible solutions. This is probably because they lack the excitement and dramatics of cure (even though this is a rare phenomenon) and they lack political attractiveness.

- *Politics and health* is a topic that is being introduced into the health education program for the first time. We have alluded to this topic in previous discussions as having significant potential for raising the level of health of the American people. Health problems of today and those anticipated for the future generally entail much more than individual health behavior and the types of health programs we are accustomed to seeing in operation. Many awesome political decisions regarding the health of people will need to be made for our national health policy, as well as for specific health issues. A health-educated populace is essential; a populace that understands the significance of political awareness and involvement. We can no longer allow political decisions about health matters to be made behind closed legislative doors. Legislators must be kept informed of the facts concerning health legislation; they must be kept aware of the needs and wishes of the people that new legislation will affect. Citizens must accept this responsibility.

Each of these content areas can be further divided into subtopics. For example, disease prevention and control may include such subtopics as the nature and prevention of chronic and degenerative diseases; this can be further subdivided into cardiovascular health (or diseases), prevention of cancer, etc. Table 4–1 provides further suggestions along these lines.

Finally, for health education to be most effective, it must include learning experiences for teachers and parents as well as for elementary and secondary school students. This is necessary because the educational impact on children and youth must be reinforced by others with whom

TABLE 4–1: Some Urgent Health Issues

Primarily Physical Health	Primarily Psychological Health	Primarily Sociological Health
Venereal disease (J,H)	Death & Dying (P,I,J,H)	Environmental Pollution (P,I,J,H)
Reproduction (P,I,J,H)	Psychosomatic disorders (J,H)	Abortion (H)
Menstruation (I,J,H)	Neurotic reaction (I,J,H)	Marriage (H)
Visual Health (P,I,J,H)	Psychotic reactions (I,J,H)	Divorce (P,I,J,H)
Auditory health (P,I,J,H)	Suicide (J,H)	Family Planning (H)
Oral health (P,I,J,H)	Sexual behavior (J,H)	Health specialists and services (P,I,J,H)
Obesity (I,J,H)	Epilepsy (I,J,H)	Health quackery (I,J,H)
Malnutrition (I,J,H)	Emotional implications human sexuality (J,H)	Dietary fads (I,J,H)
Respiratory disorders (P,I,J,H)		OTC drugs (P,I,J,H)
Hepatitis (P,I,J,H)		Health advertising (P,I,J,H)
Cardiovascular diseases (J,H)		Drug abuse (P,I,J,H)
Cerebrospinal diseases (J,H)		Alcohol abuse and alcoholism (P,I,J,H)
Rheumatic fever (I,J,H)		Smoking (P,I,J,H)
Cancer (P,I,J,H)		Prescription drugs (P,I,J,H)
Genetic health (I,J,H)		Health insurance (J,H)
		Pesticides and health (P,I,J,H)
		Radiation & health (P,I,J,H)
		Accidents (P,I,J,H)
		Human sexuality (P,I,J,H)
		The changing family (P,I,J,H)

P = Primary grades
I = Intermediate grades
J = Junior high or middle school grades
H = High school grades

they come in contact. Figure 4–5 illustrates the relationship of the informational content of health education to those who are, or should be, affected by it.

Health issues

What are health issues? How are they identified? Who do they affect? There are hundreds of health issues which need to be explored by learners at various times during their years of growth and learning. Which ones should be investigated will vary according to the criteria of "Goals of Health Education," discussed earlier. Obviously, priorities must be established by the coordinated efforts of teacher and learner.

FIGURE 4–5   The Content of Health Education
The content of health education should reflect the three dimensions of health and be directed toward all people.

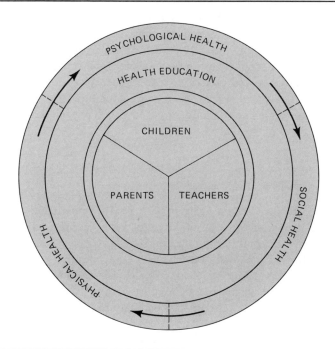

Health learning time in the school curriculum is very limited and the tendency toward content selection based solely upon attractiveness of the health issue must be avoided. Priorities must be based upon the relative importance and urgency of the health issue to the learner's over-all health behavior and societal demands. With these fundamental guideposts in mind, the teacher and learner should select those health issues that best meet their health priorities. Table 4–1 provides a listing of some health issues that can be used as a guide for setting these priorities. Note that each issue is categorized according to the dimensions of health. The references in parentheses following each issue designate the suggested grade levels at which progression should be maintained. These suggestions are based upon the level at which the greatest learner concern and educational impact is *most* likely to occur.

It must be reemphasized here that such categorization is, at best, artificial, since a health issue that is classed as "physical" may very well have significant psychological and/or sociological implications. This is probably true in the vast majority of cases. For example, the venereal diseases are fundamentally physical, caused by microorganisms and manifested in tissue destruction and dysfunction. However, there are significant emotional and social ramifications. In fact, these diseases are frequently classed as serious social health problems. This is one reason why no health issue can adequately be discussed without taking into account its total physical, psychological, and sociological impact. This points up the need for organizing health education programs on a comprehensive and sequential basis. This is clearly exemplified in regards to fitness. Usually one thinks only of physical fitness, when in reality, psychological and sociological fitness are of equal importance. It should also be noted that not all health issues are necessarily related to diseased conditions. Many are associated with the general aspects of living. For instance, marriage, family planning, and consumerism are extremely urgent issues which can and do affect the behavioral health of each individual.

Purpose of health content

To summarize, health information in terms of content has four major purposes: (1) to provide the learner with health knowledge and insight (intellectual development), (2) to provide the learner with a logical and personally acceptable foundation for health decision-making, (3) to provide the learner with health facts that can be used to clarify personal values regarding particular health issues, and (4) to provide the learner with the wisdom to behave in the most appropriate manner under a given set of circumstances. Figure 4–6 illustrates these relationships.

It is most important to understand that health issues or general informational content areas do not in themselves constitute health education. They merely identify one form of product. Of even greater importance is the specific end result these issues signify and the process used for attaining this end. The end result should be expressed in terms of behavioral or performance objectives. These are concerned with the total product of learning (cognitive, affective and psychomotor). The process (learning experiences and methodologies) of learning makes the product feasible and dynamic. Finally, the President's Committee on Health Education emphasized the importance of adequate and accurate health information when it stated that "health education is a process that bridges the gap between health information and health practices. Health education motivates the person to take the information and do something with it—to keep himself healthier by avoiding actions that are harmful and by forming habits that are beneficial."[2]

A generally overlooked purpose of health education is the development of citizen awareness of the existing political control over programs affecting societal health and the usual methods used to initiate new health programs. Executive orders, for example, may be predicated upon the advice of a small number of people. But most important is the motivation behind any executive order. Although decisions may historically be judged as valid, promoting the welfare of the people, there are many questions that need to be asked. Who are the health authorities advising

FIGURE 4–6 Purpose of Health Information

Health information should result in improved decision-making, health wisdom, and appropriate health behavior.

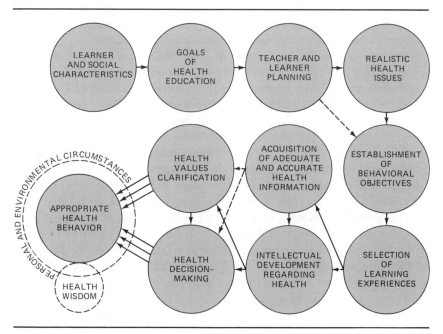

a President or governor? Upon what evidence do they base their recommendations? Is the decision based primarily on political motivation or on a genuine concern for the health of American citizens? How well informed are the American people regarding the particular health issue? Did the government make a concerted effort to provide the facts about the health issue to the people? Did the people have an opportunity to express their views to the government?

The point of this is to reveal how many health decisions made by those in power are determined on the basis of insufficient evidence, lack of factual information, political motives, prejudice, and generally questionable validity. Health is not only a concern of the medical profession or of government, but also a concern of every citizen. As such, there needs to be strict governmental monitoring of all health programs with full disclosures to the American people.

LEARNER AND TEACHER OBJECTIVES

Introduction

The developmental level and experiential background of the learner are significant criteria upon which to base the selection of the total health content. Using these criteria, the health educator will be able to choose the most relevant and worthwhile objectives to be achieved. This is one of the early steps in planning the health education course of study. Once objectives are selected, appropriate learning experiences can be provided. They must, however, be compatible, interactional, and reinforcing, and designed to influence concept development.

In view of the health issues we have been discussing, it becomes apparent that the outcomes of health education, both school and community based, are more than simply the positive alteration of individual health behavior. The health education program, its goals, organization, and processes must reflect the urgent need to provide the learner, especially the younger generation, with the health information needed to understand the complex decisions which must be made about societal health. In addition, each individual should be motivated to play an active role in these decisions. Medical technology is making advances which will profoundly affect each individual as well as our total social structure. This newfound knowledge can be used for the benefit of humanity or it may alter adversely our established way of life. The application of much of this new health knowledge can not, and indeed must not, be delegated to the judgment of only the medical profession. A health informed citizenry must play a significant and active role in future decisions.

Previous criteria no longer realistically apply to such questions as what constitutes a state of death, since it is now possible with new technology to prolong vital activity almost indefinitely. Should a parent knowingly be allowed to bring into the world a child destined to custodial care by society? Who will make this decision? Do we need a national genetic policy? Who shall make it? Who shall decide what is a defective gene? Should genetic engineering be used for the betterment of humanity? Obviously, these and many other questions can be adequately dealt with only by people who possess an abundance of accurate information, wisdom, and acceptable motivations. Therefore, the goals of health education must be relevant to *exogenous* as well as *endogenous* health factors. The development of personal integrity is becoming more and more an urgent goal of health education.

Exogenous and endogenous health factors

From the viewpoint of the health of individuals and society, the exogenous health factors are those stemming from the environment. The environment consists of natural and artificial physical and social aspects, including people, institutions, and social groups and programs, especially those created by political action, but not necessarily limited to it. The endogenous health factors are those which stem from within the individual, such as genetic potentials and normal growth and development. The expression and control of the endogenous health factors are constantly being influenced by the dynamics and quality of the exogenous health factors. The interaction between the two determines the resultant quality of individuals and societies. It is with this quality that the educational community must be most concerned. Essentially, we are referring to what the potential and the dynamic functioning of individuals and society is and what it can be in light of present and future technological development. These developments have awesome implications about the very survival of humanity.

Teacher objectives

The objectives of health education, both teacher- and learner-oriented, must illustrate insight into what has happened, what is happening, and what will happen in health. Teacher objectives are statements that describe what the teacher hopes to achieve in the health area being investigated. These objectives may imply methodology, techniques, informational content, and the like. For instance, examine the following:

1. To *show* a film on smoking behavior
2. To *discuss* the major points of the film
3. To *cover* the major concepts regarding the health hazards of smoking
4. To *give* a test on smoking and health

The first objective relates to a technique—to use a film; the second relates to a method—to discuss; the third implies that a method will be used, but does not state what it will be, that is, how the information will be covered (informational content), and the fourth objective indicates that evaluation will be made, but it does not state what kind of test (oral, written, objective, subjective, etc.) will be given. The third and fourth objectives are vague: Teacher objectives are usually not easily measured and not directly associated with learners and their needs. To overcome this unnecessary error, it is essential for the teacher and learner to plan together to determine what and how learning will take place. Learner objectives should be identified first and precisely stated in behavioral or performance terms. Teacher objectives should be identified in terms of learner outcomes and related specifically to ways in which they (the learner objectives) can best be achieved. Teacher objectives should also be suited to the competency of the teacher.

The achievement of learner objectives is dependent upon not only the capabilities of the learner, but the care with which the teacher selects objectives. These must activate the achievement of the learner objectives. Therefore, the degree to which learners achieve their objectives is dependent upon the ability of the teacher and consistency of the teacher objectives with learner objectives. The following formula illustrates this process:

TEACHER COMPETENCY → SELECTION OF LEARNER OBJECTIVES + TEACHER OBJECTIVES + LEARNING EXPERIENCES = GOAL ACHIEVEMENT

Traditionally, teacher objectives have been based on health facts and rules for health elicited from textbooks or curriculum guides. They frequently had little or no relation to learner needs and developmental levels. Just as frequently, they directed the teacher to teach unimportant health information and sometimes information that was questionable as to its relevance to health. As health education has become more defined, as health educators are being better trained, and as the educational community has begun to recognize the contribution which this discipline can make to the health of people, the health education program has gradually become more meaningful. More and more health educators are identifying their objectives in terms of the way learners can most effectively achieve objectives and goals. Consequently, teacher objectives are more likely today to be based on the following:

- The ways teachers can best assist learners.
- How material and human resources can *contribute* to learning, rather than just teaching.
- How the environment for optimal learning can be improved.
- How best to make use of such resources as audiovisual materials.
- The use of a variety of methods and techniques such as large and small group work, problem-solving, and individualized learning.
- A recognition that learner objectives exceed merely cognitive development.
- A recognition of individual differences among learners.
- The teacher's role as that of a facilitator of learning, rather than a giver of information.

Means states that "school health education today has considerable stature in the curriculum."[3] In spite of the enormous strides made in improving all aspects of health education in both the schools and public sectors, health education still remains a "step-child" in most school curricula for science, physical education, and home economics courses, none of which is equipped to achieve the goals of current health education. Health education is recognized in theory by enlightened school administrators and school boards of education, but in practice it is frequently poorly organized, taught by teachers with inadequate training, given low priority in the school's curriculum, and sometimes ignored altogether. This mismanagement perpetuates the misconception that health education is ineffective in achieving its stated goals. Unless health education is given proper status and implemented by trained health educators, it can be more harmful than beneficial.

Admittedly, health education has come a long way since its early beginnings in the late nineteenth century, but it still lags far behind what it should be in view of what is known today about health and the inherent potential value of education for health. Means goes on to explain that health education's "broad purposes, long promoted by pioneer and later leaders in the field, are perhaps more widely recognized than ever before. The variety and quality of health programs attest to progress made over the years."[4]

Progress certainly has been made since the early physiology and hygiene teachings of over a century ago. Ironically, this progress came about belatedly as a result of health crises and subsequent movements that were shut in the closet after the initial crises had appeared to pass. We find the same kind of belated responses being made today. The educational community, as well as society as a whole, seems unable to recognize and understand the value of sustaining health efforts and planning for the future so that individual and societal health can continue to improve and new crises can be prevented. Health education goes forward (and backward) in expensive and traumatic leaps and bounds.

Learner objectives—the three domains

Learner objectives are expressed in behavioral terms. They may be called behavioral, performance, educational, or instructional objectives. Regardless of the label given, a learner objective is essentially a statement that describes precisely what the learner will be doing as a result of participation in a learning experience. Learner objectives ask questions like "How will the learning experiences alter the learner's health behavior? How will the learner be different as a result of the learning experience? In other words, behavioral objectives are statements that describe what the learner will be doing to demonstrate that the goal has been achieved.

There are three basic considerations which determine what the behavioral objective will be. They are as follows:

1. An identification of the learner's total characteristics (phenotypes and genotypes).
2. An identification of learner and societal health needs.
3. An identification of short- and long-term health goals.

Once realistic and meaningful goals have been established, the various behavioral objectives can be stated. They may fall within the cognitive, affective, or psychomotor domains, depending upon the goal to be achieved. It will be recalled that the overall goals of health education are related to health knowledge, attitudes, and behavior. These are consistent with both the dimensions of health discussed earlier, and the behavioral objective domains described below. The relationship of behavioral objectives to health learning and the learner is illustrated in Figure 4–7.

There are five chief characteristics of behavioral objectives:

1. They state exactly what the learner will be doing.
2. They are measurable.
3. They are related to achieving a particular goal.

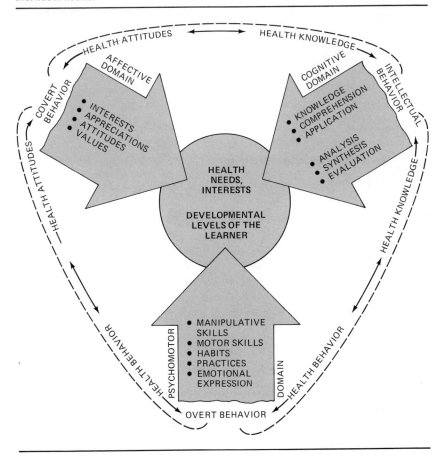

4. They fall within one of the three domains: cognitive, affective or psychomotor.
5. They state the conditions under which the new behavior will be manifested.

The *cognitive domain* is associated with any intellectual changes in the individual. It is characterized by measurable increases in health knowledge, comprehension, ability to analyze or synthesize health information, wisdom regarding health matters, and ability to apply new health information to decision-making. Bloom describes this domain as including "those objectives which deal with the recall or recognition of knowledge and the development of intellectual abilities and skill."[5]

The *affective domain* is associated with feelings and attitudes regarding health issues. It can include self-health concepts as well as social health concepts. This domain is characterized chiefly by changes relative to interests, feelings, appreciations, attitudes, and values. Health education methods stressing value clarification or similar experiences are most appropriate for achieving objectives which fall into this domain. The affective domain includes any changes in overt behavior of the individual. Since this area is concerned with emotions it is most closely allied with the psychological dimension of health.

The *psychomotor (behavioral) domain* is concerned with neuromuscular coordination, physical skills, habits and general practices. As opposed to the affective domain, it is characterized by overt health behavior. Such activities as having an annual physical examination, eating the appropriate foods, dieting when necessary, not smoking, having a Pap test, monthly breast self-examination, and the like, demonstrate achievement of these objectives. The psychomotor domain objectives are most closely related to healthful behavior.

Stating behavioral objectives

As Figure 4–8 illustrates, the three domains of objectives are interdependent, each influencing the expression of the other. For example, an individual who learns (cognitive) about the health hazards of smoking and who decides not to smoke or to quit smoking is demonstrating (behavioral or psychomotor) that the health information regarding smoking is applicable to health behavior. Consequently, we can conclude that this person has acquired certain positive attitudes (affective) regarding smoking.

Although each of the domains is different from the other, it is obvious that they are interrelated, at least to some degree. Behavioral objectives, regardless of the domain in which they fall, have certain characteristics which are common. These are summarized as follows:

- They are ends toward which the learner strives.
- They are the result of learning.
- They are stated in terms of changes in learner behavior.
- They are concerned with the product of learning rather than the process of learning (as may be true with teacher objectives).
- They establish the direction that learning will take.
- They are stated in terms of observable or measurable learner behavior.
- They are the expected end result of teaching-learning experiences.
- They describe the reaction the learner will make about the information learned.
- They describe learner behavior as related to particular environmental stimuli.
- They are associated with the learner rather than with the teacher, the content, or the approaches.

FIGURE 4–8   The Interdependency of Objective Domains
The goals of health education are interactional with the objective domains and the
dimensions of health.

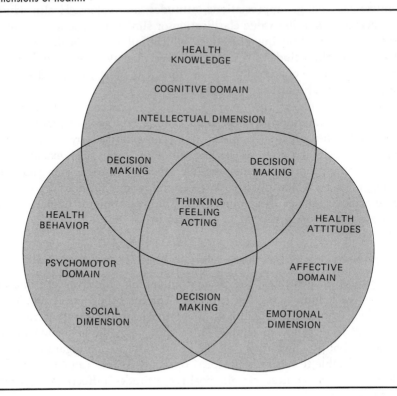

As an aid in formulating learner objectives, the following action words will be helpful (in addition, the teacher should understand that preceding each learner objective is the stated or implied phrase, "The learner will be able to . . ."): apply, use, perform, write, interpret, locate, define, differentiate, recognize, distinguish, draw, show, describe, identify, analyze, examine, demonstrate, choose, list, illustrate, prepare, develop, discriminate, construct, name, conclude, synthesize, formulate, evaluate, predict, and so on.

For example, an objective may be written as: "The learner will understand what constitutes an adequate diet." However, "understands" is nonspecific and nonmeasurable, or at least very difficult to measure. Therefore, such an objective is not a behavioral objective. An improvement would be: "The learner is able to *list* the foods one should eat to insure a balanced diet." Or, "The learner *chooses* from a variety of foods those which constitute an adequate daily diet." Obviously, the teacher and the learner must plan together precisely what the learner's behavior should be following the learning experience. And it must be possible to measure whether or not this behavior is, in fact, operable.

Some behavioral objectives fall clearly within the area of one of the three domains, while some may appear to fall within more than one domain. It is important for the teacher and learner to have a clear perception of what learning (objective) is most urgent, appropriate, and possible. From this understanding, the objective should be stated to describe (1) the precise behavior expected, (2) the domain into which the expected behavior will fall, and (3) the conditions under which the learner will demonstrate the behavior. For example, if cognition regarding cervical cancer is the priority expectation, the objective can be stated as follows: "The learner will be able to . . .

1. describe why the Pap test is important.
2. list the procedures used by a physician in giving a Pap test.
3. state when the Pap test should be given.

Each of the above objectives states exactly the cognition expectation necessary for the student to demonstrate the achievement of the objective. Each example is measurable, although the measuring technique to be used is not indicated. For instance, the description, listing, or stating could be done orally or in written form.

If, on the other hand, the priority domain is the psychomotor, the objective may be stated as: "The learner who has become sexually active will *receive* a yearly Pap test." Although this objective is measurable, it is much more difficult to do so in an educational setting since the actual demonstration by the learner occurs outside of the school and for the rest of her life.

Objectives falling within the affective domain are much more difficult to state precisely and more difficult to measure specifically, since we are dealing with attitudes, feelings, and emotions. Therefore, measurement may have to be inferred from behavioral demonstrations from the other two domains. This again attests to the wholeness of human beings. For instance, if the objective were stated as: "The learner *appreciates* the value of the Pap test for early detection and treatment of cervical cancer," and the learner did receive the Pap test yearly, we can conclude that she has acquired the expected attitude toward the Pap test.

DEFINITIVE UNDERSTANDING

Studies that have been conducted in the recent past indicate that the majority of American people lack even elementary health knowledge. This is complicated further by the multitude of health misconceptions that many people possess.

Many of our serious health problems could be alleviated and many totally prevented simply through providing people with accurate and timely health information. Some outstanding examples are glaucoma; skin, cervical, breast, and lung cancer; and many genetic disorders. As a result, the need for effective health education of all people can not logically be disputed. Each individual has a right to be thoroughly informed about health matters.

Health can be broadly defined in terms of all factors that influence the functioning ability of people. As such, the breadth of health education has no limits. Health educators, however, have the very real responsibility to identify the more urgent health issues and to establish educational priorities accordingly.

These priorities, along with the developmental levels of the learners and other individual characteristics, form the basis for the aims and goals of health education. The aim of health education is expressed in terms of its mission, which is to provide individuals with the essential ingredients necessary for effective living. The goals of health education are more defined in terms of health knowledge, attitudes, and behavior. Goals may be expressed as being either terminal or enabling. Goals, when clearly stated, provide the teacher and learner with the direction and process necessary for achieving the mission.

Health information is viewed as the factual data available. Once health information is assimilated and has influenced the predisposition to act, accommodation has taken place. At this point, we can correctly assume that the individual has a degree of health knowledge. Health knowledge is characterized by comprehension, insight, and wisdom. Its quality may be inferred from the quality of behavior. Health knowledge can be viewed in terms of three levels of application: observable adaptation, nonobservable behavior, or potentially usable information.

The content of health education includes all of the factors that affect health learning. It is the health curriculum, the total design for learning. The informational content is categorized according to the three dimensions of health: physical, psychological, and sociological.

Physical health topics are concerned with improving the learner's biological well-being. Essentially, they are (1) foods and nutrition, (2) sensory perception, (3) disease prevention and control, (4) dental health, (5) genetic health, and (6) personal safety. Psychological health deals with intellectual and emotional development and expression. The topics in this category are (1) human needs, (2) human emotions, (3) value clarification, (4) personality development, (5) coping mechanisms, (6) psychophysiological health, (7) neurotic and psychotic behavior, (8) maintenance of mental health, (9) human motivation, (10) human sexuality, and (11) grief education. Finally, sociological health is concerned with the quality of one's interpersonal relations and the effects that the physical and social environments have on this development. This is especially true in regards to "significant others." The topic areas in this category are (1) public and community health, (2) consumer health, (3) epidemiology, (4) marriage and family health, (5) safety and first aid, (6) drug education, and (7) politics and health.

These broad topic areas can be further divided into health issues or subtopics. Since there are literally hundreds of health issues, it is necessary for health education planners to establish priorities regarding those topics that are most significant and urgent. Health issues as well as topic areas usually spill over from one health dimension to another. Consequently, any categorization is intended for convenience in planning the health education program.

The purpose of health information is related chiefly to the acquisition of knowledge, decision-making, value clarification, wisdom, and political awareness. The informational content is but one form of educational product. The end result of learning is expressed in terms of behavioral objectives which will fall into the cognitive, affective, or psychomotor domains.

Selection of health education objectives will be influenced by the exogenous and endogenous factors affecting the quality of health and hence the quality of learning. Objectives may be either teacher-oriented, learner-oriented, or both. Teacher objectives state precisely what the teacher intends to do to affect the health learning of students. They must be based upon teacher competency and the nature of learner objectives. The combination of these, if effectively implemented, will direct learning toward goal achievement.

Learner objectives should be stated in behavioral, performance, or measurable terms. They state precisely what the learner will be doing following the learning experience to demonstrate that the objective has been achieved. They should indicate the way the learner's behavior is different after the learning experience. This can be measured.

PROBLEMS FOR DISCUSSION

1. Identify reasons for health education being a right of all individuals.
2. List at least ten health problems that could be eliminated if people were well-informed and behaved accordingly. Identify the cause of each health problem listed.
3. Synthesize the components which make up the breadth of health education. Show their relationships to each other.
4. Distinguish between the following: a goal and an aim; a terminal and an enabling goal; teacher and learner objective.
5. Discuss the relationship of health goals to the learner and the processes to be used.
6. List the criteria that determine the informational component of health education.
7. Describe the three dimensions of health. How do they relate to the informational content? To the three objective domains?
8. Distinguish between the product and the process of health learning.
9. Identify the chief characteristics of behavioral objectives.
10. Describe how health knowledge, attitudes, and behavior are inseparable. How does each influence the expression of the others?

11. Distinguish between health information and health knowledge. When do health facts become health knowledge? What forms does health knowledge take?
12. What are the three levels of application of health knowledge? Describe how each level is related to the three objective domains. Relate these levels to health attitudes and behavior.
13. Discuss how the "significant others" influence one's social development; one's psychological development.
14. State how health issues are different from, yet associated with, health topics.
15. What are the chief purposes of the informational content of health education?
16. Discuss the factors related to the degree to which American people should be involved in political health decisions.
17. Why is health education considered a social mandate?

REFERENCES

1. Mausner, Judith S. and Anita K. Bahn, *Epidemiology: An Introductory Text*, W. B. Saunders Company, Philadelphia, 1974, pp. 3–4.
2. U.S., Department of Health, Education and Welfare, *The Report of the President's Committee on Health Education*, 1973, p. 17.
3. Means, Richard K., *Historical Perspectives on School Health*, Charles B. Slack, Inc., New Jersey, 1975, p. 223.
4. Ibid.
5. Bloom, Benjamin, et al., *Taxonomy of Educational Objectives, Handbook I: Cognitive Domain*, David McKay Co., New York, 1956, p. 7.

Part Two

Psychological
Sociological
Perspective
of Health
Education

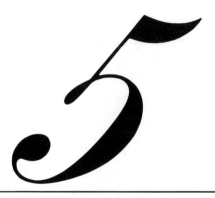

Dimensions
of Human
Health
Needs

Life is an adventure in a world
where nothing is static. . . . The very
process of living is a continual
interplay between the individual
and his environment often taking
the form of a struggle resulting in
injury or disease. The more creative
the individual the less he can hope
to avoid danger, for the stuff of
creation is made up of responses to
forces that impinge on his body
and soul.

Rene Dubos

The drama of health education
exceeds the imagination of
Shakespeare's tragedies, comedies,
and histories. Health *is* humankind!

AEB
DAB

INTRODUCTION

Bio-psycho-social needs

The dimensions of human needs are limited only by our comprehension of the nature of things. Human needs are never static: they are dynamic and ever-changing as we progress through life.

From the moment of conception, certain basic needs related to the vital processes must be satisfied if life is to continue. The prenatal needs are chiefly biological. As illustrated in Figure 5–1, they include nourishment, oxygen, and the elimination of waste. After birth, satisfaction of these needs continues to be urgent, but others associated with emotional and social growth become increasingly important. As the human organism matures, these new psychosocial needs begin to overshadow, though not to replace, the biological ones. Aside from their purely biological role, need satisfactions are essential for adequate intra– and interpersonal functioning.

Although everyone has the same basic needs, the *ways* in which they must be satisfied will vary considerably from person to person. Adequate satisfaction of all basic needs lays the foundation for healthful behavior. In addition, the satisfaction of one need may contribute to the satisfaction of others. This is especially true as one matures, since previous need satisfaction will influence the intensity of satisfaction necessary for later life. For example, a person whose emotional needs are adequately met early in life may develop a sense of security and self-worth. As a result, the need for overt recognition of accomplishments may be greatly reduced later on in life. Basic human needs are inseparably interdependent and constantly interact with each other to influence one's total behavior. As Dubos aptly emphasizes: "Because of this interdependence, anything that impinges upon [human beings] affects simultaneously both body and mind, and causes them to interact. Thus, to study the body machine and to neglect the symbolic activities which are inextricably enmeshed with it is to ignore the most characteristic aspect of man's nature."[1]

Effects of unmet needs

Needs which are left unmet or which are met in inappropriate ways can adversely affect the individual's total development and behavioral responses to the need agent. Inadequacies in one need dimension may result in a generalized and undesirable reaction in several of the dimensions of human behavior. For instance, if food is denied to an individual, unsocial behavior may result. This was exemplified in the food deprivation study conducted at the University of Minnesota in 1944: "During the semistarvation period . . . the hunger drive became the most important factor affecting the subject's behavior. The men became unsocial, frequently ignoring such amenities as table manners."[2]

FIGURE 5–1   The Relation of Basic Needs to Maturation
Initially, basic human needs are related only to survival. As one matures, new needs related to psychosocial functioning come into existence but do not replace the biological ones. Satisfaction of the biological needs contributes to satisfaction of the psychosocial ones.

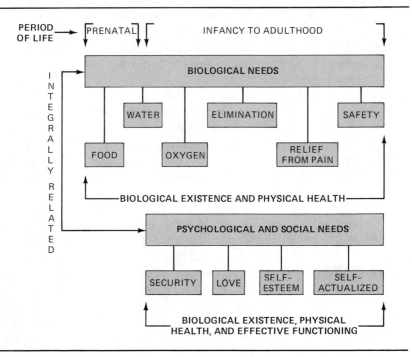

Although biological needs continue to be powerful motivators of behavior throughout life, they become less intense and less important for healthy people as they grow and develop. They can, however, interfere with the satisfaction of psychological and social needs if extreme deprivation should occur. The greatest and most crucial time for biological need satisfaction takes place during the early years. It is important to recognize not only those needs which must be satisfied, but also the ways they can best be met for maximum positive influence on the physical, emotional, social, and intellectual development of the individual.

What is a need?

A need is essentially a variety of felt urgencies related to the existence, continuation, and maintenance of life, and the enhancement of living. Needs may be at one time conscious and at other times unconscious. For example, hunger pains will bring about an awareness of the need to seek food. However, once sufficient food is taken, awareness of the need for nourishment will diminish. The more frequently and adequately needs are satisfied, the more likely their urgency will be decreased and pre-occupation with ways of satisfying them diminished, leaving the individual free to pursue more constructive forms of behavior. Conversely, a preoccupation with need satisfaction interferes with normal functioning and effectiveness as a human being.

Needs and homeostasis

Basic human needs can be divided into four convenient, though artificial, categories: biological, social, emotional, and intellectual. The biological needs are those which are necessary for the maintenance of life processes and contribute to other need satisfactions. They include the need for food, water, oxygen, and elimination of waste. The emotional needs are necessary for maintenance of behavioral homeostasis. This homeostasis implies that people can function well only if they can rapidly make adjustments to a changing environment. This adaptability is precisely defined for each organism.[3]

The social needs, which are intricately enmeshed with the emotional, allow an individual to successfully interact with others. People are social animals and dependent upon each other for the fulfillment of both emotional and social needs.[4] Finally, the intellectual needs are those which allow one to improve self-insight, self-concept, and to interact successfully with the environment through the appropriate use of knowledge, logic, and problem-solving skills. The absence of adequate environmental stimuli or the presence of inadequate stimuli, will result in a less than normally developed intelligence and a grossly atypical personality.[5] Total physiological, psychological, and sociological homeostasis is an indicator of a state of health. Homeostasis is essentially a state of balanced functioning; a state in which needs are being satisfied adequately and in the appropriate ways. Homeostasis implies that a state of health exists.

NEEDS, MATURATION, AND HEALTH

Maslow's hierarchy of needs

Maslow has developed a hierarchy of needs from the most basic, life sustaining to the most complex needs related to intra– and interpersonal functioning. These are outlined below:

- *Physiological,* which includes the need for water, oxygen, and food.
- *Safety,* which refers primarily to personal protection from hazards.
- *Love and belonging,* which relate to feelings toward others.
- *Esteem* needs, which are associated with feelings of appreciation.
- *Self-actualization,* which relates to achieving one's full potentials of growth, development, and functioning.
- *Knowledge* needs, which include the desire to know and understand.[6]

According to Maslow, a state of health can be related to one's pre-occupation with need satisfaction.[7] If people are chiefly motivated by the need to develop and actualize their fullest potentials, they are healthy, but if other basic needs are active and chronic, they are unhealthy. This concept is applicable to both physical and emotional health.

During the early years of growth, need satisfaction is relatively simple, but vital. As we progress toward maturity, many factors enter our lives to increase the complexity of this process. Children develop impressions of themselves and others, as well as of the world in general; these impressions may be inaccurate. They result in the establishment of values and personal aspirations which influence the ways basic needs must be fulfilled. In addition, simple and direct experiences take on new meanings for the individual. If past experiences are negative, erroneous impressions will have to be neutralized, overcome, or replaced.

What is the relation of needs to health learning?

The health educator must not only be aware of people's basic needs, but of the forces which have acted previously to alter the course of individual optimum development. The new learning opportunities and experiences should be determined by an assessment of the needs of each student. Such assessments will be effective only if they are relevant and meaningful. It is important also for health educators to be aware that their main responsibility should be providing learning opportunities that will assist each child to continue growth and development toward the highest level of functioning possible.

Satisfaction of the primary needs can alter not only the attitudes and behavior of the individual, but also the approaches necessary to satisfy these needs later in life. Contrary to popular belief, health education is not directed toward correcting defects that already exist in a child. This is the responsibility of the therapist. It is, however, vital that the health educator does not contribute further to the progression of negative forms of behavior, and that every effort is made to educate children according to their potentials, capabilities, needs and aspirations.

Needs according to Havighurst and Erikson

Generally speaking, the course of need satisfaction will change at various maturity levels. Both Havighurst and Erikson describe these stages in somewhat similar, but distinctive, terms emphasizing their significance in relation to individual development.

Erikson describes eight crises that each person encounters during her or his lifetime.[8] Havighurst describes the various developmental tasks that each person faces at each level of development.[9] These two theories are summarized and compared in Table 5–1. Their application to health education is also indicated.

The developmental tasks are important achievements that occur

TABLE 5–1 Application of Maturation Theories to Health Education

Erikson's Psychosocial Stages		Havighurst's Developmental Tasks		Application to Health Education	
Stages	Crises	Levels	Tasks	Educational Development	Learning Emphasis
Infancy	Trust vs mistrust	Infancy and early childhood (0–6)	Basic physical skills, foundations for social and emotional growth	Development of health awareness	Health practices
Early childhood	Autonomy vs doubt or shame				
Play age	Initiative vs guilt	Middle childhood (6–12)	Refined physical skills, peer relations, basic values and social attitudes	Development of appropriate health responses	Health attitudes and practices
School age	Industry vs inferiority				
Adolescence	Identity vs self-diffusion or negative identity	Adolescence (12–18)	Sexuality; emotional, economic and social independence	Development of health decision-making skills	Health knowledge, attitudes, and behavior, health values clarified
Young adulthood	Intimacy vs isolation	Early adulthood (18–35)	Mate relations, family relations, child rearing, civic responsibility	Development of appropriate ways of affecting health changes	Health knowledge, attitudes, and behavior
Adulthood	Generativity vs self-absorption	Middle age (35–60)	Civic and social responsibility, economic standards, new adjustments relating to parenthood	Development of serious involvement in community health affairs, political involvement	Health knowledge, attitudes, and behavior
Later life	Integrity and self-acceptance vs despair	Later maturity (60 +)	Adjustments to aging and retirement		

during various periods of growth. The more adequately people achieve a task at a given level of maturity, the more prepared they will be to face the new tasks at the next level of maturity. The developmental tasks for each maturity level include the accomplishment of the following:

- *Infancy and early childhood*—the development of simple physical skills such as walking; the development of emotional relationships with parents and siblings
- *Middle childhood*—the development of complex physical and intellectual skills; the development of wholesome attitudes toward self and society; the development of social relationships with peers.
- *Adolescence*—accepting one's sexual role; development of emotional and economic independence; the development of intellectual skills and social responsibility
- *Early adulthood*—achievements related to sexual roles, marriage, family, and children; civic and social responsibility
- *Middle age*—civic and social responsibility continues; adjustments to economic standards and to physiological changes related to aging;
- *Later maturity*—accepting the problems related to aging—accepting death of spouse

Erikson's psychosocial stages are described as developmental crises during each period of growth. As with Havighurst and Maslow, these stages are not separate and unrelated, nor do they disappear following a given growth period. Rather, they tend to be more intense and urgent at certain stages than at others. Erikson categorizes the stages and the crises for each as follows:

Infancy	trust vs mistrust
Early childhood	autonomy vs doubt or shame
Play age	initiative vs guilt
School age	industry vs inferiority
Adolescence	identity vs self-diffusion
Young adulthood	intimacy vs isolation
Adulthood	generativity vs self-absorption
Later life	integrity and self-acceptance vs despair

NEED SATISFACTION AND HEALTH EDUCATION

Introduction

The meeting of human needs is essential to the attainment and maintenance of a high level of health, and a high level of health is essential to the continuance of a society. Disease is a manifestation of the failure of the society to deal adequately with the needs of its people.

The quality of life in our society is being seriously undermined by the growing incidence of such critical health problems as drug abuse, chronic and degenerative diseases, genetic disabilities, and alcoholism. They pose a serious threat to society in terms of economy and the availability of human resources. They tend to preoccupy us with those who are ill instead of with those who are well and how they can be kept well. We must become more concerned with fostering the beneficial potentials of people. Health education can be a fundamental and vital force in this process, providing it takes into account all of the personal, social, and environmental forces that are important for human development and effectiveness.

Need satisfaction and environmental improvements

Most vital health problems can be alleviated by helping children and youth improve their life-styles, by improving the environment (including the physical, emotional, and political), and by providing youth with the knowledge necessary to deal effectively with personal and societal imperfections. It does little good to teach children how to live effectively in a society that does not exist, but we do need to provide them with the ability to make appropriate beneficial changes in the environment. In this regard, educational emphasis should be placed upon teaching how to survive in the existing society and ways in which the individual can contribute to its improvement. We need also to recognize that humans are complex creatures striving to survive in a complex world. Dubos recognized this complexity when he stated, "The history of each human being includes his private experiences and personal decisions; it encompasses also the evolutionary as well as the social past. Man's physical and mental state, in health and in disease, is always conditioned by all the multiple determinants of his nature."[10]

The urgent need for America's social institutions to take stock of its goals and procedures for assisting individuals to live better and to provide opportunities for need satisfaction is poignantly summed up in the following poem:

HE ALWAYS*

He always wanted to explain things,
But no one cared.
So he drew.
Sometimes he would draw and it wasn't anything.
He wanted to carve it in stone or write it in the sky.
He would lie out on the grass and look up at the sky;

---

* Specific source of this poem is unknown; it was handed to a grade 12 English teacher by a student who committed suicide two weeks later.

And it would be only the sky and him and the things inside him that needed
   saying.
And it was after that, he drew the picture.
It was a beautiful picture.
He kept it under his pillow, and would let no one see it.
And when it was dark, and his eyes were closed, he could see it.
And it was all of him,
And he loved it.
When he started school he brought it with him.
Not to show anyone, but just to have it with him like a friend.
It was funny about school,
He sat in a square, brown desk
Like all the other square, brown desks,
And he thought it should be red.
And his room was a square, brown room
Like all the other rooms.
And it was tight and close
And stiff.
He hated to hold the pencil and chalk,
With his arm stiff and his feet flat on the floor,
Stiff.
With the teacher watching and watching.
The teacher came and spoke to him.
She told him to wear a tie like all the other boys.
He said he didn't like them,
And she said it didn't matter.
After that they drew.
And he drew all yellow and it was the way he felt about morning;
And it was beautiful.
The teacher came and smiled at him.
"What's this? she said, "Why don't you draw something like Ken's drawing?"
"Isn't that beautiful?"
After that his mother bought him a tie.
And he always drew airplanes and rocketships like everyone else.
And he threw the old picture away.
And when he lay out alone looking at the sky,
It was big and blue and all of everything,
But he wasn't anymore.
He was square inside and brown
And his hands were stiff,
And he was like everything else.
And the things inside him that needed saying didn't need it anymore.
It had stopped pushing;
It was crushed,
Stiff,
Like everything else.

FORCES AFFECTING HEALTH NEED SATISFACTION

Genetic potentials

Essentially, the forces affecting health are *environmental*, with all of its cultural, physical, social, economic, and political influences; the *genetic potentials*; and the individual's *health knowledge, attitudes,* and *behavior.* These can not be separated, but are in continuous interaction with each other, and it is this interaction that is significant in affecting individual health. These forces can be either positive or negative.

Let us first examine the impact of genetic potentials on development and health status. Although people generally inherit similar potentials related to growth, development, and the ability to resist disease, there are considerable variations in the degree to which these innate characteristics will influence a particular person. Each person inherits certain strengths and weaknesses; these may be physical or mental.

Some individuals inherit the capacity to resist certain diseases, while others may inherit a predisposition for them. In fact, some diseases are entirely the result of heredity, while others may result from a combination of environmental and genetic factors. On the one hand, there is genetic disease, while on the other hand there is a predisposition to that disease. How this develops will depend to a very large measure upon the ability of the environment to either enhance or interfere with the disease.

FIGURE 5–2   The Forces Affecting Health Are in Continuous Interaction
Health and disease are determined by the quality of the forces acting upon the individual.

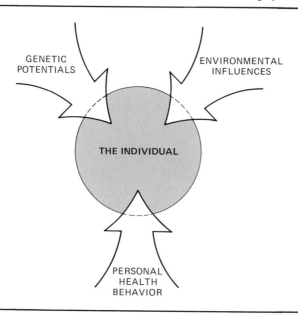

Although the term "predisposition" is usually applied to negative health conditions, it may also be used to describe positive health potentials. For example, one might inherit a predisposition for diabetes, but one could also inherit a predisposition for musical genius. A genetic potential is called *genotype*, while the expression of the genetic potential is called a *phenotype*.

Environmental influences

The environment into which one is born and subsequently grows and develops is not only an important factor in health and disease but is important in determining which of the genetic potentials will be developed and which ones will remain essentially dormant. An environment which is predominantly healthful will tend to influence the positive potentials. A healthful environment is one which provides an individual with the essential elements necessary for optimal growth as well as those elements needed to prevent the development of the negative potentials.

"Environment" is all of the factors that can not be described as genetic. It is much more than one's immediate surroundings: it includes all the factors that influence us—the physical things, the emotional climate, and the social interactions that take place. They may be concrete or abstract; they may also include one's interpretation of self, surroundings, life, as well as people, places and things.

The social aspects of the environment have the greatest influence on the development of emotional and social characteristics of the individual. The important elements of the social environment are local, state, and federal leaders, officials of social institutions, parents, teachers, and peers. People, either through direct example or through covert behavior, teach children how to perceive, interpret, and respond to the things around them. Through perception and interpretation, individual attitudes are formed; through imitation, behavioral responses and patterns are established.

As far as the attainment of health is concerned, society has a greater influence upon the quality of the environment than upon the control of genetic potentials. As indicated in Chapter 2, however, it is important to note that recent research into genetic control indicates this may not be the case in the not-too-distant future. Although we have the technology to improve the environment, we find that resources are all too frequently misdirected and that the values placed on them in relation to distribution are questionable. This problem is compounded by mismanagement of resources, the influence of vested interests, and apathy or ignorance on the part of citizens and politicians.

Children are society's most vital resource; no one will argue this point. We can predict what the future will bring by assessing the quality of the existing society and the quality of the society planned for the future, for what children experience today will determine to a great extent what they will be tomorrow. Today's social and physical environments are creating a way of life for future societies. Walt Whitman puts it in more poetic terms:

THERE WAS A CHILD WENT FORTH

There was a child went forth every day;
And the first object he look'd upon, that object he became;
And that object became part of him for the day, or a certain part of the day,
Or for many years, or stretching cycles of years.
The early lilacs became part of this child,
And grass, and white and red morning-glories, and white and red clover, and the song of the phoebe-bird,
And the third-month lambs, and the sow's pink-faint litter, and the mare's foal, and the cow's calf,
And the noisy brood of the barn-yard, or by the mire of the pond-side,
And the fish suspending themselves so curiously below there—and the beautiful curious liquid,
And the water-plants with their graceful flat heads—all became part of him.
The field-sprouts of fourth-month and fifth-month became part of him.
Winter-grain sprouts, and those of the light-yellow corn, and the succulent roots of the garden,
And the apple-trees cover'd with blossoms, and the fruit afterward, and woodberries and the commonest weeds by the road;
And the old drunkard staggering home from the out-house of the tavern, whence he had lately risen,
And the school-mistress that pass'd on her way to the school,
And the friendly boys that pass'd—and the quarrelsome boys,
And the tidy and fresh-cheek'd girls—and the barefoot negro boy and girl,
And all the changes of city and country, wherever he went.
These became part of that child who went forth every day, and who now goes, and will always go forth every day.

Personal behavior

A major force responsible for the improvement of health over the years has been individual health knowledge and appropriate behavior based upon this knowledge. Health improvement has occurred in spite of the fact that individuals are limited to some extent by genetic qualities and that societies have failed to provide an ideal environment in which to live. Even though we may possess the needed health knowledge, it does not guarantee that we will behave healthfully. However, health knowledge is an important first step toward these ends. Certainly without it we are much more likely to make mistakes, mistakes which can be crucial to our very existence.

For example, nearly everyone has the genetic predisposition for contracting typhoid fever after drinking contaminated water. If, however, we do not drink the water, or take steps to purify it, we will not contract the disease from this source. In this instance, the genetic potential and the environmental influences are overcome by health knowledge and its resultant behavior. Unfortunately, there are too many instances where people do not behave according to their knowledge of the situation, or other factors may take precedence over the health knowledge. For instance, if the thirst drive is intense, someone may drink the contaminated water with the knowledge that typhoid fever may be contracted. There are, of course, many other reasons why people may behave inappropriately. Sinacore offers the following explanation: "Part of the explanation of this is our built-in resistance to change. An additional factor involved is that when we are asked to give up something we enjoy doing, we then have to make a value judgment as to whether the possible results justify the change."[11]

Generally, people tend to avoid situations that are perceived as unpleasant or painful. However, a painful experience may be perceived as a vehicle for achieving a particular goal. For example, a cigarette advertisement may persuade a child that smoking is a sign of adulthood. Although smoking is, at least at first, an extremely unpleasant, and even painful, experience, a youngster may see it as a way to achieve manhood or womanhood (a pleasant experience). The child therefore learns to smoke and then to feel grown up. The tragic part of this is that such children may never know that becoming an adult can be a accomplished without smoking. This is where effective health education can play a vital role in helping children attain maturity.

This same principle of using an unpleasant experience as a vehicle to achieve a pleasant goal can be applied to several other situations wherein one draws false conclusions from environmental stimuli. The drinking of alcoholic beverages, initially, is unpleasant. However, one may interpret advertisements or observations of those who have been drinking as a vehicle for attaining a variety of goals: a sense of well-being, a relaxed state, maturity, social ease, etc. After drinking, the person may actually believe that the desired feeling has been achieved. This is an important misconception, since what one believes to be true is as important, in this case, as what actually is true.

The health educator can do much to assist people in examining their own values and logic. Without this assistance, people may never know that there are pleasant and constructive vehicles for attaining the same sense of pleasure.

When we relate healthful behavior to pleasure, earlier experiences may be interpreted as having been more pleasurable than is indicated by later knowledge. We need also to consider the patterns of life-styles that have been established and the attitudes associated with them. The nature of people is such that change is less likely to take place as a mode of behavior becomes more established. The new knowledge and life-styles must have a greater attraction to the individual than the former pattern of behavior; the new knowledge must be more meaningful and immediately beneficial.

As was emphasized earlier, health behavior is chiefly, if not entirely, determined by learning. It is based upon primary experiences which establish health attitudes and provide health knowledge. The mode of behavior which results is interpreted by the individual as the most desirable. This interpretation may or may not be conscious, since much of our behavior is motivated unconsciously. Some authorities refer to this behavior as "health habits," but health behavior is, and needs to be, much more than a habit, because we are often confronted with situations that require responses beyond simple habit. New and unfamiliar circumstances require new decisions. This is one of the primary purposes of health education: to provide the individual with the knowledge needed to make appropriate health decisions. Health behavior is in essence the result of the interaction of inherited potentials and environmental influences. Ruch points out that "the environment influences the development of behavior in two ways: (1) it supplies stimuli which elicit patterns of response already prepared by maturation, and (2) it presents situations that require the learning of new responses or the changing of old ones."[12]

COUNTERFORCES TO HEALTH NEED SATISFACTION

What is responsible for ill health?

The factors which cause ill health are the same as those responsible for the development of positive health, namely, the influence of heredity, environment, and personal health behavior. Just as heredity can provide us with positive potentials, it can also provide us with genetic weaknesses. Similarly, a healthful environment can influence the development of desirable potentials, while an unhealthful environment will contribute to the development of genetic abnormalities and prevent the development of desirable traits. In any case, the catalytic agent is our behavior in relation to our genetic potentials and environment. Consequently, it is vital that we understand not only our personal qualities, but the nature of the environment in which we live and how to react appropriately to its influences. It should be noted that the basis for health is determined by how well we understand the nature of the health problems that threaten us and the impact that personal behavior can have. Unless there is a recognition of the influence of these counterforces and of the need for action to correct them, disease, disability, and human suffering will remain an unfortunate fact of life.

For example, knowledge of the beneficial effects of genetic counseling can prevent many genetic diseases such as sickle-cell anemia, PKU, Tay-Sachs disease, and Down's syndrome. Genetic history is important in order for the physician to take appropriate actions regarding both the diagnosis of genetic diseases and the counseling of patients. For instance, Down's syndrome (mongolism), a form of mental retardation, can be

FIGURE 5–3   A Categorization of Counterforces to Attaining Health

The forces that adversely affect health are the environment, genetic and congenital defects, and behavior, these are interactional. How well one learns to deal with the environmental, genetic, and congenital conditions will determine to a large extent one's health.

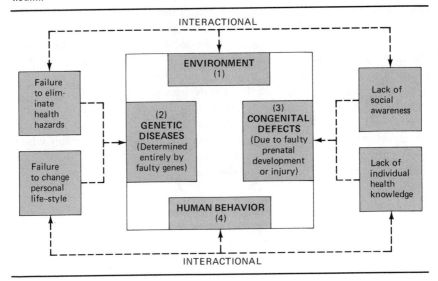

detected during pregnancy by a process known as amniocentesis. Amniocentesis is a relatively simple procedure involving the withdrawal of the amniotic fluid during the fourteenth through eighteenth weeks of pregnancy. A microscopic examination and chromosomal analysis are then made. Many genetic and congenital defects can be determined prior to the birth of the fetus. Genetic counseling is necessary to assist the prospective parents in making a decision regarding therapeutic abortion.

Apprehension based upon misconceptions can also be alleviated. This is especially true with the misconceptions surrounding the sickle-cell trait, since many people fail to distinguish between the trait and the disease.

The impact of health knowledge

As we have seen, most diseases result from poor environment, unhealthful life-style, or a combination of the two. These include communicable diseases, degenerative and constitutional diseases, and mental and emotional disorders. Such inappropriate human behavior as abuse of chemical substances (alcohol, barbiturates, amphetamines, tobacco, etc.), sexual promiscuity, and improper eating habits contribute to increases in the incidence of diseases in these and other groups. For example, most cases of lung cancer and cardiovascular diseases (the two leading causes of death in the United States) are the result of cigarette smoking; alcohol abuse can result in mental disorders such as Korsakoff's psychosis, while overeating is related to some cardiovascular diseases, as well as to social and emotional health problems.

Many health authorities believe that the primary responsibility for health rests with the individual. This is true when dealing with those diseases which the individual can control, or that result from one's personal behavior. But there are numerous diseases that are related to circumstances which the individual can not control. These include many of the genetic diseases, as well as those caused by a variety of social factors.

Everyone knows that there are certain factors essential for the attainment of health: proper nutrition, sufficient rest and exercise, clean air to breathe, pure water to drink, freedom from undue emotional stress, etc.; the list is inexhaustible. The theory has been that if one adheres to the rules for healthful living, one will indeed be healthy. But how can we account for the large numbers of people who, in spite of following a healthful regimen, still fail to attain the level of health they are capable of?

It is probably not possible to eliminate all of the health problems that exist today; however, many can be prevented or alleviated by today's medical technology. In many instances, the forces contributing to these problems have been identified, and effective procedures have been developed to eliminate them. Some health problems have simple causes, while others are much more complex. The solutions to them are quite simple in some cases, while others require massive social and personal changes. But in almost all cases the common bond is adequate health knowledge and available health care personnel and facilities. The President's Committee on Health Education supported the concept of health education as an important factor in health behavior and as a primary force for health maintenance when it stated:

> [Health] problems result, at least in part, from failure to involve the individual—and society— in health education. The degree to which each person can play an active and sometimes crucial role in his own health maintenance has not been sufficiently stressed or adequately dramatized.
>
> Controlling the controllable problems and preventing the preventable ones have received relatively little concerted attention. The health care system traditionally has been geared to short-term treatment of acute illness.
>
> Many causes of disease and death can at least be influenced, and some prevented altogether, by good health practices by the individual. The fact is, however, that good health practices are not uniformly followed or even considered. Millions of persons never think about their health until frightening signs or symptoms propel them to clinics or hospitals for possible emergency treatment.[13]

In this regard, it would be inaccurate to conclude that there is a special form of behavior that would guarantee healthy results. That is to say, there really is no such a thing as a mode of living that could be termed healthy behavior and others that are not. However, there are forms of behavior that can be termed health-related behaviors. This would include one's general style of life and specific actions called health-directed behaviors. Health-directed behaviors are those actions that one takes with a clear awareness of their effects on health. For example, one who does not smoke or who makes a conscious effort to stop smoking because of the adverse effects it can have on health is engaged in a form of health-directed behavior. Therefore, we should consider all forms of behavior as being health-related, recognizing that some behavior is deliberately health-directed.

What are the chief counterforces?

The chief counterforces to attaining health, and certainly the most numerous, fall into the environmental and personal behavior categories. Millions of Americans have only rudimentary health knowledge. Ignorance, misinformation, and superstition make the individual vulnerable to the quack and the charlatan. Moreover, our daily living pattern will be influenced by these erroneous attitudes. Once misconceptions and superstitions have been acquired, simple truth is not enough to neutralize their influence: More is needed to reverse these deep-rooted notions. It is much more productive to teach factual information at the beginning than to attempt to correct false notions later in life. Thus, personal behavior becomes an important force (or counterforce) in attaining health. Wilner et al. put individual health behavior in proper perspective when they state:

> Convincing evidence is beginning to accumulate regarding health habits, which, singly or in combination, can add up to substantially better health status and freedom from disability. Much (although not everything by any means) is known through science about likely relationships of personal habits to health status. Some way must be found to counteract the many forces at work—some cultural, some social, some personal-psychological —that interfere with attaining a health goal because of poor habits.[14]

Therefore, it is essential that health education be offered early in life and taught correctly from the beginning. In this way people will become the most important factor affecting their own health.

Compounding the situation is the inadequacy of living conditions in thousands of cities, villages, and towns, and the lack of adequate health care facilities and personnel. The individual is surrounded by forces that are counterproductive (and some downright dangerous), most of which have been created by people and many of which are ignored by those who have the power and authority to make appropriate changes for the better.

Health education, no matter how effective, can do little for those who are forced to breathe air polluted by industries; to live in substandard housing; to use unsafe appliances or other machinery; to treat their own illnesses because medical facilities are unavailable or inadequate; unless, of course, health education is related directly to helping people find solutions to these health problems.

Admittedly, health education has been (and continues to be) sorely inadequate. Health education is an area of the school curriculum and health care system that needs to be recognized for its value in preventing human suffering, but more importantly, for improving life.

In spite of the fact that modern medical technology and knowledge have advanced tremendously in very recent years to the point where many health problems are no longer serious issues, our total health care system is inadequate. Health care simply is not available to the majority of Americans. This is because many can not afford today's care, because facilities and personnel are geographically out of reach, and because many people lack sufficient knowledge about their health and the care available to seek proper attention when needed. Senator Edward Kennedy, as Chairman of the Senate Subcommittee on Health, stated:

> I am shocked to find that we in America have created a health care system that can be so callous to human suffering, so intent on high salaries and profits, and so unconcerned for the needs of our people. American families, regardless of income, are offered health care of uncertain quality, at inflated prices, and at a time and in a manner and a place more suited to the convenience and profit of the doctor and the hospital than to the needs of the patient. Our system especially victimizes Americans whose age, health, or low income leaves them less able to fight their way into the health care system. The health care industry seems by its nature to give most freedom and power to the providers of care—and very little to the people. It is an industry in which there is very little incentive to offer services responsive to the people's needs and demands. It is an industry which strongly protects the profit and rights of the provider, but only weakly protects the healing and the right of the people.[15]

DEFINITIVE UNDERSTANDINGS

The health of people is directly associated with the care taken to satisfy their bio-psycho-social needs. Although these needs are essentially the same for all people, the methods for adequately satisfying them will vary somewhat from person to person. The time when needs, especially the psychosocial ones, should be given attention will also vary with individuals. Some needs will require greater attention for some individuals at certain times than at others. Obviously, the satisfaction of needs forms the basis for human growth and development and this is related to one's health status. Finally, needs are interdependent and interactional.

Biological needs must be minimally met for the survival of the organism. These needs include food, water and oxygen. If they are inadequately satisfied, the individual's growth will be adversely affected and the attainment of optimal health impossible. The biological needs can also affect psychosocial development. All needs act as powerful motivators of behavior. All people seek their satisfaction, but the way in which they are satisfied is a learned phenomenon.

Needs are either inherited or learned internal urgencies. They are associated with biological existence and the enhancement of living. They may be conscious or unconscious. A preoccupation with their satisfaction is a manifestation of ill health.

Homeostasis is the term used to describe the tendency toward biochemical balance within the individual. It is also applied to psychosocial adjustment. If a state of homeostasis exists, the individual is enjoying good health.

Maslow states that a hierarchy of need satisfaction exists in all people. We tend to seek satisfaction of the most primitive biological needs early in life with a gradual tendency toward seeking satisfaction of the emotional ones as we grow and develop. However, biological needs are never replaced, instead, new needs come into being for the continuation of proper development.

Health education programs must take into account individual needs, the degree to which they have been satisfied, the way satisfaction has occurred, and what further needs must be met. The health educator is not a therapist, but must always be alert to the status of the learner so as not to contribute further to negative forms of behavior or development.

Havighurst and Erikson have contributed to our understanding of human growth and development by identifying certain developmental tasks and psychosocial crises, respectively. The developmental tasks are necessary achievements associated with various stages of growth; the psychosocial crises are attitudes one acquires during various stages of development. In both cases, the degree and quality of these developments are indicators of health.

Most of today's major health problems and issues are related to inadequate living environments and inappropriate individual responses to self, others, and the environment. Improvements in society's health are dependent upon the improvements that occur in all of these categories. In addition, adequate health care must be made available to more Americans than presently exists. Health is also influenced by the genetic qualities of the individual. The positive and negative qualities we possess are frequently manifestations of inherited traits; both can be influenced by the quality of the environment and our health knowledge and behavior. It is the responsibility of the health educator (or educational community) to provide everyone with the health information necessary to assist them in behaving healthfully; to make positive health decisions; to avoid known hazardous situations; and to strive to improve the environment. Only in this way can we accept our share of the responsibility for our own health. But of equal importance is the responsibility of all social and political institutions to guarantee a healthful environment for all Americans.

PROBLEMS
FOR DISCUSSION

1. Explain why human needs are never static.
2. How does the satisfaction of the basic biological needs contribute to the satisfaction of the psychosocial needs?
3. Describe how need satisfaction contributes to the improvement of health; to the improvement of society's health.
4. What are the implications of need satisfaction and need assessment to the health educator?
5. Compare Maslow's, Havighurst's, and Erikson's theories regarding growth and development in terms of their implications for individual health.
   a. How are these concepts applicable to health education?
   b. What significance does an understanding of growth and development have in regards to establishing positive health attitudes and behavior?
6. Identify the factors that are chiefly responsible for determining an individual's health.
7. Explain why genetic potentials alone do not determine a persons path of development.
8. Describe why adequate health education of parents is essential for improving the health of children.
9. Identify the environmental factors which contribute to health; those which interfere with health.
   a. What can the social institutions do to overcome adverse environmental factors?
   b. What are the implications for health education?
10. Explain why we are affected by the interactions of genetic and environmental factors.
11. Identify at least five major health problems that exist in the United States. List the criteria you used in determining this.

REFERENCES

1. Dubos, Rene, *Man Adapting*, Yale University Press, New Haven, 1965, p. 6.
2. Ruch, Floyd, *Psychology and Life*, 7th ed., Scott, Foresman and Company, Chicago, 1967, p. 383.
3. Dubos, op. cit., p. 254.
4. Ibid., p. 8.
5. Ibid., p. 22.
6. Klausmeur, Herbert J., and William Goodwin, *Learning and Human Abilities*, 2d ed., Harper & Row, New York, 1966, p. 425.
7. Maslow, A. H., and G. Murphy, eds., *Motivation and Personality*, Harper & Row, New York, 1954, p. 105.
8. Ruch, op. cit., p. 123.
9. Ibid., p. 102.
10. Dubos, op. cit., pp. 1–2.

11. Sinacore, John S., *Health: A Quality of Life*, 2nd ed., Macmillan Publishing Co., New York, 1974, p. 7.
12. Ruch, op. cit., p. 70.
13. U.S. Department of Health, Education and Welfare, *The Report of the President's Committee on Health Education*, p. 15.
14. Wilner, Daniel M., Rosabelle Price Walker and Lenor S. Goerke, *Introduction to Public Health*, 6th ed., Macmillan Publishing Company, New York, 1973, p. 14.
15. Kennedy, Edward M., *In Critical Condition: The Crisis in America's Health Care*, Simon and Schuster, New York, 1972, pp. 15–16.

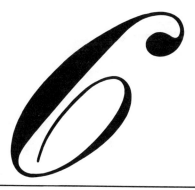

Health
and Human
Effectiveness

*The goal of self-management is
often called self-fulfillment or
self-actualization. Fulfillment seems
to be concerned with achievement,
with avoiding restraints and
discovering positive reinforcers.
Actualization seems to have more to
do with maximum genetic and
environmental histories in order
to free a person from immediate
settings. In both cases emphasis is
clearly upon the here and now, on
being or well-being or momentary
becoming.*

B. F. Skinner

To be healthy is to be effective.
To be effective is to be worthwhile.
To be worthwhile is everything
in life. And everything in life is to be
healthy.

**AEB
DAB**

DEVELOPING SELF-SUFFICIENCY

What is self-sufficiency?

In our culture there is a tendency to describe self-sufficiency in artificial terms. There is a widespread belief that success is measured by the ability to achieve according to the precepts of others. That is, one is effective (or successful) only to the extent that goals established by the social norms are achieved, rather than in terms of one's abilities, aspirations, and environmental opportunities. People should be considered effective or successful if they are achieving within the limits of their capabilities and within the confines of environmental constraints. Some individuals are capable of greater social and personal contributions than others; it is the degree to which one achieves that is important.

Dubos points out that the terms "health and disease are meaningful only when defined in terms of a given person functioning in a given physical and social environment."[1] In like manner, self-sufficiency is used to describe the capability to meet one's needs within the context of the existing circumstances. Self-sufficiency is not total independence, but rather effective dependence. To this extent, it is a manifestation of health. It is the ability to adjust to changes in the environment and to contribute constructively to society. For example, someone who is physically handicapped may be as self-sufficient within the framework of the handicap as an able-bodied person. Both health and self-sufficiency are measured in terms of these factors rather than in terms of the "greatness" of the contribution made.

The degree to which one can live adequately is a measure of self-sufficiency, and one who is self-sufficient is, in a functional sense, healthy. However, different measures of health and of self-sufficiency may not always be consistent, since a physically handicapped person may, by necessity, depend more upon others for survival, as well as for accomplishing everyday tasks. Therefore, any measure of self-sufficiency must be placed within the context of one's capabilities and the environmental factors which aid or hinder self-reliance.

For example, prosthetics and other devices can improve handicapped people's ability to do things for themselves. Even for the able-bodied an improvement in the environment can improve functioning ability. This demonstrates further that health is relative to one's capabilities and the enabling forces in the environment.

Self-sufficiency is not constant. While we may be totally self-sufficient in one environmental setting, a change in the setting may cause us to become totally dependent upon others. Self-sufficiency is not an either-or proposition. The chief factor is knowledge, application of the knowledge, and the circumstances in which we find ourselves.

Effects of health education on self-sufficiency

Environmental forces must be compatible with personal qualities for adequate expression to take place. There is a close relationship between our internal potentials and the external forces which act upon them. One of the chief functions of health education is to provide the individual with the health information needed to make appropriate health decisions that are consistent with both personal capabilities and the environmental circumstances that exist. For this to take place, we must become aware of ourselves and acquire an understanding of the nature of the environmental impact upon us and the ways we can best deal with these influencers. Since the degree of self-sufficiency we possess will vary with maturity, and since it is different for each person, health education must be a continuous process throughout life; the approaches used must take into consideration these differences and the maturation process. In this way, one is more likely to become health educated, which will result in a greater degree of self-sufficiency. Here are some of the characteristics of a health educated person:

- Possession of a sense of self-worth.
- Understanding of the environmental factors that can affect personal and social health.
- The ability to respond in appropriate ways to the various forces that can affect functioning.
- A knowledge of who can provide competent health assistance when conditions are beyond personal capabilities, and the ability to make use of this assistance.
- The ability to think through personal health concerns and issues and to come to desirable and beneficial conclusions.
- The avoidance of behavior that can adversely affect health of self and that of others.
- The capacity for responsible health behavior within the limits of personal capabilities and external constraints.

HEALTH AND SELF-SUFFICIENCY

Learning to live healthfully

"Health is an enabling value rather than a definitive purpose," states William Hubbard, Jr.[2] The quality of health knowledge that is acquired contributes to the improvement of the capacity to achieve life's purposes and, hence, to the quality of life. As stated earlier, the quality of health knowledge is determined by the realistic needs of the individual and these needs are determined by genetic potentials and personal and societal aspirations, as well as other forces.

Learning to live healthfully is, for the most part, an abstract process. It deals not only with the present, but also with the future; with demonstrable situations affecting health, as well as conceptual development; with attitudinal and behavioral development, as well as with cognition, with self, as well as with others; with comprehension and decision-making, as well as with rote learning, and with what is, as well as with what can be. In essence, learning to live healthfully is the most vital, complex, and pleasurable process we can experience during our lifetime, for it is the self in action that is an experience in living. As Reich has stated,

> The self needs, above all, privacy, liberty, and a degree of sovereignty to develop. It needs to try things, to search, to explore, to test, to err. It needs solitude—solitude to bring senses to its experiences and thereby to create a future. It needs not enforced relationships with others, rigidly categorized into groups, teams and organizations, but an opportunity to try different forms of relationships—to try them, to withdraw, to re-create.[3]

Piaget has demonstrated that abstract ideas are the most difficult to learn. Individuals should be provided with educational opportunities that will enable them to experiment and to discover, since these experiences "foster the acquisition of abstract ideas and creative abilities."[4] Health experiences must deal with the real health issues present in our society. Field experiences in health agencies such as hospitals, nursing homes, clinics, and rehabilitation centers can provide students with firsthand knowledge of the existing health problems, their causes, effects, and treatment. In this manner students can better apply new health information to their own lives. Society's health issues become the vital concern of all people, rather than remaining an abstraction; they become real and concrete.

Health and intellectual development

Human development is essentially determined by the maturation of the intellect, according to Piaget.* Intellectual development during childhood consists of four distinct stages:

1. *Sensorimotor period* (ages 0–2 years), characterized by an increased awareness of the senses, and physical development.
2. *Preoperational period* (ages 2–7 years), which is divided into the preconceptual and intuitive phases.
3. *Concrete operational period* (ages 7–11 years).
4. *Period of formal operations* (ages 11–15 years), in which the individual distinguishes between the real and the possible.[5]

---

* In an article in *Science News*, 105 (12), March 23, 1974, p. 194, Thomas R. Trabasso of Princeton University disputes Piaget's theory. Following experiments with 4- and 5-year olds, he has concluded that children can perform intellectual feats well before the age predicted by Piaget.

The two developmental concepts that form the basis of Piaget's assertions are *assimilation* and *accommodation*. Assimilation is the process of making part of the external environment a part of the self; that is, fitting an experience into the individual's existing cognitive structure. Once this process is complete, accommodation takes place. Accommodation is essentially adaptation to the assimilated "object." This total process is responsible for continual growth (maturation) and greater self-sufficiency. These two processes are related to health education in their ability to provide students with positive, meaningful health experiences which can become a part of them (assimilation), and to influence positively health attitudes and behavior (accommodation).

Self-actualization

Ultimately, the individual successful in attaining self-sufficiency will reach a point in development identified by Warga[6] as *self-actualization* (becoming one's true self). Potentials, environment, and interactions determine one's self-concept, and it is these factors which will eventually determine the kind of person that will be created. Ruch emphasized this when he said:

> As the child grows physically and psychologically, his self-concept develops into an elaborate system which includes not only his body as he knows it but all his thoughts, feelings, attitudes, values, and aspirations. This concept of self becomes, quite logically, the individual's most valued possession, and his behavior will largely be devoted to protecting or enhancing it. Whether or not his concept of self agrees with the evaluation of others, it is his real self as far as he is concerned—it is *he.* Similarly, the individual's concept of his environment is determined by his personal experiences with it.[7]

According to Warga, the self-actualized person possesses certain functional characteristics. These are summarized as follows:

- Ability to perceive reality and to be comfortable with it
- Acceptance of self and others without guilt or anxiety
- Ability to express thoughts and behavior spontaneously without extremes of unconventionalism
- Problem-centered rather than ego-centered
- Possesses a sense of cultural and environmental independence, but is not nonconformist for the sake of being different
- Capacity for deep appreciation of life's experiences
- Possesses a deep social interest and identity with humanity
- Capacity for intense interpersonal relationships
- Possesses democratic attitudes and shows respect for all people
- Discriminates between means and ends and often enjoys the means themselves
- Has a tendency toward being philosophical

- Possesses a good sense of humor
- Possesses a high degree of creativity

Emphasis must be placed on the necessity for health education to provide the *means* for promoting health and preventing the beginnings of health problems. In this manner, an improvement in the quality of life will result. We must, however, recognize that individual self-reliance will vary considerably from individual to individual, and that there is an urgent need to avoid sweeping standards of behavior for all people.

Each individual must learn how to behave within the boundaries of internal and external forces and to assimilate and accommodate the pertinent aspects of experience accordingly. People who become capable of expressing themselves fully (physically, socially, emotionally, and intellectually) are self-actualized; they are living healthfully. Therefore, no single way of living is healthy for all individuals, and no single mode of expression will result in self-actualization.

THE HOLISTIC APPROACH

What is the holistic approach?

Each person is unique and at the same time similar to all others. One factor, however, stands out: each person is an integrated whole, and the biological, psychological, and sociological qualities are in continuous interaction. Because of this, any force which affects one of these elements also affects the other two. This concept is essentially the *holistic* view of human functioning.

Viewing the individual in terms of psychobiological integration and unification is the fundamental principle underlying the holistic and psychosomatic approaches to health and disease. At least 50 percent of the people who seek medical attention are suffering from an illness associated with emotional stress. Psychophysiologic disorders are among our nation's major health problems. Any medical approach to the diagnosis and treatment of disease must take into account the holistic implications and any health education approach that is concerned with the promotion of health must consider the physical, psychological, and sociological unity of the individual, as well as the external forces affecting this unity.

There is no simple recipe for insuring that each individual will become an effective and contributing member of society. The ability to function is determined by a variety of complex, interrelated factors which may be placed into two broad categories: (1) the *internal* qualities, and (2) the *external* qualities. Both of these are associated with the capacity for healthful living. They are inseparable and in continuous interaction with each other.

Internal qualities

The internal qualities are those which determine the nature of the individual: the physical (biological), psychological (emotional and intellectual), and social (interpersonal) abilities. These are interactional components related to existence, health, and behavior. They exemplify the necessity for viewing the individual as an integrated whole. This is true whether we are considering the promotion of health or the diagnosis and treatment of disease. Oberteuffer and Beyrer stress that "man is *not* a composite of separate entities, such as body, mind and spirit, arranged in a presumed ascending order of importance. He is a multidimensional unity, with each component—chemical, physical, spiritual, intellectual, or emotional—existing within a complex of interrelationships."[8] The spiritual dimension of people mentioned by Oberteuffer and Beyrer is in reality not a separate dimension of health, but rather is an attitude which evolves from the interaction of the biological, psychological, and sociological dimensions. The spiritual aspects of health result from one's experiences and maturation. It becomes especially important as an element of human functioning that has tremendous impact upon the health of the three basic dimensions. In this regard, it is a force for health rather than a dimension of health.

External qualities

The external qualities are the forces of the social and physical environments that act on the individual. These forces are responsible for:

- enhancing or impeding physical, psychological, and social developments.
- contributing to the promotion of health and the prevention of disease and disability.
- inducing disease and disability.
- causing premature death.

Since health education is a process for improving human effectiveness, one of its primary goals is to provide people with the opportunity to develop their internal capabilities so that they can effectively deal with the external qualities of living. Health education, therefore, is concerned primarily with processes for promoting health, and with the means for preventing disease, disability, and premature death. The achievement of these goals will improve the effectiveness of the individual and the quality of society; the greater the improvement in the quality of society, the more likelihood that one's internal qualities will be more fully developed. This is obviously a cyclic phenomenon in the progress of humanity.

FIGURE 6–1   Cyclic Phenomenon of the Progress of Humanity

As individual internal qualities are improved, the quality of the environment is improved, which, in turn, acts upon individuals to further develop their internal qualities; thus, the cycle is perpetuated. If opportunities for improvement are lacking, the environmental improvements are slowed or will deteriorate.

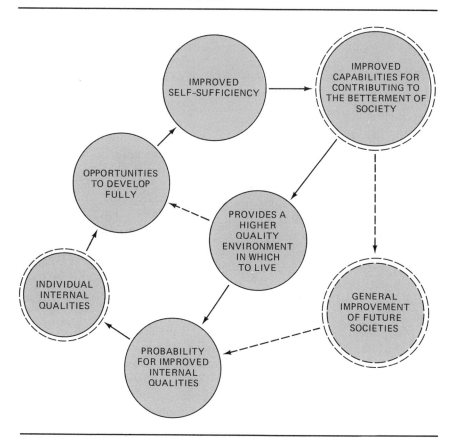

The uniqueness of individuals

As health educators, we must be concerned with the uniqueness of each individual, and with the traits that are common to all individuals. The *idiographic approach* to understanding an individual presumes that the important characteristics are those which make one different from all others. These would include unique genetic traits and those traits acquired or modified by environmental influences. The *nomothetic approach* emphasizes those elements or traits that are present to some degree in each individual.

It is important that the selection of approaches, or methodologies, to health education includes both theories. Since all individuals do possess unique qualities, health educators need to consider the value of individualized educational approaches, especially as these related to the uniqueness of one's abilities, needs, interests, inherited predispositions to disease, and potentials for optimal health status. However, it is of equal importance to recognize that those elements which are common to all individuals are the basis for the use of methodologies directed toward providing fundamental information vital to all individuals. This is one justification for large group instruction.

THEORIES OF PERSONALITY DEVELOPMENT

Introduction

An understanding of the psychological theories of individual growth and personality development is necessary in order for the health educator to provide health experiences that will be related to the uniqueness of each person, whether or not this uniqueness can be explained by the idiographic or nomothetic approaches. Most of the psychological theories that have evolved are more the result of clinical observations than the result of positive motivations directed toward health promotion; what we know about health has been learned chiefly from an analysis of disease. Once the symptoms and causes have been identified, inferences about prevention can be made. It is the responsibility of the health educator to translate this knowledge into a health orientation rather than a disease orientation.

Many theories of human development have been set forth over the years, including the psychoanalytic, analytic, individual, self-actualization, and existential schools of thought. All of these have contributed to our understanding of the processes and forces that determine how individuals learn and behave. This knowledge provides the health educator with the bases for effective health education and the areas of major health concern.

It will be helpful at this point to briefly examine some of the theories that are related to personality development and human behavior and to health education. It will be noted that all of them culminate in the holistic viewpoint. Coleman suggests that "living organisms tend to maintain their integrity—their 'wholeness'—and that this tendency appears on biological, psychological, and sociological levels."[9] These "levels" are also those with which health education is concerned.

Psychoanalytic theory

The *psychoanalytic theory* of personality formation has been one of the most influential explanations of both normal and abnormal development. Its significance in health education is apparent, despite the fact that Freud failed to recognize the importance of learning as a factor which shapes behavior (although he did stress the relationship of early experiences to later behavior). Essentially, the psychoanalytic school of thought describes the source of human behavior as being instinctive (libido); these instincts being contained in the unconscious part of the personality, the *id*. Generally speaking, these instincts are related to the basic physiological needs of the individual which require gratification. The *ego* structure regulates the pleasure seeking (pleasure principle) of the id by translating these instincts into reality (reality principle) based upon social acceptability. The *superego* is the guardian of expressed behavior; it is the value system, the conscience.

The effects that the ego and the superego have on personality development and adjustments are determined primarily by childhood learning experiences. Accordingly, the personality develops as a result of libidinal (inherent) urges that concentrate on different parts of the body through five developmental stages: the oral stage (first year of life), the anal stage (2–3 years of age), the phallic stage (3–6 years of age), the latency stage (6–12 years of age), and the genital stage (adolescence to adulthood).

The psychoanalytic theory emphasizes (1) the importance of the wholeness of people, (2) the genetic and experiential basis for mental and emotional health, and (3) the factors related to learning and intelligence that play a critical role in influencing one's effectiveness. Coleman summarizes the psychoanalytic theory in this way: "In general, then, the personality can be viewed as a composite of biological aspects, represented by the id; psychological aspects, represented by the ego; and social aspects, represented by the superego. Man's basic nature is irrational and selfish. Only social prohibitions (including his internalizations of social rules) restrains his instinctive strivings."[10]

Analytic and individual theories

Both Jung's *analytic theory* and Adler's *individual* theory of personality development stress the importance of the individual's goals and aspirations; the individual theory, however, places greater emphasis upon the social aspects of one's nature. These theories recognize the impact that one's goals and strivings to achieve them have on determining present behavior, without failing to recognize the vital role that past experiences play. Goals and strivings, then, become the basis for motivation.

Self-actualization theories

Among the more prominent theories that have been given great attention are those that are broadly classified as the *self-actualization theories*. These include Carl Roger's self theory; Abraham Maslow's self-actualization theory, and existentialism.* *Self-actualization* stresses the development of inherited potentials, placing great emphasis on the need for an appropriate environment to provide the opportunity for these potentials to express themselves. This is an orderly process occurring through stages of growth and development. It recognizes the unity of the individual and its relationship to health and disease. Ruch emphasizes this idea when he says: "The organism is a unity, and what happens in any part of it affects the whole. Organization is natural to the organism, and disorganization means disease."[11]

Existentialism

Existentialism has a direct bearing on health, and is applicable to education for health. Its central focus is on the importance of the individual in making decisions regarding life and existence. Coleman puts it this way: "Man's basic motivation is to find the best possible way of life, to actualize his potentials, and to fulfill himself as a human being."[12] Since our major health problems are essentially the result of the way people live—their life-styles—and the realization of potentials, the health educator should consider seriously the application of existentialism and self-actualization theories to the ways that health education can best assist us in deciding what kind of person we will be, since "health is an existential phenomenon."[13]

In this regard, the operant goals of health education are those concerned with:

1. *Values clarification*—providing individuals with opportunities to examine their own values within the context of personal and social goals, mores, and potentials.
2. *Decision-making*—the development of intellect and logic; providing the individual with factual information, significances, relationships, and application to various situations.
3. *Self-actualization*—a concept that has already been discussed. Suffice it to say here that opportunities to grow in all aspects of development must be provided for each individual.

The term *operant goal* is used here to describe both the end result and the process for achieving it. The term *decision-making* implies the ability to make appropriate decisions following the processes related to the development of the decision-making skills. It will become obvious that these goals are closely associated with the cognitive, affective, and psychomotor domains; the development of health knowledge, attitudes, and behavior, and intellectual, social, and emotional development. All of

---

* Credit for the development of existentialism must go to the many individuals who contributed to it. Those who stand out most prominently are Paul Tillich, Rollo May, Erich Fromm, Abraham Maslow, and Carl Rogers.

these are different ways of expressing the same thing, the achievement of which will result in promoting biological, psychological, and sociological health. Once again, we see the "wholeness" of people and the interactional nature of their elements.

HEALTH, DISEASE, AND EDUCATION

Functional and organic disease

Disease can be thought of as a failure to attain health. It can result from genetic predisposition; ignorance about health matters; inappropriate individual, social, or political responses; medical failures (lack of personnel or facilities, or misdirected efforts); and environmental forces that are detrimental to human welfare. Diseases can be organic, functional, or both. Adequate health information and its application at the right time is the primary preventive ingredient.

Since disease can be functional or organic, or a combination of the two, we can infer that health is both functional and organic. An individual who functions effectively is healthy. Any condition, either functional or organic, that interferes with our effectiveness is a disease. Specifically, a *functional disease* can be either physical or psychological and is defined as a condition which has no demonstrable organic basis or etiology. It is psychogenic, originating in the psychological domain of the individual and having no known physiological basis. In contrast, an *organic disease* is one that results from a degree of tissue alteration or destruction. Organic disorders can be a result of mechanical injury, chemical damage, infectious microorganisms, genetic aberrations, or metabolic disturbances. Disease, then, is an interruption of functional homeostasis.

Functional homeostasis is the internal mechanism which enables the individual to retain and maintain biological, psychological, and sociological identity; that is, the individual is able to adapt to the varieties of external forces in ways and at times that could disintegrate some or all of the facets of this identity. When the external force succeeds in interrupting homeostasis, illness is the result. Human effectiveness is measured in terms of the constancy of homeostasis, self-sufficiency, or adaptability. Dubos[14] relates this adaptability to health when he states, "Health can be regarded as an expression of fitness to the environment, as a state of adaptedness." He goes on to say that "homeostasis however is only a concept of the ideal. Living things do not always return exactly to their original state after responding to a stimulus." Dubos expands upon this thought by describing how the individual may respond inappropriately or excessively: "Disease is the manifestation of such inadequate responses. Health corresponds to the situation in which the organism responds adaptively while retaining its individual integrity."

The developmental processes are more significant than disease in terms of the actions required to promote and improve human health.

Optimal human development results from the interaction between genetic potentials and an environment favorable for promoting desirable qualities. Obviously, society needs to place greater emphasis on improving environment, health maintenance, education, and preventive measures. In order for this shift to take place, health professionals, especially medical personnel, must give greater attention to healthy people within a community setting, rather than focusing on sick people in therapeutic institutions. This should not be construed as advocating the abandonment of the sick; it simply means that we must begin to provide for the well with as much zeal as we have provided for the sick.

Is health education necessary?

The development of personality is dependent primarily upon the influence of the home, the community, and the educational process. Erikson, Piaget, Rogers, Freud, Maslow, and others have demonstrated the close relationship between intellectual and total personality development. Knowledge of self, of others, and of the total environment improves the likelihood of adapting to life's situations. The foundations for physical, social, and psychological growth are formed in childhood through deliberate and direct learning experiences, as well as through incidental and indirect relationships with social institutions and other environmental forces. The process of learning healthful ways to express ourselves continues throughout life.

Therefore, health education must be viewed as the basis for human effectiveness, especially when one considers the advances being made in the health sciences that will require an informed citizenry to make appropriate decisions about the application of health research. For example, genetic cloning has been achieved in frogs by a complex process involving the removal of the nucleus of an egg cell and its replacement with the nucleus from a body cell. By this process it is possible to reproduce a frog identical to the one which donated the body cell nucleus. The implications for this are obvious.* It would be possible for us to reproduce an exact copy of ourselves if so desired. As a result, awesome decisions will have to be made from both the medical and legal viewpoints; many questions and issues will need to be resolved. For instance, who will make decisions regarding human cloning? The medical profession? Legislators? Citizens? Clergy? Ausubel comments on the hazards of cloning: "Because of its potential for misapplication in a totalitarian society, cloning represents the most frightening prospect of genetic engineering. Theoretically, cloning could be used to turn out people on an assemblyline basis, each a carbon copy of the other, with whatever traits seem desirable to whoever controlled the process."[15]

However, as was emphasized earlier, a person is much more than a

---

* The reader is referred to Aldous Huxley's *Brave New World* for a science fiction account that may in 20 or 30 years be a reality.

conglomeration of genetic potentials; one's behavior is the result of the influences of the environment as stated by Ausubel, "Even if it becomes genetically possible to clone an Einstein, there is no guarantee that the products will have any of the behavioral qualities of the 'parent.' We still do not know the relative influence of environment and genetics in determining personality or behavioral traits."[16] It becomes increasingly obvious that health education is necessary for reasons that extend far beyond the simple development of individual health habits. It is very possible that the health knowledge we acquire—factual or otherwise— will be the basis for health decisions which will affect future generations; whether for good or for evil.

DEFINITIVE UNDERSTANDINGS

Individuals are self-sufficient when they are able to deal adequately with a particular situation, providing it is within the perimeters of their capabilities, maturity level, etc. More specifically, self-sufficiency is effective dependence upon the social and physical environments; it is the ability to make constructive decisions and contributions. In every case, self-sufficiency must be measured in view of ability, maturity level, complexity of the situation, and how well we make use of the available aids. Self-sufficiency or self-reliance is not total independence.

A person who is self-sufficient is essentially healthy in the functional sense. A healthy person is one who is able to contribute to the betterment of self and society. Even people burdened by handicaps can become self-sufficient to the degree to which the handicap is overcome. This may require the use of artificial aids. If these are used effectively and a constructive contribution is made, the person can become self-sufficient. Health and self-sufficiency should be measured in these terms rather than in terms of how great the contributions may be. The degree to which one is self-sufficient will vary depending upon a variety of circumstances. An individual is never self-sufficient in all situations.

Health education can provide the individual with the health information needed to make appropriate decisions. When appropriate decisions are made, the person is said to be health-educated. Health decisions are fundamentally based upon accurate and adequate knowledge and its application to the particular situation. The health-educated person possesses certain measurable characteristics.

Health knowledge will affect the quality of life only to the degree that it is applied to the individual's life-style and the resolution of problem situations. Health learning is an abstract process that is concerned with a variety of complex and continuous experiences related to improved quality of living. As such, health learning must deal with the realistic health issues, confronted during various stages of growth and development. Health learning, therefore, is need-oriented.

Piaget asserts that human development is determined by the maturation of the intellect. The intellect matures to the degree that assimilation and accommodation take place; that is, to the extent that the external environment is made a part of the self (assimilation) and to the degree of adaptation to the object (accommodation).

Self-actualization is the culminating process in which people become all that they are capable of becoming. It is associated with the development of a positively functioning concept of self. The self-concept is the self as we perceive ourselves. According to Maslow, the self-actualized person possesses a variety of identifiable characteristics. Fundamentally, these are the characteristics of a mature person; a person who possesses a high degree of positive mental health; one who can function adequately with self, others, and the society at large.

Each person is unique (in the ideographic approach) yet similar (in the nomothetic approach) to all others. Above all, each person is an integrated whole with all elements—biological, psychological, and sociological—in continuous interaction; each individual functions holistically in relation to certain internal and external qualities. These are the factors which influence, and often determine, functioning ability. The internal qualities are those associated with the biological, psychological, and sociological potentials. The external qualities are those associated with the social and physical environments and are in constant interaction with the internal qualities. How well the individual (internal) deals with the environmental forces (external) is a measure of adaptiveness.

There are a number of theories of personality development that have contributed to our understanding of people and the way they grow and develop. Among the most noteworthy are the psychoanalytic, analytic, individual, self-actualization, and existentialism. All of these are predicated upon the holistic view of human functioning. In this regard, the operant goals of health education must be concerned with values clarification, decision-making, and self-actualization. An operant goal implies both the end result and the process for achieving this end.

Health is both organic and functional. Similarly, disease is both organic and functional. Organic disease is the result of some degree of tissue alteration (such as tooth decay). Functional disease on the other hand, has no known organic etiology: it is psychogenic. Disease is an interruption of functional homeostasis. Human effectiveness is measured in terms of the constancy of homeostasis or the adaptability to external and internal forces.

Health education must deal with much more than the promotion of health of the individual to be immediately effective. Advances in the health sciences have increased the urgent need for a health-educated citizenry which can make sound judgments about the application of these new findings. It can be predicted that the fate of future societies in health matters will be dependent upon the quality of decisions being made now and those expected in the future. The quality of health decisions will be determined by how informed people are regarding health matters.

PROBLEMS
FOR DISCUSSION

1. Explain why health behavior is learned.
2. How do environmental factors influence behavioral development?
3. Discuss the relationship of self-sufficiency to health status according to the following:
    a. In what ways does the concept of self-sufficiency shed new light on an understanding of health and disease? Is health more than the absence of disease? Explain.
    b. Explain how self-sufficiency can be improved by an improvement in the environment.
    c. Describe how Piaget's and Maslow's theories of intellectual development and self-actualization, respectively, have implications for health education approaches.
4. Describe how the acquisition of health knowledge can influence positive health behavior even under adverse environmental conditions.
5. What is the significance of the use of amniocentesis in regards to the health of future generations? Discuss how this process will have an influence on the course of health education.
6. What is the significance of genetic cloning and other advances in the health sciences in the course that health education must take?
7. Show why existing health care facilities and personnel are not adequate to alleviate and control present health problems. What needs to happen?
8. Compare the idiographic and nomothetic approaches in regards to their application to health and health education.
9. Explain how the various theories of personality development are related to an understanding of the dynamics of human behavior.
10. Distinguish between the self-actualization and existential theories of personality. What is the central principle of each?
11. Health education is not only essential for the promotion of individual health, it is vital for future societal and political health decisions. Explain.
12. Discuss how the operant goals of health education are applicable to the psychological principles discussed in this chapter. (Note the cyclic phenomenon.)

REFERENCES

1. Dubos, Rene, *Man Adapting*, Yale University Press, New Haven, 1965, p. 651.
2. Hubbard, William N., Jr., "Health Knowledge," *The Health of Americans*, edited by Boisfeuillet Jones, Prentice-Hall, Inc., New Jersey, 1970, p. 93.
3. Reich, Charles A., *The Greening of America*, Bantam Books, New York, 1971, p. 150.
4. Knutson, Andie L., *The Individual, Society, and Health Behavior*, Russell Sage Foundation, New York, 1965, p. 341.

5. Longstreth, Langdon E., *Psychological Development of the Child*, Ronald Press Co., New York, 1968, pp. 137–156.
6. Warga, Richard G., *Personal Awareness: A Psychology of Adjustment*, Houghton Mifflin Co., 1974, pp. 47–48.
7. Ruch, Floyd, *Psychology and Life*, 5th ed., Scott, Foresman and Co., Chicago, 1959, p. 59.
8. Oberteuffer, Delbert, and Mary K. Beyrer, *School Health Education*, 4th ed., Harper & Row, New York, 1966, p. 9.
9. Coleman, James C., *Abnormal Psychology and Modern Life*, Scott, Foresman and Co., 1964, p. 89.
10. Ibid., p. 639.
11. Ruch, op. cit., 7th ed., p. 125.
12. Coleman, op. cit., pp. 645–646.
13. Rathbone, Frank S., and Estelle T. Rathbone, *Health and the Nature of Man*, McGraw-Hill Book Co., New York, 1972, p. 7.
14. Dubos, op. cit., p. 350.
15. Ausubel, Frederick, Jon Beckwith, and Kaaren Jenssen, "The Politics of Genetic Engineering: Who Decides Who's Defective", *Psychology Today*, June, 1974, p. 32.
16. Ibid., pp. 32–34.

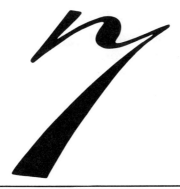

Principles
of Learning
Applied
to Health
Education

The degree of success the individual
will enjoy in society depends on
the amount of learning he consumes
and that learning about the world
is more valuable than learning
from the world.

Ivan Illich

Health educators are primarily in
the business of encouraging positive
learning experiences in health and
not solely in the business of trying to
undo the negative learning
experiences that confront everyone
in American society.

AEB
DAB

INTRODUCTION

What is learning?

Since the turn of the century, scientists have attempted to come to grips with the exact nature of learning through various types of experimentation. As a result, a variety of factors that contribute to learning have been identified. These factors have allowed psychologists to define learning in many ways. It is generally accepted that learning results in some sort of change, although what gets changed is subject to debate. Generally, definitions of learning exclude changes due to physical growth as a type of learning. Many theorists stress the importance of connections that are made between stimuli and responses, while others stress the recombination of stimuli as the key to learning. As might be expected, a variety of definitions of learning have emerged as scientists continue their search for truth. These three definitions demonstrate the differences in interpretation:

> Any change of behavior which is a result of experience, and which causes people to face later situations differently.[1]
>
> • • •
>
> Learning is the process of the formation of relatively permanent neural circuits through the simultaneous activity of the elements of the circuits-to-be; such activity is the nature of change in cell structures through growth in such a manner as to facilitate the arousal of the entire circuit when a component element is aroused or activated.[2]
>
> • • •
>
> Learning is a dynamic process. It begins with some desire, urge, or concern, or some less conscious state of tension that leads the individual to be receptive to outside stimulation. In order to learn new things he must first experience some uncertainty, or frustration or have some curiosity, perhaps, about the content or issue in which change is desired. If he trusts and is satisfied with his present facts, perceptions, values, and assumptions, he will have no need to seek new knowledge, skills, or attitudes, or to become alert to the potentialities of new ideas or alterations.[3]

Learning implies not only doing but resisting doing. In both cases the resultant action is predicated upon logic and/or feelings. Eating healthful foods, for example, is acting in accordance with a knowledge of nutrition. Avoiding excessive use of foods and alcoholic beverages is resisting doing in accordance with feelings (or attitudes) regarding the possible detrimental affects from such behavior. These feelings are learned either through direct or subliminal experiences. In any event, knowledge will be present and used as the basis for decisions being made. It is important to note that behavior can result from either factual or erroneous knowledge or simply from confusion or incomplete information which biases the decision. We simply can not ignore or separate established attitudes from the acquisition of new knowledge. How well new information will influence existing behavior is determined by how well it overcomes detrimental attitudes. In this regard, learning is any change in the individual's cognitive structure, motivation to do or not to do, feeling toward self, others and society, and any and all psychomotor or neuromuscular skills.

Two major schools of thought about learning have evolved: (1) *the associationist school* and (2) *the cognitive school.* The associationist school of thought maintains that the key to learning is a link which is created between a stimulus and a response. This link becomes stronger with repetition so that the same stimulus will produce a similar response (S–R) at a later time. In addition, associationists tend to believe that there must be action on the part of the learner for learning to take place. The major weakness of the associationist school of thought is the apparent difficulty in explaining personal social motives as factors influencing learning. There is a tendency to explain such motives as being related to internal drives similar to physiological needs.[4]

Within the associationist school of thought are two groups that view the relationship between stimuli and responses differently. One believes in *classical conditioning* while the other believes in *operant* or *instrumental conditioning.*

The work of the Russian scientist Pavlov led to the development of the classical conditioning theory through his experimentation with the salivary responses of dogs. Pavlov discovered that a dog could be made to salivate at the sound of a bell if it were first presented to the dog along with meat powder, thus establishing a link between the bell (Stimulus) and salivation (Response). The conditioning took place in the following manner:

Bell → No Reaction
Meat Powder → Salivation
Bell and Meat Powder → Salivation
Bell → Salivation[5]

It should be noted that the bell was initially the neutral stimulus because it elicited no response. The meat powder was the unconditioned stimulus because it elicited an immediate reaction. The initial salivation was the unconditioned response because it was caused by meat powder. The bell became the conditioned stimulus after being presented in conjunction with the meat powder, which resulted in the conditioned response of salivation.

Other concepts that are related to the classical conditioning theory must also be understood. These are as follows:

- *Reinforcement*—the presentation of an unconditioned stimulus with a neutral stimulus, thus establishing a connection between the neutral stimulus and the response.
- *Extinction*—occurs when the pairing of the neutral stimulus and the unconditioned stimulus is stopped or when reinforcement is halted

for a long period of time. The response will eventually no longer occur when the subject is presented with the conditioned stimulus.

- *Spontaneous Recovery*—the recurrence of the conditioned response after a period of rest with no reinforcement.
- *Generalization*—the ability of the organism to give a conditioned response to a variety of conditioned stimuli.
- *Discrimination*—the ability of an organism to limit a response to a specific stimulus.

The theory of operant or instrumental conditioning limits to a great extent the possible responses of an organism by forcing it to merely respond to conditioned and unconditioned stimuli. Operant conditioning, first to be made popular by B. F. Skinner, rewards or punishes an organism's behavior. This type of conditioning allows for the study of such reinforcement variables as the quantity of reinforcing agents, temporal factors, and sequences.[6]

Theorists of the cognitive school of learning are likely to react violently to the associationist theories because of their belief that individual differences tend to be ignored in the conditioning model. Cognitive theorists contend, therefore, that the S–R theories are too simple and incomplete. Thus, they have developed the S–O–R model; the "O" representing the organism and its perceptions, past experiences, abilities, and desires. When all of these factors are taken into consideration, the learning experience becomes more meaningful.

In regard to the process of internalization, cognitive theorists identify motivational factors that apply to learning in a problem-solving situation. (Motivation in health learning is discussed in Chapter 8, and the reader is referred especially to the discussion of P–I–S–A dealing with perception, interest, significance and application). There are five such motivational factors that are particularly important to cognitive theorists:

1. Becoming *aware* of the problem, which causes action.
2. Accumulating as much information as possible about the problem through *fact-finding*.
3. Sorting through the accumulated information through a procedure called *processing*.
4. Once processing has occurred, the information is allowed to *incubate*, which results in the *acquisition of insight*.
5. Insight provides a possible solution to the problem and results in *testing*. If the solution works, the problem is solved; if not, the process begins once again.

The association theorists and the cognitive theorists have accumulated vast amounts of information that have contributed to our understanding of the process of learning. As a result of their contributions, several basic principles of learning have emerged. These principles form the basis for learning, but especially for health learning which is concerned, ultimately, with individual self-sufficiency in all matters concerned with the health of people.

Principles of learning

The following ten principles of learning, developed by Blair,[7] are of great significance to the health educator:

1. We learn to do by doing.
2. We learn to do what we do (and not something else).
3. Without a sufficient stage of readiness, learning is inefficient and may even be harmful.
4. Without motivation, there can be no learning at all.
5. For effective learning, responses must be immediately reinforced.
6. Meaningful responses are learned better and retained longer than less meaningful responses.
7. For the greatest amount of transfer of learning, responses should be learned in the way they are going to be used.
8. People's responses will vary according to how they perceive the stimulus (situation).
9. People's responses will vary according to the atmosphere of the learning environment.
10. People will always do the only thing possible within the limits of physical inheritance, background of learning, and the forces that are acting upon them at the time.

The concept of learning to do by doing forms the basis for the experiential approach to health education. More efficient in health learning than the traditional educational approaches of memorization, recitation and the like, is the method in which the learner is directly and actively involved in the learning process. It may safely be said that the degree of learning is correlated with the amount of involvement of the learner in the learning process. This involvement includes emotional as well as physical participation.

Closely related to the above concept is the principle that we learn to do what we do and not something else. It is a fallacy to assume that a person will be able to behave healthfully through noninvolvement. For instance, learners will not acquire a positive self-concept by memorizing the various factors that constitute a positive self-concept. They will only learn how to memorize, and may retain for a time what was memorized. Until people actually become involved in developing their self-concept, learning will be incomplete.

In Chapter 5, we discussed Havighurst's developmental tasks theory which implies that various stages of readiness are passed through by individuals as they mature. Blair, et al.[8] proposed that several factors are involved in the determination of readiness in an educational setting: maturation, previous experience, relevance of the materials and methods used in the learning process, the quality of the learner's emotional attitudes, and the degree of personal adjustment which the learner attains. The determination of readiness, then, must be based upon the qualities of individuals in relation to the group. This aspect of learning provides a strong case for individualized instruction. An awareness of the need to yield to the readiness of the learner also facilitates the implementation of sequential, comprehensive health education programs.

Motivation (a topic which will be discussed later in more detail) must be taken into consideration when applying the principles of learning or there can be no learning at all. For effective learning, responses must be immediately reinforced and quite closely related. Reinforcement, or the expectation of it, is a type of motivation which stimulates behavior in certain directions. This has been clearly demonstrated through the experimentation of associationist psychologists. *Health educators, therefore, must gear the learning environment to provide for appropriate reinforcement of positive health behavior.* Behavioral examples of teachers, for instance, can be a reinforcement to children and youth.

As far back as 1885, Ebbinghaus experimented with memorization of nonsense syllables. He discovered in his experiments that meaningful material is learned better and retained longer than are less meaningful responses: When subjects memorized a series of nonsense syllables, they were retained for only a very short period of time. Obviously, no understanding or comprehension was involved because no meaningful relationships could be drawn, nor did the syllables possess any significance to the learner. *Health educators should heed these findings and design a program in which learning experiences are made meaningful to the learner.*

The degree to which learning may be transferred from one learning experience to another has been debated by psychologists for many years. Some believe that there can be no transfer of learning, while others believe that nearly total transfer should be expected from a learning situation. Regardless of the amount of transfer which occurs, however, "there is no learning which does not involve a part of a person's past experience, and in a sense all retention or remembering is a kind of transfer, because original circumstances of learning are rarely, if ever, duplicated in a new situation."[9] For health education to be most effective, health educators must attempt to create learning experiences for their students that most closely approximate the types of experiences that they will encounter outside of the formal learning environment; or better still, these external encounters can be the planned educational experiences.

Because of the variations in experience, physical attributes, and quality of the learning environment, perceptions will vary from one learner to another. Thus, the principle that responses will vary according to how one perceives the stimulus (situation) applies. The health educators must be continually aware of individual differences that contribute to such perceptual variances, and structure the learning experiences in a way that will minimize possible confusion on the part of the learner. Closely related to this principle is the concept that an individual's response will vary according to the atmosphere of the learning environment. Once again, the health educator should aid in the utilization of the existing learning environment to its greatest advantage and aid in its improvement wherever necessary.

The principle of learning that summarizes all the others is that learners do the only things they can possibly do considering their physical inheritance, their learning background, and the present forces that are acting upon them. The key here is that in the final analysis no learning is left merely to chance: it can always be explained in a logical manner. This provides the basis for educational programs in that learning can be stimulated and the results predicted through proper analysis.

Types of health learning

Health learning progresses through three levels from the concrete to the abstract and, as we have seen, is influenced by the amount and quality of learner involvement and of the internalization that takes place. These three levels—the acquisition of health facts, the development of health attitudes, and the development of values—are sometimes referred to as the *hierarchy of learning*. Health educators have continually strived to influence health attitudes and values which have the greatest impact on final health behavior. They have been quite successful in facilitating the acquisition of health facts. A problem arises, however, in that the learning of health facts does not necessarily insure proper health behavior.

In a more practical sense, Knutson[10] states that there are commonly three types of health learning situations in which public health officials are involved. The first type is the situation that requires the public to take action as specified in regulations or statutes. The aim here is that people will acquire the appropriate information and attitude to successfully adhere to these requirements. The second type of learning experience encourages the public to act upon the recommendations of authority. This is more complex, since an assumption is made that the public will act for the benefit of society through the stimulus of the recommendations as a result of attitudes and information that have already been acquired. In the third instance, the public's actions are self-directed; the public must choose its goals without the stimulus of regulations from the authorities.

Health education programs concern themselves primarily with the second and third types of learning situations since they are the result of an educational process. The first type requires little health learning in the positive sense and is an indirect means of "educating" the public.

The three types of learning situations correspond very closely to the hierarchy of learning discussed above. This is illustrated in Figure 7–1.

DYNAMICS OF COGNITIVE HEALTH LEARNING

The cognitive domain

The separation of learning into the cognitive, affective, and psychomotor domains is done basically for convenience. It is nearly impossible to classify all learning into one of these domains without also wondering what effect, if any, the learning has upon the other two. Such a system of classification, however, does serve to strengthen our understanding of the learning process and can help us gain a more objective view of the structure of the educational programs to be developed and implemented. Tanner emphasizes the interdependence of educational domains by illustrating that each domain is related holistically to individual needs

FIGURE 7–1   Public Health Learning Situations

Public health learning situations correspond to the hierarchy of learning—self-directed behavior directly affects society's health values while imposed actions result in superficial learning at best.

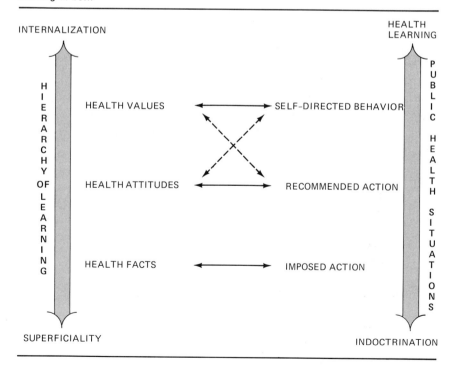

and developmental tasks. He states that "the developers of the tax-onomies of instructional objectives recognized the continuity and inter-dependence of the three domains but chose to treat them separately for purposes of focus and in view of the distinction made in classroom instruction and in curriculum materials. Yet it should be stressed that although the term *domain* implies a separation of spheres of activity, in effect learning these spheres are marked not by separation and isolation, but by continuity and interdependence."[11]

The process of learning within the cognitive domain is more than the acquisition of health facts: It includes those aspects of health learning that "deal with the recall or recognition of knowledge and the develop-ment of intellectual abilities and skills."[12] Although dealing with the cognitive domain has fallen into disfavor among many health educators in recent years through their attempts to enhance the affective aspects of learning it must not be forgotten that our behavior and feelings are based upon what we know about reality. We must not minimize the importance of cognitive learning. As Bloom states,

> knowledge . . . may be justified as an important objective or outcome of learning in many ways. Perhaps the most common justification is that with increase in knowledge or information there is a development of one's acquaintance with reality. Such reality may represent what is known by convention or definition, what are known as the findings or outcome of inquiry in the various fields, what are known as the more fruitful ways of attacking problems in the field, or what are known as the more useful ways of organizing a field. It is assumed that as the number of things known by an individual increases, his acquaintance with the world in which he lives increases.[13]

Health knowledge is discussed in Chapters 4 and 8 as it applies to the outcomes of health education in its broadest sense. However, knowl-edge and intellectual abilities and skills are composed of several ele-ments. These elements illustrate the nature and breadth of the cognitive domain.[14]

Knowledge implies an understanding of:
1. specifics
2. terminology
3. facts
4. ways and means of dealing with specifics
5. conventions
6. trends and sequences
7. classification and categories
8. criteria
9. methodology
10. universals and abstractions
11. principles and generalizations
12. theories and structures

Intellectual abilities and skills imply:
1. comprehension
2. interpretation
3. application
4. analysis and synthesis
5. evaluation

It becomes quite obvious that the cognitive domain must receive at least the same emphasis within the health education program as the affective and psychomotor domains. Although our feelings and ability to act are extremely important results of health education programs, these aspects cannot stand in a vacuum. They must be based upon our past cognitive abilities. Once again, it is not a question of what is to be learned but rather how well it is learned for miximum application. Generally, health knowledge is acquired best as a result of the affective learning experience.

Knowledge and concept development

Many educators feel that the development of sound and usable concepts is one of the most important roles of educational programs, since concepts allow the learner to adapt readily to new learning situations. Without conceptual development, the learner would have to face each learning situation as if no prior learning had occurred. As Blair, et al. point out, "concepts enable the person to generalize, discriminate, and label things appropriately so he can communicate with others."[15]

Concept formation implies the ability to categorize learning experiences in a meaningful way. We emphasize the term "experiences" here because the development of concepts is based in the cognitive realm. In addition, "conceptualization is not an all or none proposition, but a gradual attainment with experience."[16] And with further experiences, concepts can be broadened or changed. Concept development is personal; it is the way that one perceives the relationship of facts, ideas, and thoughts.

The development of concepts should be thought of as an end in the educative process, not a means to an end; that is, not a methodology. Concepts may be developed by educators as desirable outcomes of a particular program and develop means of achieving these concepts. The School Health Education Study, for instance, is an example of a *curriculum design*, not a method. And yet there seems to be some confusion among health educators about this. Read and Greene state that "problem solving is not the current method; concept development is."[17] Problem solving is a *method of learning* which *may result* in the development of appropriate concepts.

Concept formation, then, implies a generalized comprehension as a result of specific learning experiences. Health educators should design programs that emphasize experiential learning in order to foster the development of positive health concepts. Any and all methods should be considered as potential facilitators of conceptual development and utilized where appropriate. To summarize, the following may be said about health learning:

1. There are no options without knowledge.
2. Knowledge is the basic and essential element for conceptualization.
3. Conceptualization is the heart of attitude formation.
4. Attitudes direct behavior.

These principles are illustrated in Figure 7–2. It would be helpful at this point to turn to a discussion about the development of appropriate health attitudes and behavior.

Retention of health knowledge

One of the most puzzling problems confronting health educators is that of providing learning experiences for the learner that will result in a maximum amount of retention. Retention is more than remembering health facts—it extends into the areas of concept development, the ability to solve problems, and the making of appropriate decisions. The key to maximum retention is the degree of meaningfulness a particular health experience has to an individual. Rote memorization of health facts, a method that has been common in traditional health education programs, is of limited value. Such a procedure is usually unrelated to the needs of the learner and information learned in this manner is soon forgotten. On the other hand, it is suspected by some that if learning material is properly organized and meaningful to the learner, the amount of retention may actually increase with time and become the basis for further learning to occur. The lack of effectiveness of meaningless (in terms of relevance) material in health education is reflected in the results obtained when emphasis is placed upon disease conditions related to the various content areas. This constitutes a negative approach in attempting to influence health behavior. This approach has failed to make any real impact on the alleviation of disease, disability, or premature death from preventable health-related phenomena. It is a misconception to assume that certain kinds of information, no matter how accurate, will necessarily result in improved health status.

Health educators must be aware that learning in one situation may facilitate or hinder learning in subsequent learning situations. Conversely, a learning experience may facilitate or hinder the retention of previous experiences. When a learning experience hinders the retention of previous learning, it is called *retroactive inhibition*. For example, if a student were to learn the characteristics of a particular vitamin and then, at a later date, learn the characteristics of another vitamin, confusion about the properties of the first vitamin could result. On the other hand, review or clarification of material would probably result in greater reten-

FIGURE 7–2 The Influence of Health Knowledge on Health Attitudes and Behavior

Meaningful health knowledge is most likely to result in concept development, attitudinal change, and positive health behavior. Superficial health facts should be avoided since they tend to be irrelevant.

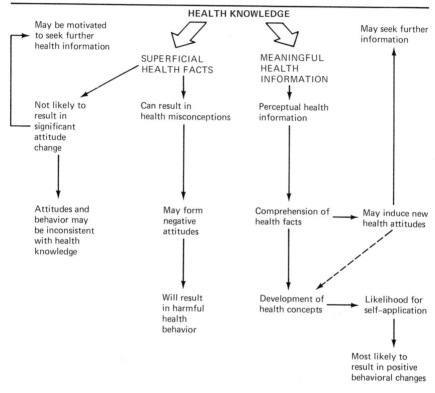

tion of a previous experience. This is called *retroactive facilitation*. The reverse of retroactive inhibition occurs when one learning experience causes later learning to be inefficient. This phenomenon is called *proactive inhibition*. If one health theory is learned, it may cause confusion in the learner with respect to theories learned at a later time. When material is presented to the learner, therefore, an effort should be made to facilitate integration of the new material with the material already learned. From a positive viewpoint, material that allows future learning to become easier is called *proactive facilitation*.

Other factors that may interfere with retention are:

1. Emotional interference, particularly when the educator creates a threatening atmosphere for learning.
2. The physical condition of learners at the time they are asked to recall what has been learned.
3. Organic defects in the neural makeup of the learner.

4. Normal distortion that results from the tendency to organize things into a stable form.

The important concept to remember with regard to retention is that the more meaningful a learning experience is to the learner, the less chance there is for confusion or distortion of information as it is perceived by the learner.

DYNAMICS OF ATTITUDINAL DEVELOPMENT

The affective domain

The affective domain involves personal interests, attitudes, and values, and the development of appreciations and adequate adjustments. Krathwohl[18] has suggested several factors involved in affective learning:

1. *Receiving*—awareness, willingness to receive controlled or selected attention
2. *Responding*—acquaintance, willingness to respond, satisfaction in response
3. *Valuing*—acceptance, preference, commitment
4. *Organization*—conceptualization of a value, organization of a value system
5. *Characterization* by a value or value complex—generalized set characterization

Attitudes can be described as the perceptions people have of things within their environment that result in a predisposition to act. These perceptions are learned and, in turn, influence behavior. Health attitudes, as with motivation, influence the direction of health behavior. The development of health attitudes is influenced largely by the development of health concepts and, as we have seen, health concepts result from comprehension and application of health knowledge.

One of the chief characteristics of attitudes is their perceptual and affective components. That is, attitudes affect *what* we see as well as *how* we see it.[19] This makes the job of the health educator much more complex in that many negative health attitudes may have to be overcome. If an individual possesses negative attitudes at the outset of a learning experience, any positive health exposure may be perceived erroneously by the individual, resulting in an ineffective learning experience. The job of the health educator would be much simpler if each individual were an "attitudinal virgin," as it were. In reality, however, the many forces acting upon an individual before, during, and after the health education experience are bound to cause some attitudinal misconceptions. Therefore, in order to enhance the likelihood of the development of positive health attitudes, the health education program must provide comprehensive experiences that are exciting, intellectually stimulating, and biologically and socially significant.

The effects of knowledge on attitudes

It should be clear by now that the acquisition of appropriate health knowledge is extremely important. The value of health knowledge alone in affecting positive behavioral change is questionable. However, one must not ignore the value of health knowledge in the development of attitudes. To a large extent what we know influences, either positively or negatively, our attitudinal development.

Some educators believe that other factors also influence attitudinal development. For instance, Kendler[20] cites three factors, in addition to knowledge, as influencing attitudes: (1) motivation and reinforcement, (2) personality, and (3) the social environment. A close look at these factors, however, results in the conclusion that even these are governed largely by what we know. What develops is a cyclical reaction in which personal motives are influenced by knowledge gleaned from experience. These motives, in turn, influence the type of attitudes developed. In addition, one's personality is influenced by what one knows which, in turn, influences the type of attitudes the individual will adopt. One's social environment limits the types of learning experiences to which one is exposed which, in turn, influences attitudinal development. This concept is illustrated in Figure 7–3.

To summarize, health knowledge forms the basis for our tendencies to behave in particular ways (attitudes). Attitudes cannot be formed in a vacuum. One learning experience may establish a deep-seated attitude. The attitude is more likely, however, to be formed through a variety of experiences, each reinforcing the other, ultimately resulting in a predisposition to behave in a given way when confronted with a similar stimulus.

Developing positive health attitudes

As with the learning of factual information, the development of attitudes is most effective when positive reinforcement is used. Children may develop the attitude that smoking is not harmful because their parents smoke. Such an attitude increases the likelihood that the child will become a smoker. Many other similar examples become readily apparent.

Most health educators are confronted with the task of encouraging the development of positive health attitudes as well as changing already existing negative ones. In either case, this is a process of persuasion; a process of convincing a learner through a variety of experiences that a particular behavioral predisposition is appropriate. Such persuasion may take a variety of forms that health educators may utilize at one time or

FIGURE 7–3   Factors Influencing Attitudes
Attitudes are an integral part of one's personality and are influenced by knowledge, motivation, and the social environment.

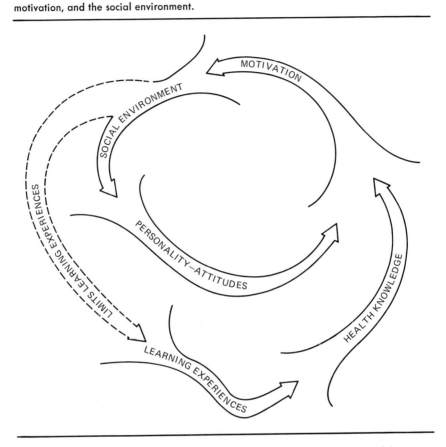

another. Kendler[21] identifies these as: (1) mass persuasion, (2) group persuasion, and (3) individual persuasion.

Mass persuasion may occur in many ways, but the one which readily comes to mind when thinking of health is the use of the mass media by large companies (pharmaceutical, tobacco, automobile, etc.) to influence the public to purchase particular products purported to improve health or to enhance an illusion of improvement. These companies spend billions of dollars annually to influence the buying public. The key factors utilized by these companies are: 1) getting the public's attention; 2) repeating the advertisement often (repetition often nearly equals truth); 3) convincing the public to purchase the product through appeals to conformity and the possibility of a better life; and 4) appearing to satisfy a basic need. Although the effectiveness of mass persuasion techniques is not fully understood, it is known that convincing even a small percentage of a population to behave in a particular way may yield large dividends to the advertiser.

One of the most common approaches employed by health educators to change attitudes is group persuasion. Health educators continually attempt to encourage their students to adopt positive health attitudes through a variety of learning experiences. It is important to note that the more positive the learning experiences are, the greater the chance of long-lasting, positive attitudinal change. The scare tactics utilized to a great extent during the drug abuse crisis of the 1960s were not effective for this reason. Research in other areas has produced similar results.* This is consistent with the basic concept that "a message's persuasiveness is inversely related to the amount of fear it generates."[22] It behooves health educators, therefore, to attempt health attitude change through positive learning experiences. By "positive" we mean those experiences the learner perceives as important in accomplishing personally relevant tasks.

Health educators as well as parents attempt to develop attitudes in people on an individual basis. This allows for stricter control of variables that may interfere with learning. In addition, learning experiences can be designed specifically in accordance with the characteristics of the learner.

When considering attitudinal change, health educators must seize the opportunity to utilize mass persuasion, group persuasion, and individual persuasion on a positive basis. Health educators cannot hope to increase their effectiveness until they acquire expertise at least equal to that of those who would exploit the vulnerability of the public.

Influence of attitudes on behavior

The development of positive health attitudes that will affect health behavior is a key factor in improving the health status of individuals and society. Only when people behave positively in accord with their health knowledge can it be said that health education has been effective. The learner must experience a sense of self-approval, self-satisfaction, and self-improvement. Artificial, educator-selected goals and activities will result in boredom, lack of motivation, and the development of negative attitudes toward health learning—pitfalls worth avoiding.

Attitudes can be imposed, resulting in behavioral change through indoctrination. We must not allow health education to degenerate to this level. Choices must remain for learners. Their attitudes, developed rationally, will positively influence behavior through the educative process. Indoctrinational attitude change or development is akin to brainwashing, and there is no place for this approach in education.

---

* Although fear or other forms of punishment may deter undesirable behavior for some individuals some of the time, positive (reward) reinforcement of desirable behavior is more powerful and more long-lasting. Health educators should strive to develop intelligent behavior rather than fear as the basis for decision-making.

DYNAMICS OF HEALTH BEHAVIOR

The psychomotor domain

The psychomotor domain includes those aspects of learning in which accumulated knowledge and attitudes are applied to particular life situations. In many respects, this is the ultimate goal of health education: the development of appropriate health behavioral patterns.

When we speak of health behavior, it is necessary to think of it as a result of an internalization process; an educative process. This type of behavior implies that the individual is able to make a choice between two or more alternatives. If no real choice exists, health education would be unnecessary.

In some cases, positive behavior may result even when no true education has taken place; that is, as a result of coercion or fear of penalty. We are confronted with these situations often in our society. For instance, a statute may restrict an individual's behavior in order to protect the health of society. The person is likely to comply with the law to avoid a fine or incarceration, but little, if any, health education has taken place, especially when viewed in terms of decision-making.

For education to effectively influence the psychomotor domain, people must behave in the learning situation the way they will be expected to behave in a life situation. It should be remembered that only rarely does an individual consistently behave as a result of the accumulation of factual information alone. Through the internalization process, concepts must be formed that influence attitudes that, in turn, give direction to the individual's behavioral patterns.

Observable and nonobservable health behavior

The component of the psychomotor domain that can be evaluated most easily is observable behavior. This type of behavior may be evaluated during or immediately after the learning experience; or it may not be possible to assess it until the learner has a chance to utilize it sometime after the learning experience in a later life situation.

Nonobservable behavior may be characterized as those instances where an individual is functioning outside of the educational setting. In this instance, inquiries must be made about the individual's activities through contacts who are aware of the individual's activities. Nonobservable behavior has also been described as those feelings and thoughts occurring within the individual.

In each case, more effective evaluation of the effectiveness of the health education program would be possible through a coordination of all providers of health within a community. This would minimize the amount of nonobservable health behavior and would make it possible to determine if those observable behavior patterns within the educational setting had been properly internalized and utilized in life situations.

Health-related and health-directed learning

Traditionally, health educators have aimed their educational programs at prevention of specific diseases and disabilities in the hope of initiating positive behavioral change. The effectiveness of this type of approach is questionable. Those behaviors that have been stressed may be identified as health-directed behaviors since they concern themselves with specific health issues.

In a broader sense, however, all behavior is influenced by one's health and vice versa. This may be identified as health-related behavior. Health educators must come to grips with this concept and design programs that focus on health-related learning. This requires an emphasis upon the individual as a whole and the individual's ability to function effectively in society.

Health education cannot be effective by dealing solely with health-directed behavior or on an intervention basis. In essence, individuals need to learn to behave in a health-related manner. Health-directed behavior, then, becomes a subcategory of health-related behavior, one which is incorporated into our life-style.

DEFINITIVE UNDERSTANDINGS

Learning has been described in a variety of ways. Theorists stress that the key to learning involves the connections that are made between stimuli and responses, while others stress a recombination of stimuli as the key to learning.

Two major schools of thought have emerged with regard to learning theory: the associationist school and the cognitive school. Associationists believe that a link must be established between a stimulus and a response in order for learning to occur; cognitive theorists stress the necessity to consider individual differences for learning to be better understood.

There are ten basic principles that may be used to describe the necessary essentials of learning. These all have significant applicability for the health educator. Learning can become maximally effective when these principles are incorporated into the health education program.

Knutson emphasizes three types of health learning experiences: 1) required behavior, 2) recommended behavior, and 3) voluntary behavior. Health education concerns itself mainly with the last two types since a certain amount of education is required to successfully carry them out.

The cognitive domain of learning is characterized by recognition and recall of knowledge, and by the development of intellectual abilities and skills. It is, therefore, much more complex than the internalization of health facts. Concepts develop as a result of proper acquisition of knowledge. Concepts enable people to generalize their learning experiences.

The key to the retention of health knowledge is the degree of meaningfulness an experience has to the individual. Health educators must be aware that learning experiences may hinder or facilitate learning at other times. Therefore, experiences should be designed to fit into the individual's existing subsumption system.

Affective learning implies the enhancement of one's interests, attitudes, and values and the development of appreciations and adequate adjustments. Health educators should keep in mind that attitudes affect what we see as well as how we see it. It must also be stressed that what we know influences our attitudinal development. Attitudes may be changed in three ways: 1) mass persuasion, 2) group persuasion, and/or 3) individual persuasion. Health educators should consider utilizing all three approaches in their efforts to educate the public.

The psychomotor domain includes those aspects of learning through which accumulated knowledge and attitudes are applied to particular life situations. Behavior resulting from education involves the internalization process. Noneducational methods may take the form of coercion or fear of penalty. Both observable and nonobservable behavior may occur. Health educators must devise means of maximizing the observability of health behavior for increased program effectiveness.

Health educators need to begin to gear their programs to deal with health-related behavior as well as with health-directed behavior. Positive behavior change is most likely to occur when the total individual is considered in the learning process.

PROBLEMS
FOR DISCUSSION

1. What is learning? Discuss the various factors involved in the learning process.
2. What elements are necessary to include in an adequate definition of learning?
3. Explain the differences between the associationist and cognitive schools of thought with regard to learning.
4. Describe how the principles of learning apply to a health education program. Give an example.
5. Explain how health education can contribute to voluntary health learning in our society.
6. Describe the importance of the development of the cognitive domain for positive health behavior.
7. What is concept formation? How does knowledge contribute to concept formation?
8. How can the health educator contribute to the retention of health knowledge?
9. What factors may interfere with retention?
10. How does knowledge contribute to the development of the affective domain?
11. What is the importance of the development of positive health attitudes?

12. Should health educators deal in mass persuasion? Why? Why not?
13. How is the psychomotor domain adequately developed in the health areas?
14. How should health educators facilitate the development of positive health-related behavior?

REFERENCES

1. Blair, Glenn Myers, R. Stewart Jones, and Ray H. Simpson, *Educational Psychology*, 3d ed., Macmillan Publishing Co., New York, 1968, p. 107.
2. Bugelski, B. R., *The Psychology of Learning*, Henry Holt, New York, 1956, p. 120.
3. Knutson, Andie L., *The Individual, Society and Health Behavior*, Russell Sage Foundation, New York, 1965, p. 389.
4. Warga, Richard G., *Personal Awareness: A Psychology of Adjustment*, Houghton Mifflin Company, 1974, p. 161.
5. Ibid., p. 162.
6. Blair, Jones, and Simpson, op. cit., p. 115.
7. Blair, Glenn Myers, "Principles of Learning," unpublished paper, 1971.
8. Blair, Jones, and Simpson, op. cit., pp. 125–135.
9. Ibid., p. 274.
10. Knutson, op. cit., p. 381.
11. Tanner, Daniel, *Using Behavioral Objectives in the Classroom*, Macmillan Publishing Co., New York, 1972, pp. 4–5.
12. Bloom, Benjamin S., et al., *Taxonomy of Educational Objectives, Handbook I, Cognitive Domain*, David McKay Company, New York, 1956, p. 7.
13. Ibid., p. 32.
14. Ibid., Part II.
15. Blair, Jones, and Simpson, op. cit., p. 240.
16. Ibid., p. 241.
17. Read, Donald A., and Walter H. Greene, *Creative Teaching in Health*, Macmillan Publishing Co., New York, 1975, p. 46.
18. Krathwohl, David R., et al., *Taxonomy of Educational Goals, Handbook II: Affective Domain*, David McKay Company, New York, 1964, p. 34.
19. Blair, Jones, and Simpson, op. cit., p. 203.
20. Kendler, Howard H., *Basic Psychology*, Appleton Century Crofts, New York, 1963, pp. 576–577.
21. Ibid., pp. 579–587.
22. Ibid., p. 586.

Life is a constant struggle to satisfy
wants, concerns, desires, hopes, or
aspirations, and to avoid, minimize,
or escape from pain, discomfort,
or injury.

Andie L. Knutson

Motivation is the force that
stimulates the child toward
achievement, success, physical and
emotional pleasure—toward
fulfillment. Fulfillment is the fruit of
life, of living. The extent to which
fulfillment is felt is a manifestation
of the quality of health attained.
How well one is living determines
the extent of fulfillment, and it,
in turn, reflects the quality of
motivation.

AEB
DAB

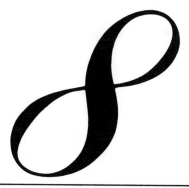

Motivating
for Health
Learning

PRINCIPLES OF MOTIVATION

What is a motive?

It is necessary to state at the outset of this discussion that the precise role that motivation plays in human behavior is still unclear. What forces, innate or environmental, impel an individual to action? A hungry person will have a tendency to seek food, but one who is not hungry will frequently show a similar tendency if the odor of food is present. On the one hand, a basic innate drive is activated; on the other hand, a learned, culturally influenced behavior is set into motion.

Simply speaking, a motive is *the internal force that compels one to behave in a certain way.* It is the causation of behavior, the reason for action or inaction. Motives arise from two chief sources: the biogenic and the sociogenic. *Motives may be conscious or unconscious, innate or learned.* For example, the tendency to seek food because of hunger is biogenic (innate and conscious), while the tendency to seek food because of an environmental stimulus such as an odor is sociogenic (learned and conscious). In addition, motivation is very personal and can take a variety of forms. It is not always possible to infer a motive from a particular action, since different motives can result in similar reactions in the same individual.

Figure 8–1 illustrates this concept in more detail. As shown, motives may be innate, learned, or a combination of both. As one matures, origin distinctions become less identifiable. It will be noted that individuals manifesting the same behavior may have different reasons (motives) for it, while individuals manifesting different behavior may do so for the same reasons; or, finally, individuals manifesting the same behavior may have the same or similar reasons. Therefore, *behavior alone cannot necessarily provide us with the motivation that caused it.* This principle has significant implications for health learning. For example, two individuals who do not smoke may have the same or different reasons. One may have experienced a close relative or friend who developed lung cancer; the other may recognize that smoking can interfere with the ability to excel in athletic endeavors and, therefore, neither one smokes. However, in both cases, the motivation is learned and conscious.

Biogenic motives

These are related directly to tissue needs: thirst, hunger, need for oxygen, etc., which are necessary for the maintenance of life and the promotion of biological growth and development. These motives are essentially innate. However, they can and do influence other, more complex forms of human behavior than merely the satisfaction of biological needs.

Motives, needs, and drives can be interpreted as synonymous. As

FIGURE 8–1   Motives and Behavior
It is not always possible to infer a motive from a particular kind of behavior since the
same motive may elicit different behavior in two individuals.

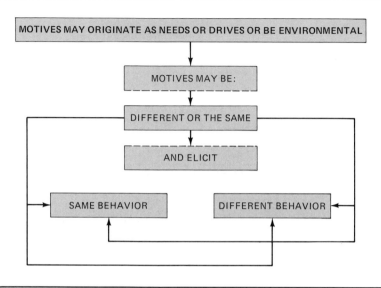

we have seen, needs are related to the bio-psycho-social aspects of human
nature and they provide the energy necessary to reduce the tension they
create. Drives are generally thought of in terms of the innate, biological
(and psychological if, indeed, they are innate) needs. The biological
needs, or drives, provide the force needed to activate the individual
toward achieving a particular goal. They may be identified as incentives
as well as motivational forces. The biological forces (or drives) manifest
themselves as *visceral* (the need for food, water, etc.); *safety* (avoidance
of bodily harm); *sex* (related to both reproduction and physical and
emotional fulfillment), and *sensory-motor* (associated with perception
and action). These drives tend toward survival of the individual, toward
biological, sociological, and psychological activation. Coleman[1] states
that "the motivation of all living organisms is based on their fundamental tendencies toward maintenance and the actualization of their
potentialities." That is to say, according to Coleman, "The individual
resists disintegration or decay and tends to develop and behave in
accordance with his genetic potentialities."

Sociogenic motives

The second group of motives emanates from the psychosocial needs.
It is thought that these motives are acquired in the process of growth
and development and are influenced, especially in terms of means for

satisfaction, by cultural mores. They are related to one's personal wants, desires, and aspirations and arise from experiences encountered during maturation. *The sociogenic motives are intellectually based in the sense that the individual, as a result of experiences, acquires insight into self and the world.* These experiences tend to become the foundation for formulating personal goals and the method for achieving them through perceived satisfactory activities. It is important to note, however, that not all the "satisfactory activities" are necessarily desirable from a cultural or social viewpoint. The sociogenic motives manifest themselves in terms of the need to achieve (1) meaning and order to life; (2) a sense of adequacy; (3) feelings of security; (4) a feeling of belonging and social approval and acceptance; (5) a sense of personal worth and self-esteem; and (6) love of self and love from others.

Satisfaction of these motives is related directly to the attainment and maintenance of one of the three dimensions of health, the psychological dimension. In this regard, it is important for the teacher and others who work directly with children to assist them to develop a positive self-image, a sense of personal worth. This can be accomplished in a variety of ways within the classroom setting. For example, the teacher can provide satisfying learning experiences for each child. Such broad methods as value clarification and individualized learning lend themselves to these kinds of outcomes.

Human motivation is so complex that motives are rarely biogenic or sociogenic in the pure form. As we have seen, human behavior is influenced as though all of its segments—physical, psychological, and social—were one. The forces behind the behavior also operate holistically. Since both the biogenic and sociogenic motives are in constant interaction, the satisfaction of a need in one category may very well contribute to the satisfaction of a need in the other.

Homeostasis as a motivating force

There is a strong tendency for the individual to maintain an equilibrium, or *homeostasis*, that is vital to total survival. In regard to motivation, the energy created by homeostasis directs one toward actions necessary for the maintenance of health and the actualization of individual potentials. These operate on two levels: the *biological level*, which is characterized by the ability to resist disease, maintain body temperature and total biological chemistry, and the *interpretive level* which is characterized by the need to establish feelings of self-worth, to interact socially, and to generally avoid those things that are identified as painful; in short, to behave in ways that result in personal satisfaction, growth and actualization. This concept is illustrated in Figure 8–2 and 8–3.

The extent to which total homeostasis is maintained will determine the degree of health or disease that results. Learning is directly related to successful balance between the biological and interpretive levels since the actions one takes can assist in the maintenance and promotion of

FIGURE 8–2   Origins of Motives and Homeostasis
Homeostasis results from motivation, but the way that it is maintained depends upon learning: the biological level or the interpretive level. The origin of both motives and homeostasis is **biogenic or sociogenic.**

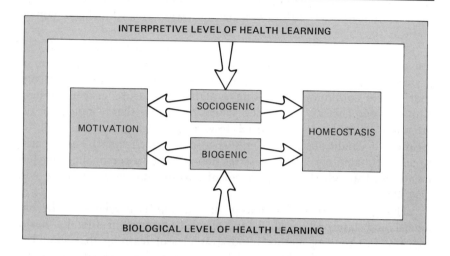

FIGURE 8–3   Homeostasis, Level of Health Learning, and Health Behavior
The level of health learning needed—biological or interpretive—is associated with the origin of homeostasis as a motivational force.

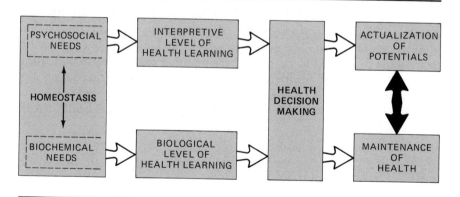

health. For example, knowledge of the importance of getting vaccinated (and actually receiving the vaccination) will help the body resist the disease for which the immunization is intended. Adequate nutritional information followed by appropriate eating behavior can result in improved health within nutritional limitations, and knowledge of self and others can improve one's mental and emotional health.

This last example will result in the individual possessing more effective intra– and interpersonal relations. In all cases, the individual learns to make vital health decisions within the realm of need satisfaction. However, the complexity of the situation and the constraints (personal or environmental) on obtaining food, for instance, will determine the nature of health knowledge necessary for achieving a homeostatic state.

Although motives are often simple and related to homeostasis, and are described as internal stresses that stimulate and regulate an individual's behavior toward a goal, it would be inaccurate to assume that one is continuously seeking a state of pleasure or contentment. Knutson emphasizes this point when he states that: "much of our attention is deliberately focused toward increasing tensions and the creating of conditions that offer suspense and excitement. The capacity to develop, maintain, and release tension is basic to personality development, and through the management of tensions one learns to cope with new life situations."[2]

The application of the concept of learning as it relates to the biological and interpretive levels is especially important for the health educator in choosing methods and strategies of learning that should be used. For example, the biological level of learning is chiefly concerned with the acquisition of basic knowledge related to maintaining physical health. Thus, the health educator needs to provide learners with experiences that will assist them in making health decisions that will result in maintaining the structure and functions of the body.

The interpretive level of learning is much more complex since it deals with health decisions related to finding the best ways of living a full, creative, and enjoyable life. This level of learning is chiefly concerned with the development of the psychological and sociological dimensions of health. The degree to which the biological level of health learning is developed has a direct bearing upon the degree to which the interpretive level of health will be developed. Once again we see the interrelatedness of all aspects of functioning and the need for the health educator to be aware of this unity when providing health learning experiences.

FACTORS THAT MOTIVATE

Intent to learn

"One of the most important motivational factors influencing learning performance of human subjects is the presence of a conscious intent to learn."[3] Intent to learn may be stimulated by external forces in the environment such as the teacher, audiovisual stimuli, etc., or may be self-imposed through aspirations, wants, and desires. *The external stimuli are incentives, while the intent to learn is the motivation.* For example, interest, curiosity, and excitement may be aroused when an individual is exposed to an attractive learning experience. This may stimulate the desire to pursue the experience, to become involved in the activity which is perceived as a vehicle for achieving a desirable goal.

For direct learning to take place, the individual must *want* to learn, and learning opportunities must be made available when *readiness* to learn is attained. Real motivation will not occur if the individual does not desire to achieve the goal or if the goal is perceived as irrelevant, meaningless, or unachievable. A question frequently asked by students is, "Why do I have to know this?" It is an indication that the students do not perceive the goal as having any particular relevance to them: There is no motivation. Unless the teacher is successful in helping students understand the importance of this new knowledge, very little significant learning will take place. At best, it is more likely to be superficial learning intended to satisfy the teacher and to reproduce the knowledge for a test rather than learning to attain any meaningful change in behavior.

Generally speaking, *the stronger the desire to learn, the more intense the motivation is and the more enthusiastically the student will become involved in the learning process.* If these factors are present, it is more likely that the new knowledge will have meaning to the student; that is, it will be internalized. When new information is internalized, it becomes a potential force for affecting future behavior and in similar decision-making situations.

Since not all goals will be perceived by all students as real, important, or achievable, not all students will be motivated to the same degree. Moreover, the intensity of motivation will vary among students who are motivated. The intensity of motivation is essentially dependent upon the arousal of interest in the goal and the learning experience and upon the student's ability to achieve. These two factors result in *reinforced motivation;* that is, awareness of the need or desire, and anticipation of achievement. However, if the goal is not real and is perceived as impossible to achieve, there will be no motivation and therefore no significant learning. As a matter of fact, a student may very well become demotivated under these circumstances.

Rewards and punishments

A sense of being successful in a given task tends to reinforce motivation. Motivation is much more intense if success is experienced rather than merely the avoidance of punishment. Therefore, reward is more desirable as an incentive than is the threat of punishment. Furthermore, if the reward is related to the satisfaction of a need, rather than being artificial, it is more likely to motivate. Artificial rewards, such as grades, gold stars, and trophies, do little to affect the quality of learning. Achievement in these circumstances is more apt to be related to acquiring the reward than to learning. Rewards as the goal for learning should be avoided. They should be incidental to, or a reinforcement of, learning, not the sole reason for learning.

Reward and punishment, however, can influence the *rate* of learning. This is especially true if a desire to learn is already present. Rewards as well as punishments may take the form of material things, such as salary, grades, or tokenism; or of abstractions, such as the feeling of success or failure, satisfaction or dissatisfaction. For example, one's own evaluation of progress can be interpreted as reward or punishment depending upon one's perception of the evaluation. A student will usually respond better to positive results (success) than to negative results (failure). Failure, as a form of punishment, tends to discourage motivation while success, as a reward, is most effective at the beginning stages of a learning process.

Students will learn more rapidly if they are continuously aware of the progress they are making. This knowledge of the results of learning is called *psychological feedback*. In essence, it is the process of keeping students aware of the correctness of their learning so that they can make appropriate adaptations to future learning. *Psychological feedback, whether negative or positive, will act as a more desirable motivating force than no feedback at all.* Students who are not provided with continuous knowledge of the results of their learning will not learn as rapidly or as well as those who are.

Finally, if the learning experience in health is inconsistent with the student's developmental level and capabilities, the threat of failure may be felt. This can result in stress. Stress under certain circumstances aids learning but under other circumstances will interfere with learning. Anxiety regarding the learning situation may reduce the ability to discriminate clearly. This is likely to result in confusion and possible misinterpretation of what is being learned. The danger in this is that the student will form misconceptions regarding the particular health issue being studied.

Incentives

External or environmental forces that activate motives are called *incentives*. Incentives are important in motivating behavior only to the extent they are associated with previous similar behavior. An incentive with which the individual is unfamiliar or whose consequences are not understood will be meaningless in motivating the present desired behavior. Basically, an incentive is something that an individual looks forward to upon completing an assigned (by self or others) task. Therefore, the task is undertaken to acquire the reward or to avoid the punishment.

Positive incentives as perceived by the individual are more desirable and usually more effective than negative ones. Positive incentives of various kinds are more likely to motivate constructive behavior while negative ones may result in devious behavior, that is, behavior that will avoid the punishment.

The strength of the incentive as perceived by the individual affects the strength of the motivation. In turn, the quality of learning usually improves as the strength of motivation increases. This is determined by the nature of the incentive and the importance the individual places on achieving the goal. *The strength of the motivation may be inferred from the speed with which learning takes place.* Conversely, strong motivation may create anxiety over possible failure and thus interfere with learning. The building of confidence through success is an essential part of the health education learning experience. Knowledge that one has learned is frequently sufficient incentive. Thus, when we speak of the factors that motivate, we are speaking primarily about incentives. When an incentive is translated by the individual into the force behind an action, it becomes a motive.

Intrinsic and extrinsic motivation

We have explored some of the basic principles of the nature, cause, and effect of human motivation. All motivation originates either within the individual or from external or environmental sources. That is to say, motivation is either *intrinsic* or *extrinsic*. An intrinsic motive is *any internal source of energy which directs an individual toward achieving a particular goal.* It is associated with basic human needs and drives. An extrinsic motive is basically an incentive; it is a *stimulus originating from the social or physical environment.* Both forms of motivation are directly related to all forms of human behavior and all forms of human behavior are directly related to the health of people. Knutson writes, "Health behavior seems so inseparably linked to motivation that logic impels one to orient any discussion of health practices to human needs and human motivation."[4]

No one would argue that healthful behavior is the ultimate achievement of health education. Health behavior is the result of two basic interacting factors: (1) *human plasticity,* or the ability to change, modify, or adapt; and (2) *human energetics,* or the variability and intensity of the response to stimuli.[5] Plasticity is the basis for learning; learning by definition is the ability to profit from experience. Energetics is related to human motivation; motivation supplies the energy needed for learning.

It is important to distinguish between intrinsic and extrinsic forms of motivation and to demonstrate their usefulness in bringing about health learning. Psychologists and other authorities generally agree that learning, as well as remembering, tends to improve when the motivation is intrinsic. When individuals feel a need to know and are active in the search for new information and answers to their questions, they will understand and remember better and longer what they learn than when the same information is simply presented for memorization.[6]

Intrinsic motivation is the result of innate and acquired needs. It is the most powerful and meaningful kind of motivation in terms of activating the individual toward satisfying needs. Ultimately, the most potent motivational force is a personal interest in achieving a potential goal. However, it is important to recognize that health learning can, and does, take place at both the subliminal and the conscious levels. Motivation does not necessarily have to be conscious or understood by the individual for effective health learning to result.

In order for extrinsic motivation to be effective, it must be closely associated with some intrinsic need. The external stimulus merely acts as the energizer. In this regard, the intrinsic need is associated with biological and psychological survival. Each individual, therefore, is seeking self-gratification for such things as hunger, thirst, relief from pain, success, and social acceptance. The *way* in which this gratification is achieved is a learned phenomenon. As with motivation, the kinds of actions one takes to achieve the goal can be contributory or defeating. They are the result of how well one has learned to achieve. For example, people seeking social acceptance may be motivated by peer pressure or misconceptions about how this acceptance can be attained. As a result, they may smoke, drink, use drugs, or become sexually promiscuous because their peers expect it. They may not have learned that there are more constructive forms of behavior to achieve the same goal. Obviously, the healthier we are physically, mentally, and socially, the more likely we are to respond to motivation and to act appropriately in achieving the goal. Health, therefore, is a means to an end, rather than the end itself. Figure 8–4 illustrates the relationship between intrinsic and extrinsic motivation, goals, actions and achievement.

INTERNALIZING INCENTIVES

P-I-S-A (perception, interest, significance, application)

Whether the specific stimulus that triggers motivation is intrinsic or extrinsic, the urge to act and the form it takes are dependent upon a variety of factors, some of which are:

- The individual's *recognition* of the presence of the stimulus.
- The individual's *interpretation* of the stimulus.
- The *value* the individual places on both the stimulus and the need to react to it.
- The individual's *knowledge* of the consequences and circumstances involved in satisfying the urge.
- The individual's *capabilities* for dealing with the urge.
- Whether or not the individual *perceives* the situation as threatening.
- The individual's *past experiences* for dealing with similar urges.
- The *environmental factors* that will aid or hinder the expression of the chosen behavior.

FIGURE 8–4   Factors that Motivate

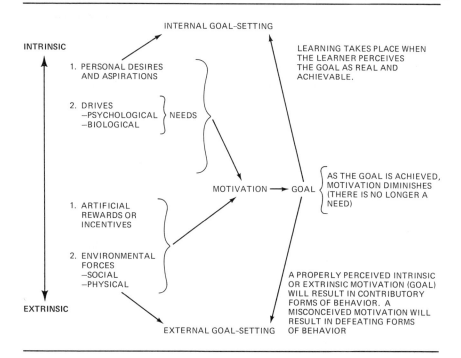

INTERNAL GOAL-SETTING

INTRINSIC

1. PERSONAL DESIRES
   AND ASPIRATIONS

2. DRIVES
   —PSYCHOLOGICAL } NEEDS
   —BIOLOGICAL

LEARNING TAKES PLACE WHEN
THE LEARNER PERCEIVES
THE GOAL AS REAL AND
ACHIEVABLE.

MOTIVATION → GOAL

AS THE GOAL IS ACHIEVED,
MOTIVATION DIMINISHES
(THERE IS NO LONGER A
NEED)

1. ARTIFICIAL
   REWARDS OR
   INCENTIVES

2. ENVIRONMENTAL
   FORCES
   —SOCIAL
   —PHYSICAL

EXTRINSIC

EXTERNAL GOAL-SETTING

A PROPERLY PERCEIVED INTRINSIC
OR EXTRINSIC MOTIVATION (GOAL)
WILL RESULT IN CONTRIBUTORY
FORMS OF BEHAVIOR. A
MISCONCEIVED MOTIVATION WILL
RESULT IN DEFEATING FORMS
OF BEHAVIOR

Obviously, motivation and its resultant behavior are inseparably tied to the physical, intellectual, and emotional capabilities of the individual, as well as the environmental circumstances that are present.

The chief motivators essential for effective health learning are *perception* of the health issues, *interest* in learning more about the health problem and its solution, *significance* of the health issue to self and society, and *application* of the knowledge of the health issue for positive adaptation of self and/or positive changes in the environment (P-I-S-A). Each of these is the result of the process of internalization of the incentives to which they relate. *Internalization is a personal process of making motives an integral part of self.* As described by Skinner, "The internalization of intellect is fully matched by that of the life of emotion and motivation."[7] Once internalization is complete, the potential for action is greatly increased.

Perception is a form of understanding, of comprehension and the ability of the individual to see the significance and relationships surrounding the health issue. Perception of the health issue may stimulate interest; on the other hand, interest in the issue and the action taken to learn about it may bring about greater perception which, in turn, reinforces the interest. These two motivational factors usually accompany each other and result in a cause and effect relationship in learning about health problems and their solutions.

Interest may take many forms; it may be interest in the nature of the health problem, the process necessary for solving it, the mysteries that may surround it, or a specific health problem may have some personal significance to the individual. Regardless of why one may have an interest in the health issue, the intensity of interest is one of the most powerful forces affecting health learning.

Significance is very closely related to perception and interest as a motivational force. It usually arises following the individual's initial explorations in the learning experience. However, many health problems have no significance to some individuals. This may be so because of a lack of real understanding of the nature of these problems and the effect they can have or because the health problem is in fact relatively unimportant or not actually a problem. This has been the case with the content of many health education programs that deal with irrelevant health matters. Instead of motivating students, such content is more likely to result in boredom and demotivation.

Application is the ultimate outcome of health learning. Health learning that influences our attitudes toward the health issue will also influence our health behavior. Application is the ability for individuals to apply their health learning to self and to society. For example, a health problem seen as adversely affecting the individual or society may result in a motivation to discover ways that it can be prevented, overcome, or controlled. Application may result in renewed interest, which begins the cycle all over again. Learning, therefore, becomes a continuous process.

Motives and behavior

Health behavior is a manifestation of the presence of one or more motives. Although the origin or specific stimulus of motivation may be either physiological, psychological, or sociological (or, more likely, a combination of these), its final translation is always psychologically internalized prior to or accompanying the resultant behavior. It is intellectually and emotionally based bringing about such behavior as thinking, feeling, or acting.

Other factors that are subordinately related to the motive described above may occur either singly or in combination to further influence existing or future motivation. Some of these factors are in themselves considered to be motives. An understanding of these is important for an understanding of the total influence of motives on human behavior. They include the following:

- The *value* placed on the health issue, goal, or learning experience.
- One's *interpretation* of self as it relates to life and living.

- How *consistent* new health experiences are with existing attitudes toward the health problem. Health misconceptions may interfere with the acquisition of new knowledge.
- *Social attitudes* that prevail toward the health problem. This is related to crisis-oriented actions by society. For example, an epidemic may motivate both social and individual action to halt it. As a result of social attitudes, individuals may develop an intense interest in the problem. The social awareness of the alcohol abuse crisis during the middle 1970s is a case in point.
- *Opportunities* for the individual to respond appropriately to the health issue. This is one of the most important responsibilities of the health educator—to provide an appropriate learning environment for each student.
- The *personal capabilities* that enable us to take advantage of the learning opportunity and to respond effectively to the related motivational forces.
- A *sense of pleasure* derived from the action being taken. If the goal is real and perceived as such, and if the individual has the capabilities and is provided the opportunity to achieve, motivation will become more intense and will be sustained until the task is complete.

PURPOSE OF MOTIVATION

Consummatory response

The *consummatory response* is behavior that indicates that the goal-seeking activity is complete. For example, the *kind* of food that one eats is the consummatory response. It results from previous learning that was motivated by the hunger drive. The consummatory response results from learning, while the drive, in this case, is innate. The more knowledge one has acquired from the learning experience, the greater the variety of responses that will be manifested. The goal-seeking activity is the action one takes following motivation; it is the pursuit of the goal.

Obviously, it is possible for a consummatory response to be based upon the acquisition of inaccurate health information or health misconceptions. For instance, if we are motivated to learn to eat healthful foods but are not taught what foods to eat, or we are influenced by food faddism, we may acquire a diet or eating patterns that are detrimental to health. The diet or eating patterns would still be the consummatory response, but the goal desired would not be achieved. Still another example is the person who fears that a lump may be cancerous but delays proper medical attention, thus failing to achieve that which is desired most: early treatment and cure. The consummatory response as it relates to health behavior should be one that represents the most desirable outcome for the individual and society. This process is illustrated in Figure 8–5.

Motivation and learning

Authorities generally agree that motivation accomplishes two chief results: (1) it provides the energy necessary for action to occur and be sustained, and (2) it determines the direction that behavior will take. As a result of our previous discussions, we can conclude that one of the chief purposes of motivation is to make learning possible. An individual, therefore, is guided through learning by the presence of a motive. Without it there is no perceived need to learn, and indeed, there will be no significant learning.

Knowledge of the cause and effect of motivation as well as the methods for motivating the learner is important to the health educator. This knowledge, when appropriately applied, can guide the teacher in providing the most rewarding learning experiences for students. Let us now summarize the relationship of motivation to the learning process:

- Learning can be motivated by a change in the sensory (learning) environment.
- Since motives determine the direction of behavior, they change one's relationship with the environment.
- The quality and quantity of learning is related to the strength of motivation.
- As motivation intensity increases, learning efficiency improves.

FIGURE 8–5   The Consummatory Response

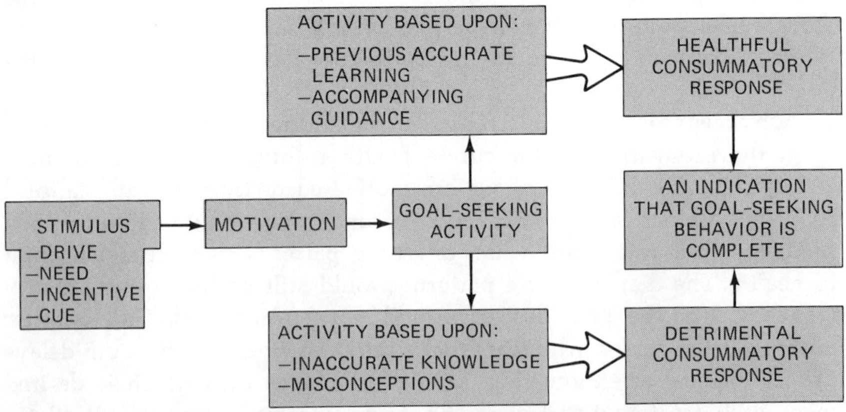

- Excessive motivation that results in anxiety or fear of failure can interfere with learning success.
- The speed with which one learns is frequently a criterion of the strength of motivation.
- Knowledge that one is learning may provide sufficient motivation.
- The influence of praise or punishment may carry from one type of performance to another. Success establishes a behavioral pattern which may be resorted to in future encounters and, in some instances, may become the generalized modus operandi.
- The use of punishment as a motivator may merely teach the learner how to avoid the punishment rather than how to achieve the goal.
- Forgetting, like learning, can be motivated. One generally remembers better those tasks that are not completed than those that have been completed. One explanation of this is that completed tasks are forgotten because the motivation was satisfied.
- Motivation is a relatively temporary factor affecting behavior. Its endurance and intensity are related to such things as the immediacy of the goal and its attainment.
- What will motivate learning in one individual may have little or no effect on another.

Results of motivation

For the most part, tissue needs can be adequately met through a basic understanding of health information and its application to life. However, many psychosocial needs can be met only through a rather profound understanding of self and others. This understanding will result only from direct involvement in meaningful learning experiences. Let us return for a moment to Figure 8–3. We note that at the biological level, physical health status can be maintained providing the biogenic needs are adequately satisfied. But at the interpretive level, innate potentials are allowed to develop, giving rise to optimal development. In both cases, health decisions are essential. For example, the hunger drive can be satisfied by the ingestion of food, but health maintenance is dependent upon the ingestion of foods necessary for energy, growth, repair of tissues, etc. Knowledge of the kinds of foods to eat and the daily amounts needed becomes essential for promoting and maintaining health.

Similarly, healthful behavior is essential for full psychosocial actualization. Individuals need to understand not only their potentials but also their limitations. Through appropriate learning experiences, an individual will become more aware of self and others, which can result in improved interpersonal relations. Health knowledge is therefore essential and fundamental at both the biological and interpretive levels for health decision-making. The maintenance of health and the actualization of potentials is the culmination of motivation for health learning.

MOTIVATION APPLIED
TO HEALTH EDUCATION

Positive vs negative approaches

Health learning takes place best when the health issues being considered are relevant and perceived by the student as personally important. In addition, the learning environment, methodologies, and learning aids being used should be consistent with previous similar learning situations, and appropriate for the developmental level of the learner. A learning experience (activity) should be initiated only after proper motivation is established. A student who is motivated is *ready to learn;* that is, a psychological set has been instituted. Readiness to learn is as important to learning success as the provision of an adequate learning environment (setting). If either the set or setting is lacking or inappropriate, learning potential is greatly reduced and very little, if any, learning will occur. Blair, et al. emphasized the importance of these factors when they stated that "coming to grips with this problem of motivation means learning how to direct appropriately the great energies of which the individual is capable. It is a first step, and perhaps the most important one in being able to control our own behavior and to teach others."[8]

Negative approaches in health education that emphasize disease rather than health, and which dictate the dos and don'ts of healthful living should be avoided since they tend to cause anxiety and stress which frequently results in demotivation for learning. The dos and don'ts of health should be student discoveries, conclusions they draw from involvement in motivated learning activities. Stressing pathological aspects of health could arouse latent hypochondriacal tendencies in some students. This may be interpreted by the teacher as a wholesome interest in the topic. A preoccupation with diseases, their symptoms, etc. should be avoided. More desirable outcomes can be achieved when the attainment of positive health is emphasized and disease, as such, is dealt with in proper perspective. Therefore, motivation should be consistent with the achievement of the goal. If the goal is to establish positive health behavior, interest in disease should not be used as the motivation.

Motivational techniques that will arouse the individual's personal desire to behave more healthfully should be used. Disease orientation should be left to the field of therapeutics. Alternative forms of behavior to such activities as drug abuse, including cigarette smoking and excessive use of alcohol, should establish the major basis of motivation in health learning. These alternatives in actuality can generate excitement, self-interest, and a desire to be healthy. Moreover, they can begin to dispel fallacious attitudes about behavior such as the belief that cigarette smoking is a sign of adulthood. Conversely, students should learn that adulthood is more appropriately characterized by responsible behavior which contributes to the betterment of self and society.

Motivational techniques that are associated with the individual's need to achieve the goal are most intense. Teachers sometimes perceive their needs (educational goals) as being equally important to students. Student needs are often quite different from those of the teacher. Positive alterations in student health behavior can not be adequately affected by systems of educational indoctrination nor by artificially established goals. In this regard, the teacher must recognize the individuality of students. What may motivate learning in one student may have little or no effect on another.

Although basic human needs are not unique to each individual, motivation for satisfaction can be. Similarly, the technique used by one person to adequately satisfy a need may be quite different from another's. This concept is supportive of the trend in education to concentrate more on individualization of learning rather than packaged learning for all.

To add to this extremely complex educational phenomenon, health educators must be cognizant of the existence of conflicting motivation. Students may be highly motivated to acquire health knowledge and greater insight into themselves but fear the consequences of peer rejection from such an achievement. One may be hungry and motivated to satisfy this hunger appropriately, but be influenced more strongly by the urge to satisfy immediate taste pleasures. The need to fulfill emotional pleasures may overshadow knowledge and logic.

Motives are dynamic. They may have an intellectual, emotional, social, or biological basis, or any combination of these. One may take precedence over the others in spite of the consequences and the individual's knowledge of them. To emphasize only the intellectual aspect of health education is to invite failure in actually improving health behavior and health status.

In health education, the achievement of one goal should lead to the formation of new ones. This is the basic principle that distinguishes inductive learning from deductive learning. Essentially, inductive learning involves the problem-solving approach. It is progression from the specific to the general. This will be discussed in more detail in Chapter 12.

Cue function

As children begin to mature, they soon recognize certain signs in the environment that provide clues to the ways in which they should react. Children's actions are either praised or punished; these consequences supply some indication of how they should behave in future encounters. As a resurt, these environmental stimuli may act as cues to behavior when they occur. As was stated earlier, motivation is the reason for action, but it also provides the direction the action should take. Whenever motivation possesses this direction, it is said to provide a *cue function*. Cue function is *the element of motivation that provides signs or signals indicating the direction behavior must take to satisfy the need or to achieve the goal.* For instance, the odor of cooking food may stimulate the desire to satisfy the hunger drive and, at the same time, provide a clue as to the location of the food.

Motivation for health learning should stimulate the desire to act (interest in the learning experience) as well as providing a cue function. The cue function in this regard would indicate how health learning could best take place. The cue function may, for example, be the methodology to be used. The student may infer the course of action from previous and similar experiences, or the teacher (or some other source) may provide specific instructions regarding the course of action to be taken. When students' responses to the motive result in a reduction of the need for goal achievement, they perceive the form of behavior used as adequate. When similar feelings (needs) arise, the student is likely to resort to the same kind of behavior. The need reduction acts as a reinforcement for the action, while the presence of the need is the cue. The need and action together constitute the cue function.

DEFINITIVE UNDERSTANDINGS

A motive is an internal source of energy that directs the individual toward the achievement of a predetermined goal; it is the causation of behavior. A drive is a motive. The origin of motives may be either biogenic or sociogenic. The biogenic motives are associated with tissue needs while the sociogenic motives are associated with psychosocial needs.

Homeostasis, the tendency to maintain a chemical and psychological equilibrium, acts as a motivating force. This tendency operates at the biological and interpretive levels. The biological level is associated with survival and the maintenance of health through a satisfaction of tissue needs. The interpretive level is associated with learned behavior that is directed toward the actualization of individual potentials. When homeostasis is complete, it is likely that optimal health status will be reached. An interference with homeostasis results in less than optimal functioning of the individual and, if extreme, disease or death may result.

There are a variety of factors that motivate an individual. Some of these factors are in themselves motives. The most important motive affecting learning is a conscious intent to learn. Learning takes place best when people want to learn, when the learning experience is consistent with their developmental level, and when the goal is perceived as relevant and achievable.

Rewards and punishments can act as reinforcers of learning. Rewards are more powerful incentives than punishments. They are more effective if they are real rather than artificial. The use of punishment as an incentive may result in behavior that is directed toward avoidance of the punishment rather than achievement of the goal. Reward and punishment should be used primarily to increase the rate of learning; they should not be used as the goal.

Psychological feedback is an evaluative technique that keeps students continuously informed of the success of their learning. A person who is receiving psychological feedback will learn more rapidly and thoroughly than one who is not. Psychological feedback can be a powerful incentive to learning.

An incentive is an external factor that activates motivation. It is effective only to the extent that the learner is familiar with it and understands its consequences if obtained. Positive incentives are more desirable than negative ones. They tend to result in constructive forms of behavior; negative ones tend to result in avoidance behavior.

Motivation may be either intrinsic or extrinsic. The intrinsic motives are those internal sources of energy that direct one toward a specific goal. They are true motives related to both innate and acquired needs. Intrinsic motivation is associated with biological and psychological survival. The way in which the goal is achieved is learned and, as such, is closely associated with the development of health behavior. Health behavior is related to human adaptability and human energetics. It is a manifestation of the presence of a motive. The extrinsic motives are essentially external stimuli; they are incentives.

Recognition, interpretation, value structure, knowledge, capabilities, perceptiveness, and past experiences influence how well the stimulus will bring about motivation. The stimulus must be internalized. Internalization takes place when an individual perceives the significance of the health issue; is interested in some phase of the health issue, and is willing to apply the new health learning to affect a change in health behavior regarding self or society (P–I–S–A). Consistency, social attitudes, opportunities to respond, and a sense of pleasure affect the intensity or success of motivation to alter behavior.

The change in behavior resulting from motivated learning is called the consummatory response. The kind of food one eats, for instance, is the consummatory response. It results from previous learning experience about foods. It is important to recognize that a consummatory response can be based upon inappropriate experiences or inaccurate information. The development of health misconceptions may result in a consummatory response that is detrimental to health.

The quality and intensity of motivation affect health learning by providing the needed energy and direction that learning requires. The health educator can improve learning through an appreciation of the factors that motivate the learning process. Learning experiences will be effective if proper motivation has been achieved. A motivated student is ready to learn; therefore, opportunities for this learning should be made available. These two factors constitute both a set and a setting for learning. Motivation is seldom pure, however. Frequently, conflicting motives may be present which interfere with the new learning experience.

External environmental stimuli may trigger a form of behavior previously learned. The stimulus accompanied by the behavior is called a cue function. A cue function may be valuable to the health educator by bringing about new learning through application of the cue.

PROBLEMS
FOR DISCUSSION

1. Describe how motives are related to human needs and drives.
2. Distinguish between biogenic and sociogenic motives. Which are essentially innate and which are essentially learned?
3. Knowing that the origin of motives is biogenic or sociogenic, describe several ways that individuals may behave to achieve goals associated with each.
4. Distinguish between the biological and interpretative levels of homeostasis.
   a. Do both have application for health learning? Explain.
   b. Describe how health learning at both levels affects the quality of one's health decisions.
   c. How can a knowledge of human homeostasis influence techniques of motivating health learning?
   d. Which level is dependent primarily upon attitudinal change or development? Explain why.
5. Describe the relationship between incentives and motivation.
6. List, in order of importance, five factors that will bring about learning.
7. Describe how psychological feedback during a learning experience can help sustain motivation.
8. Distinguish between extrinsic and intrinsic motivation.
   a. Which one will influence the rate as well as the quality of learning most? Explain.
   b. Intrinsic motivation is true motivation. Explain.
   c. Describe what must be present to make extrinsic motivation effective.
   d. List two forms of intrinsic motivation and two forms of extrinsic motivation.
9. List the processes necessary for incentives to become internalized.
10. Relate internalization of incentives to motivation. Discuss the factors that influence the process.
11. Motives affect behavior during goal-seeking and following goal achievement. Explain these processes and how they are significant to learning and the resultant health behavior.
12. Describe the two factors that make health behavior possible.
13. Distinguish between a cue function and a consummatory response. How are they related?
14. Describe how motivation affects learning. How can it interfere with learning?
15. Identify a health goal. Describe the techniques that can be used to motivate students to achieve this goal.
    a. What fundamental factors related to the students must be taken into consideration?
    b. What factors related to the goal must be considered?

16. Explain why negative approaches to health learning and motivation should be avoided.

REFERENCES

1. Coleman, James C., *Abnormal Psychology and Modern Life*, 3d ed., Scott, Foresman and Company, Chicago, 1964, p. 70.
2. Knutson, Andie L., *The Individual, Society, and Health Behavior*, Russell Sage Foundation, New York, 1965, p. 203.
3. Ruch, Floyd L., *Psychology and Life*, 7th ed., Scott, Foresman and Company, Chicago, 1967, p. 221.
4. Knutson, op. cit., p. 212.
5. Ruch, op. cit., p. 375.
6. Ibid., p. 223.
7. Skinner, B. F., *About Behaviorism*, Alfred A. Knopf, New York, 1974, p. 165.
8. Blair, Glenn Meyers, R. Stewart Jones, and Ray H. Simpson, *Educational Psychology*, 3d ed., Macmillan Publishing Co., New York, p. 166.

Part Three

The School/
Community
Health
Education
Program

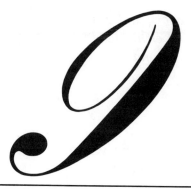

Professional
Preparation
of the Health
Educator

*Health education theory and practice
must change . . . and either lead
the way or be left behind.*

Howard S. Hoyman

University officials must be willing
to take bold actions in order to
achieve bold results in the
professional preparation of the
health educator. This will result in an
impact on America's health care
system never before experienced.

AEB
DAB

WHO IS A HEALTH EDUCATOR?

Introduction

Is there more than one kind of health educator? Although health education as a recognized discipline is still in its infancy, there have emerged three basic types of health educators. Currently we see them functioning within the health care system (and sometimes outside the health care system) in separate and sometimes autonomous professions. There is some evidence, however, of a gradual movement toward a single profession with three major spheres of concentration. This movement is encouraging since it will bring us closer to the establishment of comprehensive and coordinated health education programs. Hoyman aptly pointed out the urgency of this change when he stated that "the results of our asinine splintering of health education into community and school sectors is a grim reminder of the dangers of separation in public health."[1] With the coming of the patient health educator, we need to be even more cautious that this profession too is not isolated.

In one sense , everyone is a health educator—parents, siblings, peers, relatives, etc. Despite the fact that the quality of health education from these sources is too frequently of questionable quality, we need to recognize that health education of one kind or another can and does happen in a variety of settings and through the influences of the various media forms. These modes of acquiring health information, regardless of their haphazard manner, do have significant impact on the health attitudes and behavior of people. One needs only to point to the numerous health misconceptions communicated daily through television advertisements. In some (perhaps many) instances, this is the only significant health education some may receive. Consequently, it has become imperative for children, youth, and adults to be exposed to health information that is accurate and relevant. This can take place only with the guidance of those who are adequately trained in health matters in an environmental setting that is conductive to health learning.

There have evolved over the years three kinds of health educators: (1) the school health educator, (2) the community or public health educator, and (3) the patient or clinical health educator, who has appeared only within the past few years. In many respects, the training and the approaches each may use are similar, but they each possess a functional uniqueness. Certainly, modes of functioning are founded upon identical philosophical principles. They are distinguished chiefly by the nature of the learning environment in which they must practice and by the nature of the learners with whom they are concerned.

The most significant similarity of the three health educators, regardless of their labels, is that they are all attempting to improve health through the use of the educational process. Their approaches must by necessity, however, be quite distinct, since their students' needs and goals will vary. For instance, the clinical health educator deals primarily with patients recovering from a disease, while the school health educator is concerned with those who are essentially well. The community health educator must be concerned with the general population which represents all levels of socioeconomic and health status. Figure 9–1 illustrates the relationship between the three types of health educators. It becomes apparent that if health education is to be effective, there must be a continuing cooperation and interaction between all who are concerned with the health of people. This includes those employed in the treatment and rehabilitation realm as well as in all other areas of the health care system.

FIGURE 9–1   The Relationship of the Three Types of Health Educators
Although each type of health educator is responsible to a particular group of people, they should interact and reinforce each other's efforts for greatest effectiveness.

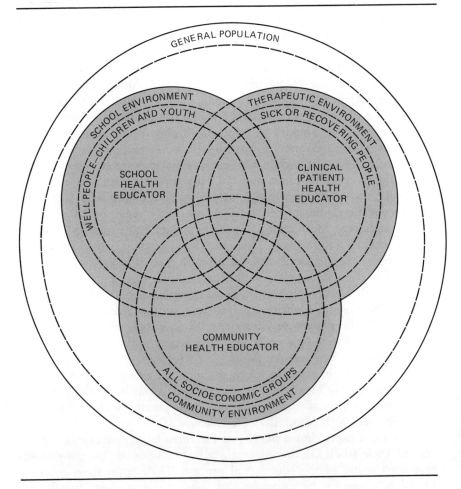

The school health educator

During the early 1960s, health educators, school administrators, school boards of education, parent groups, the medical and dental professions, and state departments of education, along with other groups, were awakened to the need to reevaluate the practices taking place in school health education. Some of the questions being asked were:

1. How effective are teachers of health education in actually improving the health knowledge, attitudes, and behavior of children?
2. How effective are health education methodologies, techniques, strategies and learning aids?
3. How effective is the design of the health curriculum? What changes must be made?
4. How effective is the informational content of the health program in promoting health and preventing disease or other health problems?
5. What priority should health education have in the school's educational program?
6. What are the health needs of children and society?
7. How can the health needs of children and society best be met?

It was not until the late 1960s that these concerns began to be reflected in state laws and subsequently in teacher training programs at both the school and university levels.

The school health educator assumes a great deal of responsibility for contributing positively to the health and well-being of the developing child. The school health education program is directed toward primary prevention of ill health through the promotion of growth and development. This can best be achieved through viable comprehensive health education programs conducted by teachers who are adequately prepared in the health sciences and the educational process. This concept has been reiterated often by a variety of organizations concerned with school health. The following resolution by the American Nurses' Association as adopted in 1974 is typical of current thought regarding the need for comprehensive health education programs:

Whereas, Each school-aged child and adolescent in the United States should have the opportunity to develop his/her potential to the fullest; and

Whereas, Education for personal health and health citizenship assists the individual to make his/her maximum contribution to the welfare of his/her community and country; and

Whereas, Advances in health sciences can only be utilized when people are properly informed about them; and

Whereas, In many schools, health education programs are fragmented and crisis oriented to meet a current need, as veneral disease, drug abuse, etc., therefore, be it

Resolved, That the American Nurses' Association promote and support a unified, integrated, sequential approach for comprehensive school health education program, grades K through 12; and be it

Resolved, That ANA promote and support health education programs as a basic segment of college curriculum, and be it further

Resolved, That ANA, state and local nurses' associations work cooperatively with the NEA and other appropriate educational officials and agencies and representatives of federal, state and local governments to secure legislation and funding for school health education programs.[2]

The public health educator

The public (community) health educator traditionally has had the awesome responsibility of developing health education programs for the community at large, for people with varying degrees of health status, representing a myriad of sociocultural backgrounds, all of which must be taken into consideration in the process of planning and conducting community health education programs.

Community health educators are typically employed by either governmental or voluntary health agencies. It is quite common for governmental agencies to require the public health educator to possess a graduate degree (M.P.H. or Dr.P.H.) from a school of public health that has been accredited by the American Public Health Association. These requirements, in addition to the lack of emphasis placed upon health education in most schools of public health and in the health agencies themselves, have contributed to a disproportionately low number of health educators in the field of public health. As Milio points out, of the more than four million health workers in the United States, "those personnel whose task emphasis is counseling and education of ill or healthy consumers comprise the smallest proportion, less than 5 percent. . . . These include social workers, health educators, and dieticians."[3] This is a grim reminder of the emphasis placed upon treatment of disease while the promotion of health is virtually ignored. Such an emphasis only contributes to the argument that in modern idustrialized nations the citizens "are presumed sick until proven healthy."[4]

Many public health agencies also employ as community health educators those who have been trained as school health educators. This practice may have long-term benefits in that a person trained in school health and working in the community sector can facilitate the coordination of effort between school and community which is so urgently needed. In addition, many public health agencies will provide on-the-job training for those not adequately prepared or they may subsidize graduate training for their employees.

In the past, it was quite common for a community health educator to do little more than develop pamphlets describing the available services of a particular agency or describing the ramifications of various health problems. Little direct contact was made with the public. It is now becoming common practice for community health educators to have direct interaction with the public through more elaborate health education programs. There are at least two problems however, that become apparent: (1) Community health educators do not receive, as a rule, in-depth training in educational theory and methodology; and (2) There is little coordination between the health education programs of the various health agencies, resulting in a fragmentation of community effort.

Community health educators need to receive better preparation in educational theory and methodology as part of their preservice training. They do receive adequate training, for instance, in epidemiology and in the functioning of the health care system, but surprisingly little in how to apply health principles to a community setting beyond adapting programs to the value system of a given culture. As the health education profession becomes less and less fragmented, those traditionally trained as community health educators must become more educationally oriented—a change that necessitates revisions in the community health education training programs. The evolution of the various segments of health education into three closely related realms is shown in Figure 9–2.

Community health educators, representing a variety of health agencies, continue to function rather independently of each other. This has resulted in a duplication of effort in many instances. Means are being developed, however, to aid in the resolution of this problem; this will be discussed later in more detail when we discuss the functions of the health administrator.

The patient (clinical) health educator

The most significant development recently in health education is the introduction of the patient or clinical health educator. These professional health educators focus primarily on patients and their families to facilitate recovery from a disease or disability and to minimize the likelihood of a recurrence of the same or related health problems in the future. The appearance of the patient health educator signals a shift of emphasis from a complete reliance on treatment to a recognition of the importance of prevention. The patient health educator is an essential addition to the health team for individuals who fall within the intermediate and secondary levels of health status as described in Chapter 2.

In a broader sense, the patient health educator serves as a consumer advocate. Conant described this function when he wrote:

> The health care system needs reorganization. Health educators should see themselves as a catalyst in changing this system as they function with and on behalf of the patient and the community. His job is to help assure that whatever system evolves will function in accordance with consumer expectations and be accountable on that basis.[5]

FIGURE 9–2 The Evolution of the Health Education Profession
Traditionally, the three types of health educators have functioned independently of each
other—as indicated by the outer circle in the diagram. There is evidence, however, that
they are evolving into interacting segments of a single profession—as indicated by the
inner circle.

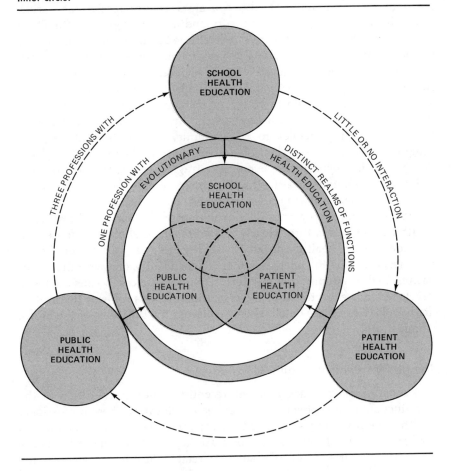

More specifically, patient health education is designed to meet several
objectives aimed not only at aiding the patient in the recovery process,
but also at improving the efficiency of the health care system. These
objectives are: (1) more accurate knowledge of patient problems, interests, and attitudes; (2) improved communication between all those
individuals and agencies concerned with patient care; and (3) improved
patient care as expressed by patients' ability to help control their illness.

The advent of the clinical health educator as a new component of
the health education profession is exciting because they will function
in close proximity to those who are involved in treatment. This will

provide a necessary vehicle for the promotion of the health education profession within the boundaries of a therapeutically oriented health care system. Furthermore, it can add the ingredient so long ignored by the medical profession—helping patients to understand more fully the nature and consequences of their illness and what to do about it.

This new profession also creates challenges for those who are directing the professional preparation of health educators in general. It seems clear that clinical health educators are in the mainstream of the health care system. They will eventually be the individuals who will make programs for prevention of disease and maintenance of a health-oriented health care system work. To this end, the clinical health educator should be trained along with other health professionals—medical, dental, nursing, and allied health personnel[7]—and should receive the same in-depth educational training as the school and community health educator. The health education center concept to be discussed later in this chapter provides a logical arena within which such training can effectively take place.

Certainly the clinical health educator should not replace anyone within the health care system, nor should any educational responsibilities be relinquished by other health professionals. As Zimmering and McTernan point out,

> the health educator joins the [health care] team to bring the previously lacking expertise which leads to positive behavioral changes on the part of the patient, and to increase the effectiveness of the professional-patient interaction. Thus, although the clinical health educator will directly plan, supervise, and perhaps conduct a wide variety of educational programs aimed directly at the patient (or potential patient), his family, and other consumers; perhaps one of the most important roles of the new professional will be to assist the other members of the team in understanding, enhancing, and improving the effectiveness of their own roles as educators —as well as therapists.[8]

HEALTH EDUCATION TRAINING PROGRAMS

What constitutes professionalism?

One of the major problems confronting the health education profession is unification around a particular, acceptable set of standards that explicitly governs the functioning of the profession—standards for the training of health educators, standards of professional ethics, standards of practice, standards of definitions, and standards of goals and philosophy. Professionalism can be defined as "the methods, manner, or spirit of a profession."[9] Although attempts have been made by a number of individuals and organizations in recent years, the establishment of accepted standards of professionalism does not as yet exist for health education. What has evolved is that the field of health education continues to be divided into a variety of factions separated by variances in philosophy, quality of training, and modes of practice.

Possibly one of the major factors stifling the growth of health education as a profession has been the frightfully slow development of activities in the political arena by both individuals and professional health organizations. Politics is used here in the broadest sense to include activities influencing legislation and participation in the development of health educaton programs supported by state and local departments of education and health. Professional health organizations need to further develop a political awareness and astuteness among their membership. They need to accept unconditionally the leadership responsibility that is theirs since only the health education profession possesses the expertise for this leadership. Neither legislators nor state departments of education should be relied upon to provide the high quality of guidance and direction so desperately needed without advice and counsel from the professional organizations. They simply do not possess the understanding or experience to make appropriate judgments about health education professional practices. This has been convincingly evident over the decades.

An excellent case in point is the failure of the profession to provide guidance and leadership for those states allowing certification of school health educators possessing only a minor in health education, or health education certification through the use of proficiency examinations. Such practices are indictments of both the profession for allowing it to happen and of the state departments of education for imposing them. Such practices do little to improve the standards of the profession. Haro justly expressed great concern when he so strongly argued, "Why does the profession of health education—if indeed it is a profession—stand idly by and let "proficiency health educators" and "minor health educators" . . . usurp the potential job market from the most qualified and interested of the profession's potential product."[10]

The concept of professionalism, indeed, does extend to setting standards for professional training. These standards must come from within the profession rather than being imposed by those outside the profession. Health education is just beginning to reach an evolutionary level that will allow for internal governance of professional training and practice standards that will result in increased professionalism for those claiming to be health educators. It behooves the professional health organizations to become the vehicle for establishing acceptable professional standards. Historically, the major difficulty has been the lack of a single national organization to speak for health educators as a group. There is an urgent and critical need for a national organization devoted *solely* to the requirements of the entire health education profession; one which can concentrate on promoting effective health education legislation, developing a canon of professional ethics, establishing standards for accreditation of institutions training health educators, and disseminating pertinent information to its members. Until such an organization exists, the attainment of true professionalism in the field of health education will continue to be retarded.

Universal standards

Closely related to the concept of the establishment of a national association devoted solely to the promotion of health education professionalism is the founding of universal standards for professional preparation. There currently exist national standards as set forth by the American Public Health Association for the accreditation of community health educators, and a growing number of states have established standards for the accreditation of training programs for school health educators. There remains, however, a large divergence in standards from institution to institution and from state to state as far as required course content and field work experiences, types of required student teaching experiences, faculty preparation, library holdings, etc., which has resulted in health educators being graduated with a variety of functioning abilities (competencies) in the community and school settings. Moreover, nearly no training standards have been established at either the state or national levels with regard to patient health educators.

As with the resolution of the American Nurses' Association cited earlier, there have been similar resolutions regarding professional preparation in health education. A typical one was adopted (1970) by the NEA–AMA Joint Committee on Health Problems in Education as follows:

> Whereas, Major health problems affecting this country have placed renewed emphasis on health education, and
> Whereas, Effective personal and group action are enhanced by precise knowledge, positive attitudes and practices, and
> Whereas, All elementary and secondary teachers and administrators share responsibility with parents and medical advisors for the health education of students, and
> Whereas, The Joint Committee has frequently expressed its support of effective health education in schools supported by sound teacher preparation since 1911; therefore be it
> Resolved, That the Committee reaffirm its resolutions urging a sound sequential health education program, for grades kindergarten through 12, and be it further
> Resolved, That all prospective teachers and administrators be required to participate in professional courses of health education in order to qualify for certification recommendation, and be it further
> Resolved, That in-service training programs be offered in the various school districts to supplement and update the education of teachers and administrators currently in the profession.[77]

Such resolutions, although positive in their recognition of the need for high standards of professional preparation and programmatic organization, are of little benefit to the profession unless adopted into law by the various state legislatures. The health education profession has been only minimally successful in the attainment of these ends.

What is needed are professional standards recognized by the profession as a whole, which if not met by individuals or institutions will risk having sanctions placed upon them by the profession itself in the form of nonsupport and/or nonrecognition as a qualified health educator or qualified health education training institution. This is closely akin to the previous discussion on professionalism and must be pursued if high standards are to be attained and professionalism promoted.

Current role of colleges

Since there are no universal standards that guide the professional training of health educators in the United States, each state establishes certain minimal criteria and each training institution decides for itself how far it will go in excess of these criteria. This is especially true in regard to health education programs at the undergraduate level. At the graduate level the training standards tend to be more uniform, especially in the area of community health education where such standards have been adopted by the profession and, in many instances, incorporated into law by state governments.

The lack of consistency in standards at the undergraduate level is alarming. In some states, for instance, a major is required in health education for teacher certification, while in other states certification is granted with a major in another discipline with perhaps only one or two health courses being required for certification in health education. It is heartening to note that most states that have enacted health education mandates do require a major in health education for certification.

It has become the norm at the undergraduate level in those institutions offering a health education major to provide students with the option of majoring in school health or community health. Until very recently, the differences in such options tended to be quite profound. The trend is to make content courses for each option as similar as possible with the basic difference being a community health practicum for the community health option and student teaching for the school health option.

Some colleges have even gone one step further in offering a combined major in which a student would receive both practicum experience in the community and student teaching experience in the school. This aids both the student and the college by making the student with such a major more marketable. In addition, such an opportunity conforms more closely with current health education philosophy as to the interrelationship between the various types of health educators.

One of the most pressing problems confronting colleges today in the area of professional preparation is their role in the training of the patient health educator. Several questions in this area are currently being grappled with:

1. What types of special learning experiences are required to qualify one to be a patient health educator?
2. Are schools of public health or those traditionally emphasizing school health best equipped to train patient health educators?
3. Should states or the health education profession establish minimum standards for the licensure of patient health educators?
4. Should patient health educators be more highly trained than the typical school or community health educator? If so, in what respect?
5. Which agency is sufficiently qualified to rule on the accreditation of patient health education training programs?
6. Should training be essentially pathological or health oriented or a balance between the two?
7. How can the educational principles be altered to apply to the one-to-one ratio practiced by the patient health educator?
8. What principles of training for the social worker and psychologist should be applied to the patient health educator?

The need for change

Significant changes in the way that training programs are conducted is indicated to establish the quality of health education programs that are so desperately needed. Mere modification of current course content or course offerings will have little effect on improving the quality of health educators. The commonalities between the various types of health educators far outweigh their differences. They should be trained with this in mind, while respecting their differences and magnifying their similarities.

The health education center concept and the competency-based teacher education concept, although still in their experimental stages, hold the promise of a future with a greatly improved health education professional training model. There is probably no one solution to this problem, but we know it will not come by reordering past deficiencies.

RECENT INNOVATIONS

Establishing new criteria

The trend in American education toward an emphasis on behavioral objectives has led educational leaders to search for a means of demonstrating the worth of education in general as a mainstay of society. The development of competency-based teacher education (CBTE) is one means of demonstrating accountability and has been sweeping across the country in very recent years. Since we need to begin to think of new ways to prepare professional health educators and more importantly, to devise new ways of evaluating their potential for success, the establishment of competency-based teacher education may provide us with the means for achieving these ends. Gone are the days when we could take comfort in a student passing a few content courses and serving a practicum for a few weeks and being called a qualified health educator. New criteria for professional preparation that take into account recent technological advances in society, the current philosophy of health education, and the future importance it will have within the national health care system must be established. This is beginning to happen in many colleges and state education departments.

Figure 9–3 illustrates in simplified form the relationship of training criteria to the implementation of professional education experiences. The learning experiences provided by the college for the potential health educator are determined by the criteria established. These experiences are not limited only to the college setting, but may very well extent into hospitals, research centers, and other related health settings. Students in the future will not be restricted to exposure only to the instructors present on campuses. On the contrary, they will most likely, through media, visitations, and field work, obtain the benefits of some of the most prestigious authorities in the health sciences. Health education students will be recognized as professional health educators only when they demonstrate capabilities to function in accordance with the established criteria for basic competencies.

Competencies of health educators

Despite the noted differences of each of the three areas of health education, there are basic competencies common to all. In general terms, they may be expressed as those associated with (1) a profound knowledge and comprehension of all health matters affecting individuals and society, (2) a demonstrated possession of positive attitudes (feelings, values, and emotions) connected with all health issues, (3) a motivation to act and react healthfully, (4) a demonstrated dedication to the welfare of people, and (5) an ability to apply what is known about health to the improvement of the health of people.

More specifically, the qualified, professional health educator must be able to demonstrate proficiency in the following ways*:

- Identifies patterns of normal human growth and development related to biological, sociological, intellectual, and psychological patterns.
- Applies knowledge of human growth and development to the planning of appropriate learning experiences that will meet the specific and/or special needs of the learner.
- Provides effective motivation for learning related to the planned educational experience.

---

* These competencies are adapted from those developed by the Department of Health Education, York College, City University of New York, 1976.

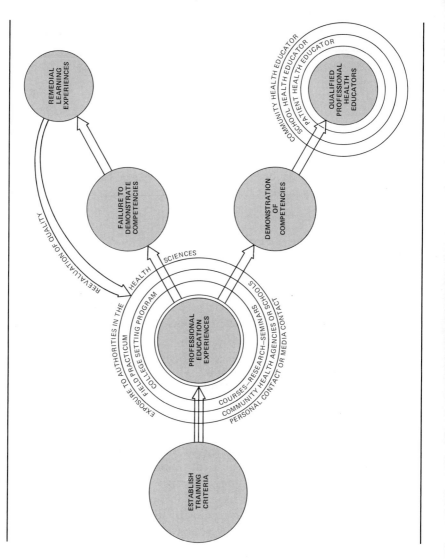

FIGURE 9–3 The Relationship of Training Criteria to the Professional Preparation Program Professional education experiences for the health educator must be associated with the achievement of predetermined competencies. When this happens, health educators will be better qualified to assume their professional responsibilities.

- Demonstrates knowledge of, attitudes toward, and skills in interpersonal relations with a variety of people.
- Demonstrates skill in assisting the learner in analyzing and synthesizing facts regarding health issues.
- Provides health learning experiences consistent with the·learner's needs and concerns, abilities and experiential background, and in accord with available learning resources and environmental constraints.
- Provides an educational environment that will motivate learning.
- Recognizes the need and makes provision for a variety of learning experiences to meet the needs of individual learners.
- Makes use of a variety of evaluative procedures and techniques to determine learner progress and to alter the learning process in accordance with the data obtained.
- Evaluates the usability of learning aids and selects those which are most appropriate to assist the learner in achieving the predetermined goals.
- Recognizes the value of achieving short-term goals as a step toward achieving long-term goals and provides for learning experiences accordingly.
- Is functionally familiar with the principles of learning and uses approaches for health learning that have been shown to be sound.
- Participates in school/community health planning and implementation meetings and discussions.
- Demonstrates the ability to plan effective health education programs for the intended learner.
- Describes the similarities and differences associated with school, community, and patient health education.
- Demonstrates responsible behavior within the limitations of laws and regulations governing health education.
- Demonstrates an understanding of the importance of health education for parents and other adults, as well as for children and youth.
- Applies personal and professional ethical conduct in all matters concerned with the health and education of people.
- Identifies and uses appropriately the varieties of community health resources, both material and human.
- Seeks continuous professional growth.
- Demonstrates a sensitivity for the health, safety, and general welfare of the learner.
- Actively participates in professional organizations for the improvement of the health education profession and recognizes values in regard to the ultimate health of people.

What is competency-based teacher education (CBTE)? Competency-based teacher education is a relatively new educational reorganization designed to promote accountability within the education profession. The basic premise behind the concept is that a potential teacher must demonstrate proficiency in numerous established competencies in order to become certified, rather than merely receiving passing grades in a set number of courses. With CBTE, the need for distinct courses, in the traditional sense, is eliminated or greatly reduced; they are replaced by a program leading to the attainment of competencies on a more or less individualized basis. Such an evolution, however, will be extremely slow in becoming reality. Presently, program changes have typically amounted to nothing more than a reorganization on paper of the existing course structure.

At the risk of oversimplifying a very complex educational change, we can define CBTE as predetermined criteria-referenced educational experiences designed for the development of a variety of functional abilities and skills to assist learners in most efficiently becoming health educated. Essentially, the criteria that are formulated are associated with training health educators in such a way that there is some guarantee that they can and will facilitate the achievement of learner objectives when called upon to do so as professionals. Such a process of teacher training recognizes the application of professional practices, rather than simply the demonstration of academic or intellectual skills, as the important outcome of the training program.

Most educators would not argue with the philosophy behind CBTE: Educators should be able to demonstrate competency in their given areas of specialty. Although the concept has been abused, as has been the case with many significant educational innovations, the establishment of teacher competencies in health education should not be viewed negatively. The development of health education competencies could have a very positive result, facilitating a unification of the total educational process.

A NEW LOOK AT AN OLD PROBLEM

The quality of training of secondary school health educators

The quality of the training of secondary school health educators has always been questionable. There are still many states that certify school health educators with very little health course work required. In those states that have, in recent years, increased the requirements for health certification, there is a problem of finding enough qualified health educators to fill the potential available positions. Two measures have been employed to overcome this deficit: (1) retraining teachers for health education who are already certified to teach in another subject area, and (2) administering proficiency examinations that, if passed, will at least partially fulfill certification requirements. In some cases, these examinations fulfill certification requirements in their entirety. This is true, for example, in New York State, where a battery of three examinations have been developed. Each will provide twelve college credit hours toward New York State certification in health education. New York State currently requires 36 credit hours in the health sciences for certification, in addition to the 12 credit hours in the educational courses and student teaching practicum. Anyone possessing a baccalaureate degree that passes all three of the examinations may be awarded 36 credit hours in health sciences for provisional certification in health education.

Both of these measures should be considered stop-gap approaches insuring that minimum state mandate requirements are met. If they are utilized as a means to fulfilling certification requirements, many problems can result. Some of these problems are:

- Graduates of formal training programs may be denied access to the job market because of the existence of an ample supply of less trained and less qualified people. Program quality will suffer as a result and children will be penalized by being deprived of the health education that is their right.
- As a result of the administrative desire to comply with state mandates and the need to minimize school district expenditures, teachers already on the staff may be required to become certified in order to retain their teaching position even though they may have little or no interest in teaching health education. Again, program quality suffers, children suffer, and in the long run, society suffers when a person who lacks interest and dedication to the discipline is required to teach health education.
- In the future, the number and quality of persons seeking training through bona fide programs may be greatly reduced. The impact on the profession in subsequent years will most likely be detrimental to the whole field of health education since it will be oversupplied with individuals having less than desirable training and interest in contributing to the improvement of health education.

The typical training programs conducted in colleges for health education majors emphasize content courses in the health sciences with the expectation that the information acquired by the student will automatically be applied to produce effective teachers of health education. It has only been recently that some colleges have adopted a philosophy of providing prospective health educators with as much practical experiences as possible with an emphasis upon a broad and deep understanding of health information and health values and their application to the teaching-learning process.

There are paradoxes in the training of secondary health educators. For example, comprehensive health education programs are stressed philosophically while little, if any, contact is made by students in training with others in the health care system on a functional level; and experiential learning is stressed philosophically with little true experiential learning, aside from student teaching, taking place. Other paradoxes exist as well. They serve to exemplify the cultural lag between what is believed to be and what is actually happening in practice. However, the gap between theory and practice will be narrowed as the health education profession evolves into a discipline comprised of highly trained and dedicated individuals.

What about the elementary school teacher?

There is an urgent need to require health education courses for elementary school teachers during their preservice education. Although health education is required at the elementary school level in most states, little training in health education is offered to elementary education majors. In some instances, however, prospective elementary school teachers are encouraged to take one or two health education courses on a elective basis. Authorities generally agree that the development of health attitudes and practices can best be developed early in a child's school experience. This dictates the necessity for preparing the elementary school teacher for accepting this enormous responsibility.

For those already employed in elementary schools, the best method of providing them with the training they need is through in-service programs designed to supply them with basic health knowledge and the methods to be used with their pupils to achieve the desired objectives. (In-service training programs will be discussed in Chapter 10.)

As a further aid to the elementary school teacher, the creation of the position of elementary school health education specialist has been proposed. Their role would be to function as health educators in the elementary school, relieving the classroom teacher of the responsibility for health education. Although at first glance this may seem desirable, in reality it would place elementary school health education outside of the normal functioning of the classroom teacher and preclude interdisciplinary approaches, integration in other disciplines, and correlation with other subjects. There is the danger of isolating health from other aspects of life. Special efforts would have to be made to relate health learning with other areas of the curriculum. Therefore, elementary health specialists should be employed only in schools where each subject is taught by specialists. Team teaching approaches could then be used to overcome some of the drawbacks to the use of a specialist.

The school nurse-teacher's role

It has been common practice to regard the school nurse-teacher solely at a part of the health services department with little responsibility for health education. Since the chief responsibility of the school is education, all those associated with it should perform some form of educational function. In fact, the American Nurses' Association stressed this important role in a resolution adopted in 1974:

Whereas, School nursing is a specialized service contributing to the process of education; and

Whereas, Nursing provided as a part of the school program for children is a direct, constructive and effective contribution to building a healthful and dynamic society; and

Whereas, The health status of children has a direct influence upon their educational achievement; and

Whereas, For many children in the United States, the school nurse is the only contact the child has with the health care system; and

Whereas, The professional school nurse, with his/her experience and knowledge of growth and behavioral patterns of children, is in a unique position in the school setting to assist children in acquiring health knowledge, in developing attitudes conducive to healthful living and in meeting their needs resulting from disease, accidents, congenital defects and/or psycho-social maladjustments; therefore, be it

Resolved, That the ANA actively seek legislation to mandate nursing services as an integral part of every school's basic services; and, be it

Resolved, That school nurses participate in school health education programs both in teaching segments of the curriculum and as a resource to teachers and administrators in the school system; and, be it further

Resolved, That ANA and its constituent Associations work with institutions of higher learning to provide opportunities for school nurses to supplement and update their preparation in health education so that they may actively participate in school health education programs.[12]

It is quite apparent that the school nurse-teacher has a much greater responsibility than has been assumed. The nurse's role is a key factor in the success of a comprehensive health education program. One of the chief problems associated with the school nurse-teacher is a widespread lack of support by school boards and administrators. This generally results from the way school boards and administrators perceive the nurse, not from the way nurses perceive themselves. Consequently, school nurses are plagued by the stigma of being a frill in the school's program and are frequently the first to suffer elimination or reduction during economic crises. Obviously, school nurse-teachers must not only be highly trained to assume the increased responsibility; school administrators must begin to be trained to recognize the importance of the school nurse-teacher within the school's organizational structure and program.

Future expectations

The training of health educators has reached a significant turning point in its evolution. The spearhead is the tendency to change the process of training so that there is but one health education discipline with a variety of areas of concentration. This will best facilitate the attainment of increased status and effectiveness within the health care system that the profession so desperately needs. With this change, new emphasis will need to be placed upon (1) increased practical experiences for students in training, (2) increased contact with health professionals of all kinds, (3) training for medical, nursing, dental, and other health students, and (4) an increased involvement of health educators in training to find solutions to prevalent health problems.

In order to accomplish this, the method that shows the most promise is the health education center concept. This approach makes use of an already established vehicle. Programs can be incorporated into the health education center with a minimum of disruption of current training programs. In essence, the center provides a link between the traditional college training program and the health care system. It serves to facilitate the training of health educators who have appropriate informational background as well as the ability to function as effective health professionals along with other health professionals.

THE HEALTH EDUCATION CENTER CONCEPT

What is a health education center?

Originally conceived by John S. Sinacore in 1964*, the health education center concept takes a giant step toward effectively integrating health education into the total health care system and coordinating the health education efforts of the school and the community on a regional basis. The chief goal of regional health education centers is to coordinate the educational efforts of the schools, official and voluntary health agencies, community service groups, and the health professions. The major driving force behind the establishment of these centers is the economy of the times. With spiralling health care costs in the treatment realm, the delivery of health education to the public has become critical. Through these preventive efforts the cost of health care will better be controlled, yielding greater dividends for our investment in health.

From an educational point of view, the creation of health education centers goes one step beyond the traditional health education programs by providing a means for continuous evaluation of the health education programs being conducted by the various segments of the health care system within the region. This will result in closing the gap between new discoveries in the health sciences and their application to the people they affect.

---

* Dr. John S. Sinacore was at this time Chairman of the Department of Health Education at the State University of New York at Cortland. He served from 1967 to 1974 in the New York State Education Department as Director of Health and Drug Education Services and is presently Professor and Chairman of the Department of Health Science, State University College of New York at Brockport.

A regional health education center should not be perceived as a "building" or a similar structural confinement. Neither should it be perceived as being a part of a larger organization. Rather, it should be viewed as a focal point for the health education efforts of a region; it should be autonomous, providing services where needed to facilitate the effectiveness of health education programs. It is a concept of services for planning, implementing, evaluating, and communicating in relationship to health education and health educators.

The five components

The health education center's programmatic units and their functions can be summed up this way:

1. *Research and evaluation.* This unit is concerned with providing expertise in conducting research in health education. This includes the evaluation of current health education programs, the development of instruments to effectively evaluate new health education procedures, and assisting in the development of appropriate evaluation designs, upon request, for use in self-evaluation projects. The logical result of such activities is the accumulation of a large number of valid evaluative instruments and procedures that have been sorely lacking in the health education area in the past.
2. *Personnel development.* The primary purpose of this component is the training of both professional and lay health personnel. The training of professional health educators is done in conjunction with a department of health education at a college in the region. The training of lay personnel would be conducted through workshops and institutes in cooperation with continuing education departments of the college. The training of both groups would be coordinated by the health education center in cooperation with the college, based on the health needs of the region.
3. *Community service.* The regional health education center is inherently community service oriented since its basic goal is to coordinate the health education efforts of the various communities within the region. The center serves as a clearinghouse for the health education resources of the region, such as journals, pamphlets, newsletters, agency directories and the like. In addition, the center's personnel serve as consultants to community organizations, consumer groups, and individuals concerned with the promotion of health.
4. *Communication and media development.* One of the most vital functions of the health education center is the development of media resources to be used as tools in the health education of the public. In addition, the center develops media packages for use by colleges and public and private schools.
5. *Program development.* This component actually encompasses many of the functions of the other units. Functions of this unit include the

development of school health education curricula with recommendations for implementation and evaluation. This type of curriculum development could be done for either local school districts or for state departments of education. Similar programs can also be developed in the community health education and patient health education realms. In this regard, the center's function is one of coordination of health education programs among the schools, official (governmental) agencies, and voluntary community health agencies. By means of this component, the center can make valuable contributions through the development of mass media programs.

Organization of the center

There is a danger of the regional health education center functioning in a vacuum unless the needs of the various providers of health education are known. In this regard, proper organization can be accomplished only after careful consideration of the perceived needs of both providers and potential providers. These can be ascertained by the use of health education surveys designed to elicit responses about the various types of programs offered. In addition, the survey can serve to indicate the types of assistance that is or will be needed.

Depending upon the size of the region and its programmatic needs, the center should be staffed by no more than seven health education professionals in addition to support personnel. The organizational structure of the center is illustrated in Figure 9–4. A key feature of the center is its organizational flexibility, making it possible to respond to regional expectations rapidly and effectively. In addition to the full-time professional and support staff, the center would make use of other expertise available in the region and, if need be, outside the region.

The functioning of the center is, in large measure, determined by several advisory committees located in various parts of the region. These committees are composed of representatives of civic organizations, industry, clergy, and the like. Recommendations are submitted to the center, where they are screened. Those that are accepted are then carried out by the staff of the center. It must be noted that much of the functioning of the center is greatly influenced by the Health Systems Agency* of the region, which is charged by law with coordination of the efforts of the entire health care system of the region.

The importance of health education centers

Never before in the history of health education has there been a single development as important for its advancement than the health education

---

* The Health Systems Agency (HSA) is discussed further in the final section of this chapter. See also Appendix C.

FIGURE 9–4 Organizational Structure of the Health Education Center

The health education center provides for continuous services to the community or region, based upon their perceived health education needs. The community or region provides the center with continuous feedback for immediate need adaptations.

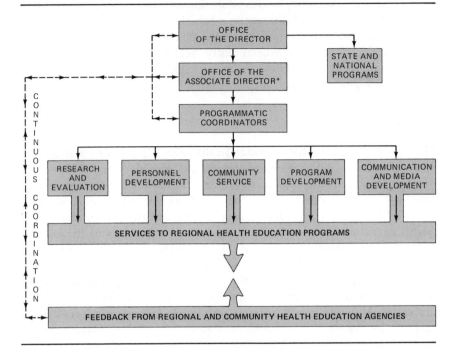

center concept. The very nature of its organizational structure makes it inherently efficient in meeting challenges as they arise. The center is designed to provide the model, assure the quality, and set the standards for health education programs within the region.[13] The establishment of a center, however, is not without its obstacles. Its initiation, like its implementation, must be predicated upon cooperation by those who possess similar ideas about health education and its potential for improving the health of society. The same obstacles present in any major social change will be present in the initiation of a health education center concept, and must be dealt with in the planning stages.

One of the long-term effects of the health education center will be to motivate and direct the establishment of comprehensive health education programs throughout the region and to require that a functional merger take place between health education and the health care system. Traditionally, health education programs have been conducted in a more or less haphazard manner, with little or no coordination of efforts among the providers of health education. When the health education center is fully operational, this inefficient practice will be all but eliminated. The establishment of regional health education centers, therefore, is a vital factor in the improvement of health education programs across the nation.

Relation of health education centers to the health care system

The development of regional health education centers is consistent with the recent organizational patterns of other segments of the health care system. In fact, the current trend was first proposed by the National Health Assembly[14], which issued a report calling for regionalization of the treatment realm in 1948! More recent developments include the Partnership for Health Act during President Johnson's administration; and the act calling for the establishment of Health Maintenance Organizations (HMOs) during the Nixon administration. Most recently, Congress enacted a law[15] calling for the establishment of Health Systems Agencies, the boundaries of which are determined by the states. The functions of the HSA will be to coordinate all of the delivery of health services throughout a given region. The HSA is governed by advisory committees made up of 51 percent laypersons and 49 percent health professionals.

From our viewpoint, a key aspect of the HSA legislation is its requirement of provision of health education programs as an integral component of the health care system. A logical first step toward fulfilling this requirement is the establishment of regional health education centers, the boundaries of which will correspond to the boundaries of the HSA. This will facilitate the coordination of effort between the health education center and the HSA.

The President's Committee on Health Education[16] recommended the establishment of two national health education components: a national center for health education funded through the private sector and a bureau of health education within the Department of Health, Education, and Welfare. The national center for health education has been established under the coordination of the National Health Council.

Within the federal government, the Bureau of Health Education is an integral component of the Center for Disease Control of the United States Public Health Service which, in turn, is a part of the Department of Health, Education, and Welfare. The Bureau of Health Education was established in September, 1974. Its mission is "to provide for the prevention of disease, disability, premature death, and undesirable and unnecessary health problems."[17]

The Bureau of Health Education consists of (1) the office of the Director, (2) the National Clearinghouse for Smoking and Health, (3) the Community Program Development Division, and (4) the Professional Services and Consultant Division. Although each section of the Bureau has specific responsibilities, the overall action priorities[18] are to:

- help assure that health education is appropriately included in major developments on the national health scene, such as health resources planning and development and national health insurance.
- continue and, where possible, strengthen the effectiveness of activities designed to reduce the health consequences of smoking.
- develop and maintain a useful data base on health education efforts in HEW and in other selected Federal agencies.
- stimulate cooperation between federal agency health education programs that are directed toward common target populations or share mutual educational goals.
- encourage development of effective mechanisms for collaboration among voluntary, professional, industrial, and other private sector groups with health education interests.
- select specific projects for direct intervention and support that are designed for population groups in specific need of health education (e.g., ethnic and linguistic priorities, youth, rural and inner city communities, the aged, and the handicapped).
- provide, within financial and staff constraints, technical assistance and consultation to public and private agencies and groups.

An important action taken was the establishment of the Interdepartmental Panel for Health Education of the Public. It was authorized by the Secretary of HEW in May, 1974, under the National Health Education Action Plan. The purpose of the Panel is "to establish a central focus for the development and promulgation of Department-wide health education policies, and to facilitate the implementation of multiagency health education activities."[19] In this regard, the panel's functions[20] are to:

- develop and recommend throughout the Department a set of policies related to health education of the public.
- recommend that appropriate attention be given to health education within each agency's program.
- identify educational goals common to two or more agencies and develop and recommend methods for interagency cooperation in accomplishing these purposes.
- recommend appropriate consideration of health education in the implementation of major departmental initiatives.
- conduct liaison activities with other federal departments and agencies and with the private sector in relation to health education programs.

There exists an organizational foundation for the implementation of comprehensive health education programs throughout the United States, with two agencies coordinating the national effort. The HSA legislation and health education center concept provide the means for implementing coordination between the treatment and prevention efforts of the health care system at the grassroots level.

DEFINITIVE UNDERSTANDINGS

As the health education profession has evolved, three types of health educators have come into being. They are the school health educator, the community health educator, and the patient (clinical) health educator. These should not be considered three separate disciplines but rather one profession with three spheres of influence. The common factors uniting them are much greater and important than their functional differences.

One of the chief factors inhibiting the growth of health education as a profession has been its inability to unite around a particular set of standards that can serve as guidelines for its functioning. Political apathy and/or misdirection has also been an inhibiting element in the attainment of professionalism. It is imperative that a national professional organization be founded to represent the interests and philosophies of all health educators. It should be so designed that it can and will establish and maintain professional standards and function as a political advocate for members of the profession.

Universal standards of professional preparation must be formulated to maintain continuity and ultimately to be recognized by the states as the principles governing the functioning of the profession. This must be done through the political advocacy of professional associations.

Basic structural changes must be made in health education training programs to coincide with current health education philosophy, including the provision of learning experiences for those being trained in the other health sciences. This will result in cooperation and understanding between health educators and the other health professionals after their initial training is complete.

In order to demonstrate accountability in health education, new ways of preparing health educators must be developed. One way currently being tested is the development of competencies which prospective health educators must meet as a prerequisite for certification. This implies a basic reorganization of current teacher education programs so that they will be geared toward the attainment of competencies rather than the mere fulfillment of course work.

The deficit in qualified health educators has been met in some instances through the use of proficiency examinations and a "retreading" of teachers certified in another area. When abused, both methods can result in problems for the profession. Emphasis should be placed upon an upgrading of existing teacher training programs to facilitate the implementation of state mandates.

At the elementary school level, the most efficient method of training teachers for health education responsibilities who are already in practice is through in-service training programs. Colleges must meet their responsibility for training elementary education majors in health education during their preservice education.

The school nurse-teacher must be thought of as a major part of a comprehensive school health education program, rather than merely a member of the health services team. The nurse's role can be especially valuable at the elementary school level by providing technical expertise, conducting in-service training programs, and participating in the activities of the various health education classes.

One of the most significant developments in health education in recent years has been the establishment of health education centers. Such centers serve as the focal point for the health education efforts of a given region. In essence, the health education center functions as the coordinators of health education programs for that region. It provides a variety of essential services such as research and evaluation, personnel development, community service, communication and media development, and program development.

The health education center is a key factor in facilitating an increased status of health education within the health care system. It is imperative that health educators be trained by exposure to all health professionals in order that they may function within the health care system after formal training is complete.

The enactment of federal laws and the initiation of a variety of national programs are consistent with many of the policies and recommendations of several professional health and health education associations. As these programs are brought more into focus and become more functional, it is important that the whole concept of preparing health educators be changed accordingly.

PROBLEMS
FOR DISCUSSION

1. Describe how the three types of health educators are similar in their functioning responsibilities.
2. Show how health education is a single, unified profession.
3. Distinguish between the functional variations of the three types of health educators.
4. Explain why the three types of health educators should be trained together as a single profession.
5. Distinguish between the professional preparation and functions of the three types of health educators as they now exist and how they are evolving.
6. Discuss how the introduction of the patient health educator may very well be a key factor in changing the focus of the entire health care delivery system.
7. Outline the general areas to be considered in establishing standards for health education professionalism. How are they similar to, or different from, other professions?
8. Develop a philosophy of health education professionalism.
9. List at least five general practices of traditional training of health educators that are likely to be eliminated as health education training programs begin to implement the concept of competency-based teacher education programs (CBTE).

10. Is it possible to establish universal standards for professional preparation of health educators? Explain.
11. In what ways is the establishment of competencies for prospective health educators different from traditional modes of preparation?
12. Develop competencies for the school health educator; for the community health educator; for the patient health educator. Analyze the three lists. What can be concluded?
13. Analyze the quality of preparation of present-day health educators. What are its strengths? Weaknesses? How would you change this preparation to reflect realistic improvements in their preparation?
14. Describe why the health education preparation of elementary school education majors must be strengthened.
15. Explain the emerging role of the school nurse-teacher in the health education program.
16. Discuss the advantages and disadvantages of elementary school health education specialists.
17. Describe how the development of the health education center concept will revolutionize the training and functions of health educators. What impact can this concept have on the training of other health professionals?
18. Show how each of the five components (programmatic units) of the health education center concept are integrally related to each other.
19. List the chief functions or purposes of the health education center concept.
20. List some of the important national movements in recent years that have or are affecting the nature of the health care system.
21. What is a comprehensive health education program?

REFERENCES

1. Hoyman, Howard S., "New Frontiers in Health Education," *Journal of School Health*, vol. XLIII (7), p. 423.
2. The American Nurses' Association, "Resolution on Comprehensive School Health Education Programs," 1974.
3. Milio, Nancy, *The Care of Health in Communities*, Macmillan Publishing Co., N.Y., 1975, p. 143.
4. Woodward, Kenneth L., "The Morbid Society," *Newsweek*, vol. LXXXVII (23), June 7, 1976, p. 87.
5. Conant, Richard K., et al., "Health Education—A Bridge to the Community," *American Journal of Public Health*, vol. 62 (9), September 1972, p. 1244.
6. Ibid., p. 1239.
7. Zimmering, Stanley, and Edmund J. McTernan, "A New Player on the Allied Health Team: The Clinical Health Educator," unpublished paper, 1975, p. 10.
8. Ibid., p. 9.
9. *Standard Dictionary of the English Language*, International Edition, Funk & Wagnalls, New York, 1974, p. 1006.
10. Haro, Michael S., "School Health Revisited," *Journal of School Health*, vol. XLIV, (7), Sept. 1974, p. 367.
11. Joint Committee on Health Problems in Education, "Teacher Preparation in Health Education," Resolution, National Education Association—American Medical Association, 1970.
12. American Nurses' Association, "Resolution on School Health Nursing," 1974.
13. Ad Hoc Committee on Consumer Health Education, "Consumer Health Education: A Priority Whose Time Has Come," unpublished document, 1974, p. 2.

14. The National Health Assembly, *America's Health: A Report to the Nation*, Harper and Brothers, New York, 1949.
15. National Health Planning and Resources Development Act of 1974, Public Law 93–641, January 4, 1975.
16. U.S. Department of Health, Education and Welfare, *Report of the President's Committee on Health Education*, 1973.
17. Bureau of Health Education, HEW, *Facts*, Atlanta, August, 1975, p. 1.
18. Ibid., p. 2.
19. Interdepartmental Panel for Health Education of the Public, *Charter*, March 26, 1975.
20. Ibid.

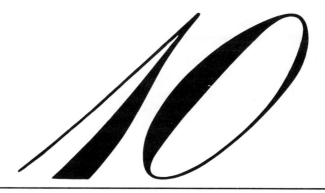

Organizing
for Health
Education/
Theory
and Practice

- Basic Principles of Organization and Administration
- The School Health Education Administrator
- Administrative Techniques
- School/Community Relations
- The School Health Program
- Definitive Understandings
- Problems for Discussion
- References

We do not reject our traditions, but are willing to adapt to changing circumstances. We are willing to suffer the discomfort of change in order to achieve a better future.

The Hon. Barbara Jordan

Health education programs will never be successful, nor will they ever be comprehensive, without proper organization and competent administration. Although not easily attainable, such a goal for health education must not be put off any longer.

AEB
DAB

BASIC PRINCIPLES OF
ORGANIZATION AND ADMINISTRATION

Purpose of organization

Organizing for health education is a fundamental and necessary process. Its basic purpose is to facilitate health learning of children, youth, and adults. Organization brings into focus such key elements as intraprogram communications, school/community interaction, program coordination, and employment of qualified teachers. As a result, learning experiences are less likely to be offered in a haphazard manner and in places and at times that will do little to benefit the learner. In addition, duplication of effort will be avoided, preventing inefficiency and ineffectiveness.

Unfortunately, many erroneous conclusions have been made about the ability for health education to favorably influence health attitudes, knowledge, and behavior of learners with poorly organized, administered, and staffed programs that do not recognize the fact that they are inherently doomed to failure. It is somewhat comparable to attempting a moon landing with a parachute.

On the other hand, adequate organization and administration guarantees a coordinated effort in terms of the timing of various program components, who will offer them, and where in the community they will be most worthwhile and effective. According to Miller[1], some basic questions must be answered when planning the organizational design of the health educational program:

1. *Who is to be educated?* That is to say, to what target population will the program be offered? What are their demographic characteristics? What are their particular health needs?
2. *How shall they be educated?* Once the target population is identified, what methods will best be suited to meetings the learners' health needs based upon their ages, socioeconomic and experiential backgrounds?
3. *How shall the program be staffed?* Staffing is best achieved by employing personnel that can work efficiently with the agency's or school's target population, rather than attempting to mold the learner to the desires of the staff.
4. *What physical facilities shall be required?* Based upon program needs, the health education administrator must decide what facilities are required to implement the program most effectively. In addition, means for securing the necessary facilities must be determined. This will include funds and location.
5. *How shall the program be supported financially and how will it be managed?* Consideration must be given to locating operating funds. Sources include both the private and public sectors. In addition, the people best equipped to administer the program must be identified.

6. *What shall be the structure of the program?* Determination must be made as to what constitutes a comprehensive health education program, how the school and community can interact effectively, what specific educational experiences will be offered and when, and how the program will be coordinated with others.

Finally, the activities of an organized health education program—whether the setting is a governmental or voluntary health agency, the school, or a treatment center—are identical. They consist of *planning, structuring, administering, evaluating,* and *adapting.* All of these activities are the primary responsibility of the health education administrator, who may be advised by individuals or committees.

The need for organized health education programs

One of the first tasks of the health education administrator is to identify the real health goals of the learners and the health education program. These should always stem from the existing or anticipated health issues within the community and school environments. There are usually a variety of health agencies and educational institutions, all of which might be working toward the achievement of their own goals with little regard for those of the other agencies. This is likely to result in inefficient duplication of services and the creation of large program gaps. However, with the establishment of the health systems agencies, it is becoming more feasible to formulate and implement broad organizational and administrative structures that are designed to codify the health education endeavors of all health-related agencies. The introduction of the health education centers throughout the nation will expedite this process. As a result, a comprehensive health education program which addresses the health needs of the community and is aimed at conserving human resources will evolve.

Once programmatic goals have been identified and educational procedures established, health personnel can be assigned to various tasks. Qualified health educators can accept responsibilities and perform duties that will mesh with those of other health personnel. *Organization for health consists of a group of competent people in a network of working relationships combining their abilities and energies to accomplish a purpose which no one of them could do alone.* The health education administrator's role is to provide direction, leadership, and coordination so that goals can be achieved with maximum efficiency and minimum expenditure of human energy.

How well the health education program is organized and administered will determine how well it can achieve its purposes. No health education program that is not organized appropriately under the leadership of a competent health education administrator can survive very long. The need for a strong organizational and administrative structure is further indicated when we remember that the promotion and maintenance of health are dependent upon effective interaction of *all* segments of the health care system. None of these segments can effectively or economically function in a vacuum. Proper leadership in health education provides the means for improving communications and solidifying cooperation between all health-related program directors.

Meeting the organizational needs of health education will allow programs to move in a logical progression and to incorporate idealism and pragmatism. Of equal importance is the ability of programs to adapt to the changing health needs of society so that health education can move away from being crisis-oriented, reacting belatedly to health problems of short-term significance, toward being health promotive-oriented. This requires a permanent, but flexible, organization and administration structure.

Over the years, few exemplary comprehensive health education programs have been established in the United States in either the school or community sectors. On the infrequent occasions when qualified health education administrators have been employed, and where community support has existed, it has been possible to develop some significant segments of a comprehensive program; some of a truly admirable nature. There are many other factors that must be considered when attempting to initiate and develop these programs. Health education has moved from rather simple goals and approaches to extremely sophisticated purposes and multiple methodologies. Hochbaum described some of the reasons for this:

> Traditionally health education has addressed itself, by its very nature, primarily to those determinants of health behavior that are responses to *educational* intervention: knowledge, attitudes, perceived needs, motivation, and the like. But by now we have come to recognize and appreciate the extent to which behavior is directly determined by factors that are *not* responsive to traditional educational intervention: social, political, economic, and environmental conditions as well as conditions in the delivery of health services themselves. In short, a multitude of factors impinge on people's daily lives, pushing them into actions they may not wish to take, or making actions they do wish to take difficult or impossible.[2]

Such changes make it imperative for programs to be organized and administered by those who recognize these changes and are capable of doing something about them. However, even in these instances when a qualified and capable health education administrator is available, the program is usually understaffed, with a limited budget and insufficient community support. Not until these deficiencies and constraints are overcome can even the best health education administrator expect to establish a totally worthwhile comprehensive health education program. Moreover, the health education profession is faced with numerous developments that challenge the profession, society, and government—developments that challenge the very nature of humanity. Health educators and administrators must be aware of these developments and their significance to health education and the resultant change in people's attitudes and behavior. Hochbaum describes the situation: "Among those developments that impinge on health education from the outside is the stress on consumer rights; there is the upheaval in the health care system; there is the proliferation of new allied professions and greater utilization of sub– and even non-professionals in the health field; there is the growing crisis of medical care cost; and there is the dramatic spurt of appreciation for the importance of people's health behavior to the effective and efficient delivery of health care."[3]

One of the major factors impeding the progress of the development of effective health education programs that we are grappling with is a general lack of organization and/or mismanagement. For example, many school health education programs are organized within the department of pupil personnel services under the "leadership" of a director of this area; or, more frequently, they are placed within the physical education department under the "leadership" of a director of physical education or athletics. Although these individuals are usually competent administrators in their area of expertise, they frequently either do not possess an understanding of the purpose and processes of health education or have other interests or priorities occupying their time and efforts. Consequently, many health education programs are deprived of the attention and prestige they must have to be effective.

Health education administrators should possess training and experience in the principles of organization and administration and, equally important, they should possess a profound understanding of health education philosophy and practice. Further, they must have a working knowledge of health education in the settings outside their primary area of responsibility. For example, the school health administrator must understand the problems of patient educators as well as community health educators and be able to relate positively with them. Finally, the health education administrator must understand the interrelationships of health education as an integral and functional component of the health care system. Mayshark and Shaw assert that the art of administration is rapidly evolving:

> Two fundamental truths that have paramount importance for the administration of school health programs are evident in that evolution. The first is that no one can ultimately administer such a program without detailed knowledge about its substance, but it does not follow that one with such knowledge can administer effectively unless he also knows, understands, and can selectively apply many of the concepts and techniques of modern organization and management. The second is that whatever the responsibilities and duties of an administrative position in a school health program might be, its occupant will share universal problems in common with all other administrators in all other kinds of organizations.[4]

Factors affecting organization

There are numerous forces that play vital roles in influencing the organizational growth and administrative expediency of health education programs in both the community and school sectors. Most authorities generally agree that these forces can be placed within the confines of five general areas: (1) political pressures and resultant actions, (2) social demands, (3) economic and budgetary constraints, (4) the activities of all health-related organizations, and (5) the talents of the administrators of health education programs. These influences are not mutually exclusive, but tend to be interdependent and interactional.

Political pressure pervades nearly every aspect of societal functioning. Administrators of social institutions tend to view their ability to function in the best interests of society as paramount. This results in a breakdown in communications, with each institution or agency exerting pressure upon the others to deal with the needs of society differently. Further, this has often resulted in the creation of a kind of sacred territory with artificial boundaries of functioning. When this happens, the ability to interact with each other is hampered. For example, legislative action sometimes recognizes the services that one segment of the health care system can provide while excluding other segments that have a vital part of play in efficiently providing this service or a portion of it. If legislators were to recognize the need to provide funds to conduct a large-scale immunization program without providing adequate funds to carry out public education efforts, the program would be less effective; that is, it would reach fewer people.

In the area of health education, pressures are often exerted upon program administrators to place emphasis upon areas of crisis that will capture the attention of the community. In addition, health educators often stress those areas of concern that will result in a positive response from community leaders. We have alluded to the need for health educators to become more politically astute, to have the ability to recognize when the political system is threatening, and to be able to utilize the resources of the political system to the advantage of the program and its services. Political involvement is an inherent part of being a health educator and administrator.

Many social factors affect the organization and administration of health education programs. Society has a variety of health needs that must be met. Paradoxically, the fulfillment of these needs may not be recognized as a benefit and instead, society may demand that others be satisfied. Ideally, community health needs as well as those of society as a whole should be met. In discussing the role of the schools in this regard, Miller states, "The school system becomes a place where the individual seeks to understand and to find his best self in a kind of world that fits him. It is concurrently the place where society seeks to shape and condition individuals to fit its needs and values."[5]

Working with and for people in various situations is one of the most fundamental activities in which the health education administrator will become engaged. This relationship may take the form of line or staff within the organizational structure. A *line relationship* implies that a person in an authoritative position must interact with subordinates. This brings about a process known as supervision. A *staff relationship* implies consultant and advisory activities between persons of equal or near equal authority within the organization and outside as well. These are extremely important for cooperation and interaction between individuals concerned with health-related activities. Whether the relations of people are internal and external, their quality is vital to the smooth development and implementation of health education programs. It is generally agreed among administrative authorities that most administrative problems stem from inadequate relationships between people. They usually develop from differences in program philosophy, poor communication, personality differences, or the inability of the administrator to motivate people to action, efficiently direct their activities, or coordinate individual and group functions.

A perennial force affecting the establishment of health education programs is budgetary constraints. This is especially true during times of economic crises. The health education administrator can do much to relieve this problem by seeking funds beyond those available through the usual channels of local tax sources or donations. It may also be possible for the health education administrator to initiate a reordering of existing program priorities of the total educational program within the community. This may result in a release of funds from nonessential expenditures that can be applied to the health education program. However, the administrator will need to be prepared to provide substantial evidence of the value of health education for negotiations with school administrators, boards of education, or governing bodies of health agencies.

Although organizational structure is influenced by the qualities of health education administrators, the structure, in turn, influences how well they can carry out their responsibilities. However, the organizational structure is meaningless unless the administrator is effective in organizing, planning, coordinating, conducting, supervising, communicating and evaluating. The extent to which these leadership qualities are manifested will determine the extent to which health education gains the respect of other health professionals and the community and whether it achieves its goals and final purposes.

School/community communications

Effective communication requires direct involvement in all community health affairs. It is more than a public relations effort or an exchange of resources persons at social or educational functions. Instead, it is a continuous process of informational exchange and direct interaction among all those concerned with health. Programs emanating from the school must take the initiative toward removing any barriers to effective interaction by taking advantage of the wealth of resources available. There are three chief reasons why this is necessary: (1) the school's health resources are no longer adequate to meet the health needs of children living in today's complex society, (2) the school is the educational leader of the community, and (3) community involvement with the school's program allows for greater learner and professional participation within the health care system. In this way, the school's health education program becomes a part of the community rather than being a group of activities which merely test the values of the community from time to time.

According to various sociologists, social workers, and community organization authorities, health administrators have three options when attempting to stimulate school/community communications. They are: (1) *locality development*, which is changing the activities of a community through participation of the people affected, (2) *social planning*, which is placing an emphasis upon professional cooperation and planning, and (3) *social action*, which is enlisting the participation of potentially militant factions to change the organization of disadvantaged segments of the community.

The health administrator may choose to use any of these approaches or a combination of them in order to achieve the goals of the program. The important factor is that community and school cooperation is essential. The health education program must be organized and administered accordingly.

THE SCHOOL HEALTH EDUCATION ADMINISTRATOR

Professional preparation

With the rapid development of health education programs within the school systems of many states in recent years, a need has been created for qualified school health education administrators to organize health education programs on a district-wide or regional basis. It has been common practice for the administration of health education programs to fall within the purview of individuals whose main area of interest is *not* health education. This has come about as a result of the unwillingness of school administrators to allocate additional funds for the administrator of health education, and the lack of health educators with administrative qualifications. Consequently, many health education programs that appear to be well-coordinated are, in fact, coordinated only on a part-time basis in a manner not conducive to their promotion.

Many colleges and universities have recognized the lack of qualified health education administrators and have designed programs that combine basic health education content, philosophy, and methodology courses with others in educational administration. These programs are typically offered at the graduate level, many leading to a master's degree in health education or an administrator's certificate. Because of the increasing need for school/community interaction, many of these health administrator programs require a practicum in community health education to facilitate this interaction once the administrator is placed in the field. Some authorities suggest that the health administrator should possess at least six general characteristics:

1. Training and experience in both public and school health education.
2. A complete understanding of the principles of learning and how to apply them to health education.
3. The ability to communicate effectively with all kinds of people in a variety of settings.
4. The ability to organize.
5. The ability to establish realistic health goals and to achieve them.
6. An in-depth knowledge of current health problems and issues and how to solve them.[6]

The emphasis on training of health education administrators is a relatively recent approach that has introduced a whole new era in health education that was not possible in the past. The first such training program was initiated in 1972 by New York University as a result of a grant from the New York State Education Department. With additional funds being made available to the Education Department, it was possible to place 27 highly trained health education administrators in several New York State Boards of Cooperative Educational Services (BOCES)* and in four of the large city school districts—Buffalo, Rochester, Syracuse, and Yonkers. Many of these individuals completed the innovative health education administrator's training program at New York University. Unfortunately, most of these positions were eliminated in 1975 when the New York State Legislature chose to discontinue their funding. This demonstrates once again the importance of political action in the growth or continuance of essential health services. Although economic difficulties may retard the growth of the numbers of health education administrators employed by school districts, the main concern of the health education profession is convincing school administrators and legislators of the importance of properly administrating health education programs by individuals who are competent in both health education and administration.

Functions and responsibilities

Effective communications is the most important strategy available to the health education administrator for initiating and administering the

---

* BOCES are intermediate administrative school districts whose primary purpose is achieved through cooperative shared funding for special educational services by participating school districts.

health education program. This is demonstrated by the "awareness-action-reaction cycle" introduced by Bedworth and D'Elia[7] in 1973. They stated, "Recognizing that health problems . . . occur in communities, it is imperative that health education programs consider community demands for action." They amplify this when they state that "the demands of the community are motivated by an awareness of the existent health problems and their interference with normal social living." The health education administrator must be effective in communicating the school's awareness of the community's reactions to these demands. This not only initiates the cycle but also continues it as long as communications are sustained and actions and reactions are appropriate.

The specific function of the health education administrator fall into seven general categories:

1. *Planning.* This includes all of the preliminary activities related to designing the comprehensive program. It should take into account the ways in which each segment of the program relates to and influences other segments. Effective planning is necessary for program success.
2. *Structuring.* Organizing is usually an integral component of planning. It anticipates how the elements of the program relate to the people affected and the step-by-step actions needed to initiate, develop, and implement each. Organization and administration are inseparable.
3. *Administering.* This includes coordinating, conducting, and supervising.

   Coordinating. Since many activities will be going on at the same time and will be conducted by many people, it is vital that they all be related with the philosophy and organizational plan. This requires continuous communications with both the intra– and extraschool people engaged in health education. The health education administrator has the awesome responsibility of insuring smooth functioning and avoiding duplicated efforts.

   Conducting. Many aspects of the health education program must be conducted by the health education administrator, while other phases must be administered. For example, the health education administrator frequently conducts in-service training programs.

   Supervising. This is closely allied with coordinating; but supervision implies authority. Coordination is more a matter of providing advice, although some supervision may be necessary. For instance, the health education administrator is responsible for supervising the activities of the health educators as they teach.
4. *Communicating.* Lines of communication must be established between all those engaged in any phase of health education. This essentially involves public relations strategies, as well as relations with staff.
5. *Evaluating.* This is related to all aspects of the program and influences what is to be planned and implemented.

Although it is probably not possible to elucidate all of the functions of the health education administrator, some attempts have been made along these lines. The following list is an adaptation from a bulletin issued by the New York State Education Department* in 1971:

1. Organizes the entire school/community health education program including the medical and psychological service aspects.
2. Provides leadership in developing appropriate health education philosophy and methodology based upon accepted educational principles.
3. Establishes mechanisms for the continuous supervision of the teaching of health education.
4. Coordinates the review and evaluation of all learning resources by learning resource committee.
5. Provides expertise in the development of appropriate evaluation criteria.
6. Initiates and maintains continuous contact with all agencies that are concerned and/or involved with health education and coordinates their involvement in the health education program.
7. Participates in the development of criteria for the selection of health education resources and makes recommendations to the school's administration relative to selection.
8. Gives assistance in the interpretation of laws, policies, regulations, and procedures governing health programs to concerned individuals and agencies.
9. Takes the lead in securing adequate funds for the financing of health education programs.
10. Coordinates and supervises in-service training programs for elementary school teachers, health educators, school administrators, and other school personnel involved in the health education program.
11. Coordinates continual evaluation of health education programs and adapts the program accordingly for the attainment of the most viable program possible.
12. Organizes and supervises a variety of community health education programs including workshops, discussion groups, seminars, lectures, and research programs.
13. Organizes and chairs four basic committees:
    a. the health education advisory committee
    b. the health education program and instruction committee
    c. the learning resource and evaluation committee
    d. the teaching teams
14. Establishes a health education learning center for use by both teachers and students. In addition, the coordinator provides for the

---

* "Suggested Responsibilities of the Health Education Coordinator," New York State Education Department, Special Unit on Health and Drug Education, Albany, 1971.

continuous evaluation of materials in the center to insure their appropriateness and currency.

15. Cooperates with other committees in the development of a kindergarten through adult health education program based on student interest and needs.
16. Organizes the school community health education efforts to alleviate current health problems.
17. Coordinates the health education efforts between various levels and departments within the school system.
18. Maintains contact with building administrators and those responsible for the development of curricula to insure the proper application and priority of the health education curriculum.
19. Consults with various community agencies (governmental and voluntary) and gives educational advice to facilitate the coordination of health efforts.
20. Serves as a consultant for groups within the school system engaged in health activities.
21. Contacts and encourages parent groups to participate in the health education program and to assist in future program development.
22. Participates as a consultant and resource in the classroom setting.
23. Initiates and maintains ongoing public relations and information procedures.
24. Utilizes mass media to best advantage for the health education program.
25. Coordinates the provision of community awareness programs.
26. Establishes and coordinates a speakers' bureau for use by civic organizations (e.g., church organizations, parent-teacher groups, fraternal organizations, etc.).

At this point, one could conclude that *the most important element influencing the success of health education programs is the quality of the people responsible for it.*

ADMINISTRATIVE TECHNIQUES

General considerations

There are several basic principles of administrative functioning. The following list was compiled by Zimmerli,* and suggests the most effective techniques the health education administrator may use to facilitate implementation of the health education program:

---

* Dr. William Zimmerli was Chairman of the Department of Health Science, State University College of New York at Brockport at the time this list was compiled. The principles listed are those used in health education programs directed by him.

1. The successful administrator will attempt to involve the most qualified people available in the health education program. This involves the identification of the most competent resource people both inside and outside of the organization to assist in the actualization of the institution's objectives and goals. Therefore, administrators will employ individuals best able to perform the duties of the position in question, even at a salary greater than their own.

2. Administrators must be generalists. That is, they should be knowledgeable about all facets of administration and be aware of *what* needs to be accomplished, not necessarily *how* to accomplish the task. It is also necessary for the administrator to possess a working knowledge of educational philosophy, curriculum design, methodology, and evaluation.

3. The successful administrator will deal equally and fairly with all constituents—students, faculty and staff, other administrators, and community members. Dealing in favoritism threatens the success of a program.

4. A properly administered program will operate within a defined organizational structure. The structure may be horizontal, vertical, or funnel-shaped. The important concept is that there should be clearly defined channels of communication.

5. The administrator will establish a productive environment in which a communication system facilitates a free flow of ideas and two-way communication. This necessitates an open means of communication for students, teachers, community members, and administrators.

6. The successful administrator will follow an operational model that incorporates the functions of planning, implementing, assessing the product, evaluating, and adjusting the program accordingly.

7. The administrator will develop the program along the lines of established principles, policies, procedures, and rules that are clearly delineated for all institutional constituencies—students, teachers, community members, and administrators.

8. Successful administrators will understand the various principles of community organization (structure and process). They will be knowledgeable about social, economic, and political aspects of the community and will know how to utilize the power structure.

9. Administrators will be able to generate support for ideas among students, teachers, administrators, and community members. In addition, they will also be able to motivate them to actively participate in the educational process.

10. The successful administrators will operate by consensus whenever possible through the use of compromise, and negotiations; and democracy (majority rule) whenever necessary.

11. The administrator will operate within established criteria following the policies of the organization, utilizing the structure of the institution and implementing the desired operational model.

12. The successful administrator will utilize appropriate decision-making

skills and procedures when a process of consensus-democracy is not possible.

    a. In any decision-making process, those who will be affected by the decision should be informed and, if possible, consulted. The goal is to help all who are involved in the institution feel that the institution's business is basically their business.

    b. The students, faculty and staff, and administrators should be the first to hear about important decisions and developments. Although they may have had adequate participation in the process, the nature and timing of the announcement of the final decisions are important.

    c. The people who are consulted when a decision is being sought should be helped to understand the way in which their advice or counsel will be used. Failure to understand how the decision-making process works, who is involved, and who makes the final decision is a source of much misunderstanding. If given the proper information, most people will accept the fact that they, or the committee of which they are working members, are a part of a complex and sometimes lengthy process. Understanding is the key here: Individuals or committees should understand as clearly as possible the limits and extent of their role and responsibilities.

13. The successful administrator delegates responsibility and the authority that goes with it. When responsibility is delegated (as it should be in any organization), corresponding authority should be delegated within reasonable limits. Few things are more destructive to morale than giving a person responsibility for doing a task or solving a problem and then neglecting to give, or at some point withdraw, the authority to do the job. Of course, in very sensitive areas, authority may have to be limited or in rare cases, withdrawn. But if this is practiced consistently, the delegation of responsibility becomes impossible and administrators find themselves burdened with all responsibility—a highly destructive situation for the administrator and for the institution.

14. In order to most efficiently solve problems, the administrator should, as a general rule, allow the person closest to the problem make the decision. However, it may sometimes be necessary to involve others. This applies to teachers as individuals, teaching teams, departments, etc. The further the decision is from those immediately involved, the greater the likelihood that the decision will not be appropriate.

15. The successful administrator will make an effort to insure that those involved in the educational community understand that there must be a relationship between responsibility and competence—that individuals can be given responsibility only in areas where they have established their competence. To put it another way, the boundaries of competence and responsibility should coincide. The effectiveness of any academic organization rests on respect for

competence and the adjusting of responsibility to competence. The administrator should keep and eye out for competence, talent, and special skills and should utilize them whenever possible.

16. It is imperative that the administrator keep all segments of the educational community—board of education, students, faculty, staff, administrators, and community members—informed of the central theme, goals, and objectives for which the educational institution was created.

Establishing advisory committees

No administrator can function effectively for very long without making use of available expertise. One technique frequently used is the establishment of basic committees related to the major functional areas of the program. Since the health education program is concerned with both school and community communications and actions, committees will fall into internal and external organizational categories. The *internal committees* consist of individuals within the organization that possess special expertise in areas such as curriculum development, while the *external committees* consist of individuals from community health-related agencies who have direct contact with and awareness of the health issues that exist or may be evolving.

Generally, there is a need for only one external committee. It is usually called the school/community health education advisory committee, and is made up of representatives from governmental and voluntary health agencies, civic and service groups, professional health associations (medical and dental societies, for example), parent groups, and clergy. Since the individuals that comprise this committee represent a cross-section of the community's population, as well as specialized areas concerned with the health of the people, its purposes are chiefly: (1) to identify the health needs of the community, (2) to anticipate areas of possible concern in the future, (3) to coordinate the health activities of both the community and school, and (4) to establish a system of effective communications between all who are concerned with health education. This committee should be chaired by the health education administrator, who acts as the liaison between the school and community.

Essentially, the school/community health education advisory committee provides the health education administrator with advice, counsel, guidance, and technical information that can be applied to developing action programs in health education. This committee does not get involved in curriculum development, however, but may very well provide the basis for new or revised curricula. It may also review and react to existing curricula and make recommendations for its improvement. Promotional and preventive health education efforts can be tailored to specific health needs as well as to specific populations within the community as a result of the advice from this committee. In essence, this committee is the "health barometer" of the school and the community at large.

From time to time, it may be necessary for one or more subcommittees to be formed to investigate and report on special health issues. For example, it may be valuable to investigate the epidemiological nature of drug abuse in the community so that preventive programs can be launched that will reach the affected segments of the population before it becomes a crisis.

The internal committees should be designed to put into action the advice from the school/community health education advisory committee. There is a need for at least three ongoing committees: a health education program and curriculum committee, a learning resources and evaluation committee, and a teaching/learning team. The health education administrator can chair each of these committees or function in an exofficio capacity to assure proper coordination of their activities with the school/community health education advisory committee.

The *health education program and curriculum committee* is the primary program action committee since it establishes the basis for curriculum development. This committee should consist of a broad representation from the school's staff—health educators, elementary school teachers, school administrator, medical and psychological services, and students. Since this is an action committee, representation should be limited to a functioning number, and a division of labor established in its early organizational phases. Some may function best as advisors or consultants while others wi'l design and write the curriculum. The effectiveness of the committee is dependent on the quality of information from the school/community health education advisory committee and its ability to respond to their recommendations. These recommendations may apply to curriculum development for any or all phases of the comprehensive health education program; for learners in grades K–12, teacher in-service programs, or adult health education programs.

The *learning resources and evaluation committee* has three major functions: (1) to review, evaluate, and make recommendations about the varieties of learning resources available, (2) to assist in the development of the evaluation program, and (3) to make recommendations about policies for the selection and use of resources. This committee must function in close cooperation with the program and curriculum committee since evaluation and the use of learning resources are inherent components of curriculum and the health education program. It may be advisable for these two committees to meet periodically to share their progress and to advise each other about new directions that are needed.

The *teaching/learning teams* culminate the activities of all other committees by implementing the programs developed by them. The very nature of many of the health issues that are identified may require expertise beyond that possessed by the health educator or elementary school classroom teacher. To overcome this problem, teams of teachers may be formed to combine knowledge and experience about complex health issues, improving the health learning experiences for students. For example, science and social studies teachers could team with health educators to motivate learning of genetic health issues from the viewpoint of the science of genetics, the health implications of genetic counseling, and the political and legal ramifications of genetic engineering. In addition, students could be trained in peer teaching and become a part of a teaching team with teachers, or conduct peer teaching sessions with other students.

Interdisciplinary approaches should be used when appropriate; however, they do require extensive team planning and follow-up procedures in order to be effective. These methods are discussed in more detail in Chapter 12.

Dealing with the board of education

The board of education is the legally constituted body for setting policies governing the school district. The health education administrator and other members of the health education team recognize that positive interaction with the school board is a key factor in the establishment of productive school/community relations. As Sumption and Engstrom point out: "It is important to good school-community relations that the school board be recognized as having comprehensive and final authority, subject to the limitations imposed by the state. All other citizens serve as advisors, counselors, guides, resource people, and executors. School boards almost without exception are composed of lay citizens, so that in effect the decisions made are those of lay people."[8] However, school boards are not necessarily representative of the community as a whole and may not yield to the demands of the public. Therefore, public relations with the board, although vitally important, should not be considered all-inclusive. Every effort must be made by the health professionals in the community interested in health education to develop positive relations with as many elements in the community as possible to help insure the establishment of the best possible health education program within the jurisdiction of the school.

In addition to the various school community techniques discussed earlier, the health education administrator should also communicate with the various subcommittees of the board of education and attempt to gain representation on these committees where appropriate to aid in the development of community understanding of the health education program. Because of the direct access these committees have to the whole board, any health education representation will add to the stature of health education in the eyes of the board. It may be possible to organize the school/community health education advisory committee as a subcommittee of the board of education. This would result in direct communication with the board, expediting their work and that of the health education administrator.

Relation to other school disciplines

Other authorities have often stressed the desirability of integrating health education into other areas of the school's curriculum, especially at the elementary school level. The value of such an integration cannot be disputed considering the difficulty of establishing the viability of health education in some school districts. Traditionally, health education has been placed in school districts in whatever manner was possible (often the integration approach), in hopes that the program would prove itself and subsequently be recognized by the central administration. However, we have progressed beyond this point as a profession.

The health education profession must now stand by the philosophy that health topics should be covered by other disciplines only to enhance the quality of those fields of study. If any true integration is to occur, it should take the form of other disciplines being integrated into the health education program. In essence, the health education program should become the basis for all curricular activities of a school system. The occurrence of such a phenomenon is made possible through the activities of the health education administrator.

The establishment of teaching teams enhances the possibility of opening up the lines of communication between the health education program and other curricular areas within the school system. It is refreshing to note that such communications are initiated by health educators and not vice versa. One of the key factors in establishing credibility within a school district and enhancing the concept of professionalism is achieving a status equal to that of any other discipline. If the health educator takes the lead to enhance the curricular offerings for students, then the health education program will gain the respect of other educators in the school district.

Obviously, little can be done on a district-wide basis to promote interdisciplinary communications that result in any productive programmatic enhancement without such leadership. However, in terms of offering a systematic interdisciplinary approach spanning grade levels and schools, a health education administrator is required so that the program may be observed in a more or less panoramic view.

SCHOOL/COMMUNITY RELATIONS

Public relations

Communication is the foundation for public relations. A lack of effective public relations by the health education profession has been in evidence for many years. Health educators simply have failed to communicate their message to the general public. It seems as though health education has been intended for the health educator rather than for the health needs of people. Hanlon is emphatic about this situation: "It is self-evident that health education has been regarded too much in the past as private preserve by the professionals in public health, medicine, and education; to be perfectly honest, they have tended to be stuffy, overly didactic, and lacking in understanding of what really worries the average and less educated components of the population."[9]

Effective public relations requires a thorough knowledge of the community. Based upon this knowledge, an effective communications structure can be established that will aid in the dissemination of information to the community as well as providing a means for meaningful community involvement in the health education program. It may be necessary to study the community to determine what avenues of communications are available and/or possible. Sumption and Engstrom indicate that the following questions should be answered to secure necessary information about the community:

> What is the educational level of the people in the community?
>
> What proportion of the population is at each school-interest level?
>
> What organizations are interested in education, and how large is their membership?
>
> How well developed is the power structure?
>
> What school liaison groups exist, and how effective are they?
>
> What media of communication does the school community possess?
>
> How effective are these media?
>
> Which are available to the school, and which might be made available?[10]

Very often, chief school administrators of school districts delegate the responsibility for public relations to a member of their staff. If such a person exists, it behooves the health education administrator to utilize this resource, both to enhance intraschool communications and to eliminate the unnecessary task of studying certain elements of the community that have already been cultivated by the central administration. This does not mean that all public relations efforts stop here, however. It is necessary for health education administrators to cultivate their own community resources, since one central public relations office cannot meet the needs of *each* program within the school system.

Public relations implies more than just informing the public of the activities of the health education program. In its total sense, public relations is the involvement of the community in the planning, organization, and implementation of the program in a concerted and coordinated effort. The effective utilization of advisory committees as personal contacts with other health agencies and the board of education are all part of an effective public relations effort.

Working with community health agencies

In addition to working with community health agencies through their representation on the health education advisory committee, it is necessary for the health education administrator to assess the types of educational activities being conducted by these agencies. Communications with them will aid in the coordination of the health education efforts of the school and community. For example, it may be possible to involve students in hypertensive screening programs coordinated by the local heart association, or in the activities of nursing homes and hospitals. In this way, students can contribute significantly to the promotion of health within the community, as well as acquiring greater insight into the health issue.

It may very well be that through sound health education programs emanating from the school, health agencies not currently offering much in the way of health education will begin to become involved after observing the benefits that result from such programs. In essence, the health education program will have as much educational value for the various health agencies as it does for the community as a whole, ultimately benefiting all concerned.

Adult health education

The major emphasis of traditional health education programs has been the education of children and youth. The adult population has been largely ignored by schools until very recently. Yet exposing adults to health education can be one of the most valuable public relations tools available to the health educator, as well as reinforcing other health education endeavors.

Ideally, these programs should be made available through the continuing education department of the school district. However, other options include the public health agencies as well as civic and church groups. In some instances, nearby colleges have established courses, seminars, and institutes on various health issues. Since health matters affect all segments of the population, it is important to make use of a variety of avenues available to insure that most of the citizenry have the opportunity to become health educated. Health education for adults should be directed toward: (1) encouraging awareness of the health problems prevalent in the community, (2) disseminating factual health information and dispelling misconceptions, (3) teaching the value of the health education being offered by the school and community health agencies, (4) motivating adults to support health education programs, (5) offering opportunities to share experiences with others concerning certain health issues, and (6) teaching new ways to communicate with their children, other adults, and health agencies.

Political considerations

One of the most important concepts that health educators must grasp is that knowledge of the political makeup of the community is essential for effective functioning. This goes beyond the party system and beyond the statutes that govern our nation, states, and communities. Those who make the decisions, particularly at the local level, are not necessarily elected officials, but in fact are people whose power supercedes that of the authority structure—power that is often used for the satisfaction of personal interests.[11] This group is often referred to as the "power structure" of the community.

Of course, it is possible for the authority structure and the power structure to coincide. However, health educators must be aware that the two may exist separately. For a program to be successful, it may be necessary to gain the support of both groups. A health educator may also have to consider whether dealing with the power structure at the expense of the authority structure is ethical. Such support may make a beneficial program possible; but is the program so important that it warrants ignoring the authority of the elected officials of the community?

In any case, dealing with these two structures at least indirectly is inevitable. It requires extremely astute educators who are aware of the consequences of their actions. It is quite possible for one aspect of a program—such as sex education—to offend one powerful segment of the community, resulting in the elimination of an entire program. Careful planning and effective public relations are necessary along with community involvement to minimize the impact of relatively small segments of the community that may threaten the democratic principle of majority rule.

In quite another vein, effective school/community relations can come as a result of programmatic involvement in the political arena. Very often legislation that will either enhance or hinder the health education efforts of a community is proposed. It is both educationally beneficial and a positive public relations technique to promote student and community involvement in the political process as it may affect the health of the people. Such activities generate support for the program and provide health learning experiences for both the students and the adult community.

THE SCHOOL HEALTH PROGRAM

Organization and administration

Any organization consists of a structure, functions, and the relationship of the people who achieve its purposes. Each individual must have responsibilities for various aspects of the program and the authority to function within understood boundaries. Frequently, human relations problems arise not because of the people involved but rather because the organizational purposes are confusing or in conflict or the individuals do not clearly understand their role as it relates to others. The organization, therefore, is incomplete unless some person is given responsibility and authority for the entire program. Through appropriate leadership, the people involved are more likely to understand what is expected of them, how they are to work, and their working relationships with others. Without competent leadership, individuals will be unable to perform efficiently simply because of the impractical nature of the organization (or complete lack of it).

Effective organization of the health education program is characterized by efficient working relationships among the people involved, attention to all essential tasks, and a minimum of duplicated effort and expenditure of human energy. In short, a well organized health education program runs smoothly through efficient coordination efforts by the health education administrator.

The result of effective organization is educational productivity. Productivity is measured in terms of the progress that is made toward achieving the purposes of the program as established in the initial stages of planning and development. *The extent to which productivity is achieved with a minimum of effort determines the efficiency of the organization.* Frequently efficiency suffers because of ineffective planning, lack of working skills (or inappropriate delegation of responsibility), and poor coordination.

Attention must be paid to both the physiology and anatomy of the organization. On the one hand, we should be concerned with ideas (philosophy), on the other, we should be concerned with actions. The organization of health education is first conceptualized, then followed by specific programs of functioning. These actions are directed toward all elements of the health education program—curriculum development, teacher training, resource development and selection, methodology, and evaluation. In addition, there must be continuous review of the goals, activities, organizational structure, supervisory strategies, skills, and abilities of the teachers, and review of the ability for the program to respond rapidly to new needs and demands. These must all be accomplished with the knowledge that they must facilitate the implementation of health education for students in grades K–12, adults, teachers, and nonteaching personnel.

Since it is teachers who must implement the health education program, it is important that in-service training opportunities are made available. This is especially true for elementary school teachers, who must teach children in the most formative years. In-service training is important for the following reasons:

1. The curriculum of many teacher training institutions was inadequate to prepare teachers for health education responsibilities at the time they were preparing to be teachers.

2. There is usually a loss of knowledge during the time between college learning and teaching.
3. Continual scientific developments, changing concepts, facilities, and resources necessitate constant study and reevaluation of present knowledge and concepts.
4. The teacher can be given assistance while in service to make adaptations in health education to meet the changing needs of communities and teachers.
5. Teachers and individuals seldom concern themselves with health conditions and problems until faced with specific crisis situations.
6. Teachers with limited training and experience in health education need special in-service training.
7. Teachers with special responsibilities for health education need to be kept informed of changing health education patterns.
8. In-service education helps to improve and maintain the mental, physical, and emotional health of teachers, pupils and the community, as well as developing broader understanding.
9. In-service training in all phases of education brings about more effective cooperation and communication between teachers and the community.
10. In-service training helps teachers become more aware of their role within the health education program.

Health education for students with handicaps

Health education is as important for students with physical or mental handicaps as it is for those without serious disabilities. It should be emphasized that the goals for these students should be the same as for those in the normal population. As one authority has pointed out, we must realize that despite disabilities, "the mentally handicapped child or adult is not very different from any other human being. First, this individual is a human being, and only secondly does he have a handicap. His basic needs are as great is anyone else's, but his difficulties in learning, relating and coping may be greater. His behavioral manifestations may be inappropriate and because of this so-called negative behavior, his problems are great."[12]

Any efforts that the school makes in the area of health education for students with handicapping conditions must be coordinated with the other areas of health education within the district. The comprehensiveness of the program will determine how this will be accomplished. In addition, the program must be coordinated with the psychological and medical services of the community and school as are the other aspects of health education.

For the physically handicapped, the health education program can play a key role in assuring that the school adopts the physical facilities accordingly: accessible doorways that will accommodate wheel chairs, ramps in addition to stairs, and accessible toilet facilities, for example.

In the final analysis, the health education program for the physically and mentally impaired has as its major goal the enhancement of the quality of life for these individuals so that they may achieve the greatest effectiveness of which they are capable; they too can achieve optimal health.

The role of school health and medical services

The health and medical services components of the health education program is made up of medical and dental services and psychological services, and should fall under the administrative leadership of the health education administrator. They perform the screening and intervention functions traditionally assigned to them, but because they function within the school setting, they also become involved in the health education program. This area has both intra– and extraschool components; the intraschool components are composed of medical and dental personnel (school physician, school nurse-teacher, dental hygiene teacher, and supervising dentist) and the psychological services (school psychologist, school social worker, and guidance counselors). The extraschool components include community referral to medical and public health services, mental health and psychological services, and family counseling services.

Anderson and Creswell[13] indicate that school health services include appraisal, health guidance and supervision, prevention and control of communicable diseases, remedial measures, and facilities for carrying out these functions. Although this does summarize these services adequately, we must not lose sight of the effects that personal contact by the health services personnel can have on students' health behavior.

DEFINITIVE UNDERSTANDINGS

Organizing for health education is a fundamental process necessary for its success in serving the people of a community. The activities of organized health education include planning, structuring, administering, evaluating, and adapting under the leadership of a competent health education administrator. The health education administrator must be prepared in both health education and administration.

Organized health education tends to facilitate the health education of children, youth, and adults. Mismanagement and lack of funds, facilities, and personnel all have a retarding effect on the growth of health education programs. The result is lowered status and decreased effectiveness. Adequate organization and administration guarantees coordination of programs directed toward health need satisfaction.

The initial step in planning for organization is answering the following questions: (1) Who is to be educated? (2) How shall they be educated? (3) How shall the program be staffed? (4) What physical facilities shall be required? (5) How shall the program be supported and managed? and (6) What shall be the structure of the program?

The promotion and maintenance of health are dependent upon the interaction of all segments of the health care system. This requires a strong organizational structure and administration. These will provide the means for improving communication and cooperation between health-related program directors.

Organized health education is most effective when it consists of a variety of people combining their talents to accomplish tasks that no one of them could do alone. The health education administrator provides direction, leadership, and coordination. Such an arrangement tends to effectively combine idealism with pragmatism and perpetuates comprehensive and progressive health education activities that are health promotive rather than being crisis-oriented.

There are essentially five forces that influence organization and administration of health education programs: (1) political pressures, (2) social pressures, (3) budgetary constraints, (4) activities of school/community health organizations, and (5) talents of the health education administrator. These are not mutually exclusive; they tend to be interactional and interdependent.

An effective school/community communications network is basic to program functioning. It must be planned and continuous, with a two-way flow of information. School health education administrators should take the initiative in establishing the communications network. They have three options available for stimulating school/community communications: (1) locality development, (2) social planning, and (3) social action.

With the rapid development of health education programs in recent years, a need for qualified leadership has been created. Many colleges have responded to the need by offering programs that combine health education and administration. Overall, the health administrator should possess at least six characteristics: (1) training and experience in both public and school health education, (2) an understanding of the principles of learning, (3) the ability to communicate effectively, (4) the ability to organize, (5) the ability to identify health goals, and (6) an in-depth knowledge of current health problems and how education can contribute to their solution.

The functions and responsibilities of the health education administrator are numerous and varied. They can be categorically identified as planning, organizing, coordinating, conducting and administering, supervising, communicating, and evaluating. Probably the most fundamental activity of the administrator, and one that permeates all others, is communicating effectively. Within each of these categories are numerous basic strategies that the administrator uses to achieve the purposes of the health education program. However, the success of the program is dependent chiefly upon the quality of the people responsible for the activities being conducted.

There are sixteen successful administrative techniques available to the health education administrator. They are: (1) involving qualified people in program development, (2) becoming a generalist who is knowledgeable about all facets of administration, (3) treating all personnel equally and fairly, (4) defining the organizational structure, (5) establishing a productive environment and communication system, (6) following an operational model, (7) utilizing established principles in administering the program, (8) making effective use of community organizations, (9) generating support for the program, (10) using a democratic style in administering the program, (11) functioning within the policies of the organization, (12) using the best decision-making skills available and involving those who are affected by the decision, (13) delegating responsibility to the appropriate authority, (14) allowing those who are closest to the problem make decisions regarding it, (15) delegating responsibility to those who are competent to follow through, (16) establishing an effective continuous communications network.

The use of advisory committees can do much to facilitate the achievement of goals through the use of resource people who possess experience and expertise in a variety of health areas. At least four such committees should be considered: (1) a school/community advisory committee made up of people from outside the organization, (2) a health education program and curriculum committee consisting of teachers, administrators, and nonteaching personnel, (3) a learning resources and evaluation committee made up of teachers and students, (4) teaching/learning teams composed of teachers who can implement an interdisciplinary approach and students trained in peer education. Activities of all committees should be coordinated by the health education administrator.

It is important to establish lines of communication with the board of education. The health education administrator should act in a consultation and advisory capacity to the board. Suggesting that the school/community health education advisory committee be organized as a subcommittee of the board of education could be an initial step in establishing effective lines of communication.

It is important that the health education program utilizes the talents of other teachers in other disciplines through interdisciplinary approaches when appropriate. However, other disciplines should be integrated into the health education program rather than health being integrated into other disciplines. Ideally, all other disciplines should evolve from health education, since it is concerned with all elements of life influencing individual effectiveness.

The establishment of school/community relations is fundamental to the successful functioning of any health education program. This cooperation can be accomplished through public relations programs consisting of working relationships with community health agencies, offering adult health education programs, and making appropriate use of the political structure. The basis for effective public relations is the development of continuous communication with key people in the community as well as with the general population. The use of the various media can be a most effective vehicle for initiating a school/community communications network, as well as personal contacts with agency directors and serving on boards of directors or other community health committees.

Organization depends on structure, functions, and people to achieve its purposes. In addition, the organization must have a person who is responsible for administering all phases of the organization and supervising the activities of the people involved. This insures that individuals work well together and that there is a minimum of duplicated effort. This will result in educational productivity, which is measured in terms of the progress being made. Productivity is indicative of efficiency. Essentially, health education organization is concerned with actions that will make ideas a reality.

The elements of the health education program are: curriculum development, teacher training, selection of resources, methodology, and evaluation. It is especially important to develop and implement continuous in-service training programs for elementary school teachers since many did not receive adequate health education during preservice training.

Health education should be offered for students with handicapping conditions as well as for all others in grades K–12. Adult health education is also essential to insure that concepts developed by children and youth are reinforced in the home and community.

Personnel in health and medical services have much to offer the health education program. The basic activities of health services fall into three general areas: (1) appraisal, (2) health guidance and supervision, and (3) prevention and remedial measures.

PROBLEMS
FOR DISCUSSION

1. Identify the guiding principles of organizing for health education.
2. Why is it important to organize the health education program under the leadership of a trained health education administrator?
3. What qualities should the health education administrator possess to insure proper and successful organization and administration of the health education program?
4. List the factors that influence the organization and administration of health education. Describe how each affects organization and administration.
5. Discuss the importance of effective communication for both the internal and external aspects of the health education program.
6. Outline the functions and responsibilities of the health education administrator.
7. Describe the functions of various committees as they relate to smooth coordination of the health education program.
8. List the groups that the health education administrator must communicate

effectively with and state why this interaction is essential for the success of the program.

9. Describe how the health education administrator can relate the health program to other disciplines and why this relationship is important.
10. List the chief components of a well organized health education program and state the learning audience with whom each component is primarily concerned.
11. Develop a philosophy of health education organization and administration. Include purposes, goals of the programs, components, strategies for initiating programs and for implementing them, and how the health education administrator can work with other groups or agencies.
12. State why it is important to organize and implement special health education programs for students with handicapping conditions.
13. Identify the social forces that impinge upon the health education program. What are the implications for the future of health education?
14. Outline the directions that health education should be taking in the next ten years and justify each.

REFERENCES

1. Miller, Van, *The Public Administration of American School Systems*, Macmillan Publishing Co., New York, 1965, pp. 66–68.
2. Hochbaum, Godfrey M., "At the Threshold of a New Era," *Health Education*, American Alliance for Health, Physical Education and Recreation, Washington, July–August, 1976, vol. 7, no. 4, p. 3.
3. Ibid.
4. Mayshark, Cyrus, and Donald B. Shaw, *Administration of School Health Programs: Its Theory and Practice*, C. V. Mosby Company, Saint Louis, 1967, pp. 51–52.
5. Miller, op. cit., pp. 65–66.
6. Bedworth, Albert E., and Joseph A. D'Elia, *Basics of Drug Education*, Baywood Publishing Company, Farmingdale, New York, 1973, p. 30.
7. Ibid., p. 31.
8. Sumption, Merle R., and Yvonne Engstrom, *School-Community Relations*, McGraw-Hill Book Company, New York, 1966, p. 159.
9. Hanlon, John J., *Public Health: Administration and Practice*, 6th ed., C. V. Mosby Company, Saint Louis, 1974, p. 671.
10. Sumption and Engstrom, op. cit., p. 130.
11. Ibid., p. 13.
12. Dippo, Jeanette, *Health Education for Special Children, A Curriculum Guide*, Cortland-Madison Board of Cooperative Educational Services, New York, 1976.
13. Anderson, C. L., and William H. Creswell, Jr., *School Health Practice*, 6th ed., C. V. Mosby Company, Saint Louis, 1976, pp. 95–97.

*Three characteristics of the time
directly affect curricular reform:
the rapid advance of knowledge, the
prodigious growth of population,
the prevalence of violence and
catalysmic social change.*

Sidney Sulkin

The time has come for the health
education profession to take a
backward look at the health
education curriculum. This is
necessary so that we can forge ahead
to new levels of curriculum design
that will reflect the health concerns
of children and youth rather than
those of the teacher of health and
the school administration.

AEB
DAB

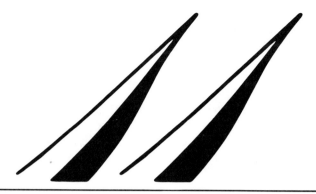

Curriculum
Development
in Health
Education

INTRODUCTION: ORIENTATION
TO CURRICULUM DEVELOPMENT

What is curriculum?

During the national economic crunch of 1975, several state departments of education began to make a concerted effort toward "returning to the basics of education." It is assumed that by "basics", they meant reading, writing, and arithmetic. This was a misconception for several reasons. First, the so called "basics" have never been removed from the curriculum. Second, what is more *basic* than the health of children and youth? And, finally, what did these educators perceive curriculum to be?

Health education has never actually been removed from the curriculum, nor can it be. It is only disguised by different labels, deemphasized, and moved down on the list of priorities. It can not be removed from the curriculum as long as teachers view and treat their pupils as human beings; as long as teachers are concerned for the welfare of children; as long as learning, any kind of learning, affects the way children view themselves, others, and the world in which they live; as long as learning takes place wherever and whenever children are in touch with their environment; and as long as the curriculum can not be restricted solely to the school environment.

In 1971, the Connecticut State Board of Education published *Connecticut Citizens Response to Education Goals, 1971–72,* which cited six main goals:

1. Each student learns to communicate effectively.
2. Each student accepts learning as a lifelong continuing process of self-development.
3. Each student develops the skills, knowledge, and values necessary for responsible citizenship.
4. Each student increases his ability to understand himself and to function in his environment.
5. Each student acquires habits and attitudes which have proven value for health and family life.
6. Each student applies his accumulated knowledge and skills to present day living.

Each of the above goals were divided into "subgoals" totalling 80 in all. Public response to these goals and subgoals was then solicited. School administrators felt that family, health, and career goals were most important, while parents had only an average response to these. Below is a summary of health-related goals for students and the percent of respondents that considered them most important.

- 69.3%—increasing the ability to understand oneself and to function in one's environment

- 68.1%—taking responsibility for personal development and obligations
- 66.7%—recognizing and accepting strengths and weaknesses and developing personal goals accordingly
- 66.4%—accepting changes and adapting to changing situations
- 65.8%—acquiring an understanding of the extent of control over one's body, mind, and future
- 65.7%—acquiring habits and attitudes that have proven value for health and family life
- 65.7%—recognizing feelings and emotions as a component of life situations
- 65.0%—applying accumulated knowledge and skills to everyday life
- 62.0%—becoming aware of the potential harm caused by excessive use of alcohol and/or tobacco
- 61.8%—acquiring an understanding of the interdependence of people
- 61.2%—valuing self and others positively
- 59.8%—developing ethical, social, and spiritual values and using them in establishing personal goals
- 59.4%—acquiring the ability to act as an intelligent consumer
- 58.5%—acquiring good safety habits
- 53.3%—understanding the relationship between health and physical activity

The goal considered most important by most respondents was learning to communicate effectively (87.2%).

Curriculum is any and all things that influence learning in any way. It can be planned and deliberate, or unplanned and haphazard. The school health curriculum should be viewed in terms of a philosophical base and planned as a cohesive and progressive process of health learning. Koopman defined curriculum development as "that aspect of teaching and administration that designedly, systematically, cooperatively and continuously seeks to improve the teaching-learning process."[1] Curriculum development in health education, as with teaching and learning, is a continuous process embracing initial construction, evaluation, reorganization, revision, experimentation, administration, and all other elements of the school and community that influences the quality of learning and teaching. The health education curriculum, although planned and organized, reflects the importance of the contributions to health learning from unplanned and unforeseen experiences within the school and community settings. We are beginning to eliminate such labels as extracurricular or cocurricular experiences since many of these do contribute to the achievement of the goals of health education and are, therefore, an integral part of the health education program that should be taken into consideration when planning the health curriculum.

We have heard a lot over the past ten to twenty years about humanizing education. Health education lends itself to this process more readily than any other discipline in the school's curricular offerings. As a matter of fact, humanization is the ultimate goal of the health education curriculum and, as such, it must reflect this in its design, as well as in everything else it attempts to accomplish. Most importantly, the teacher must play the humanizing role to facilitate this endeavor. The teacher, therefore, must understand the full potential of humanity both from the individual's viewpoint and from that of his or her society. By humanizing the health education curriculum, we mean that it must be designed as a way of helping children to become successful people. It must be, as Wilhelm states, "warm, accepting, helping."[2]

The purpose of curriculum guides

A curriculum guide is, according to Saylor and Alexander,[3] "a written curriculum plan." They go on to say that it is "used to describe many types of written materials designed to give guidance to teachers and others in the final development of the curriculum in learning situations." Essentially, the health education curriculum guide is the culminating document of evaluation and planning related to the health education needs of the learner. It is a tool to assist teachers and learners in systematically achieving health goals through predetermined processes. Curriculum guides take several forms—from the master plan to the course of study. Each of these will be described in detail later on in this chapter.

The curriculum guide establishes the framework for communications between the learner and teachers or other sources of learning to insure efficiency of learning. It documents the thinking of the curriculum committee, the goals they feel are important, the most effective ways of achieving them, the sequence of learning and its boundaries, and ways to ascertain program effectiveness and learner progress.

The basic principles of curriculum development

Although there is no single ideal way of developing the health education curriculum, there are certain basic concepts and procedures that seem to apply to all curriculum development efforts. Curriculum development should be undertaken only when it has been found that a need exists and that this need can be at least partially fulfilled through the education process. Having established this, the next step is to begin to plan the curriculum, its development, and its implementation.

Planning the health education curriculum should involve the participation of many people. The establishment of a curriculum development committee with appropriate representation from the varieties of health areas for which the curriculum is intended will facilitate this effort. The health education curriculum must possess certain basic characteristics if it is to be effective. For instance, it must be so designed that it is *dynamic* and lends itself to change as new developments in the health sciences and educational process arise. Planning must be *continuous* as long as there is a need for the area in the school's total educational program. Development and implementation procedures should be consistent with the general philosophy and goals of the school's educational program and those of the community. Evaluation of effectiveness should be a planned and integral component of any curriculum development design. Once these factors have been clarified, curriculum guides can be developed.

THE VARIETIES OF CURRICULUM GUIDES

Introduction: statement of philosophy

The development of curriculum guides should proceed from general premises to specific procedures that will favorably affect the health learning of children and youth. The guide should provide guidance in the scope of learning and the progressive sequence that it should take. To accomplish this, it is necessary to first establish clearly the program aim; that is, the overall mission of the health program.

Once the program aim is stated, the general goals must be identified. These will describe how the learners will be different following their experiences resulting from participation in the program. Goals are further defined by the identification of both terminal and enabling objectives. These form the basis for curriculum guide design and development. They establish the boundaries and suggest the procedures for health learning.

Figure 11–1 illustrates the relationship between program development and curriculum guide development. The guides should evolve as necessary tools for implementing the program. As a result, it is important to establish the purposes of the guides as they relate to helping the teacher and the learner to achieve the program goals. The following preliminary questions will be helpful in providing guidance throughout the stages of curriculum development:

Suggested preliminary questions for curriculum development
1. What evidence is available to support and justify the program?
2. How will the curriculum materials favorably affect initiation and completion of the program aim?
3. What is the program aim?
4. How will achievement of the aim promote health and prevent disease, disability, and/or premature death?
5. What goals must the learner achieve to accomplish the aim?
6. What do the curricular guides intend to accomplish?
7. How will they achieve the purpose?
8. What design of the curriculum is most likely to provide the teacher with the most efficient ways to initiate and implement the program?
9. What terminal objectives will result in the learner reaching the goals?

FIGURE 11–1 Curriculum Development in Health Education

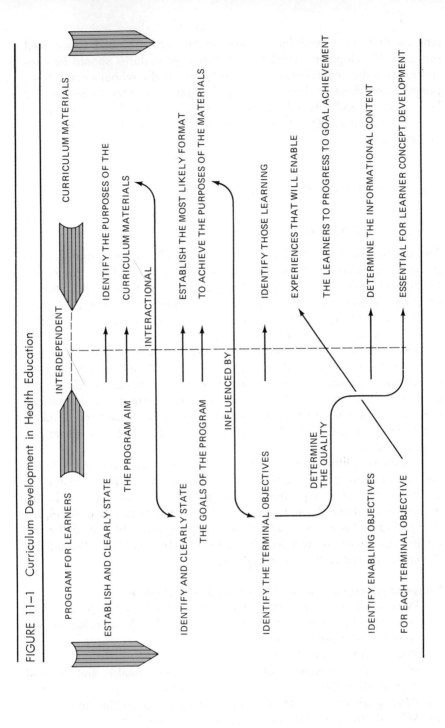

10. What enabling objectives must be achieved by the learner to achieve the terminal objectives?
11. What learning experiences are necessary to assist the learner in achieving the enabling objectives?
12. What information does the teacher need to effectively assist the learner through the learning experiences?
13. What informational content will assist the learner to develop appropriate concepts relative to the health area?

The resource guide

Once the preliminary steps have been taken in establishing the aim and goals, it is usually useful to develop a resource guide as the next step. The *resource guide* is a list of all the people, materials, and other resources available within the school or community that can be used as aids in implementing the program once it is completely developed. In developing the resource guide, it is not necessary to evaluate the effectiveness of the resources available. This process will, however, be necessary when developing the course of study.

The resource guide can take a variety of forms. Some merely list all resources as they are discovered without any particular categorizations. The most useful format appears to be where the resources are placed into two general classes: (1) human resources and (2) material resources, which are further subdivided according to acceptable classifications. For example, human resources could be classified as intraschool and community. These can be further subdivided into functional categories such as speakers, consultants, and so on.

Material resources should be identified in a similar manner, indicating those available in the school and in the community and where they can be found. As curriculum guidelines are being developed, it will prove helpful if the material resources have been listed according to their type (e.g., films, slides, posters, pamphlets, and so on). Many resource guides also list the materials according to health topic areas (e.g., alcohol, mental health, nutrition, etc.). Organizing the resource guide in this manner will make it more useable when it becomes time to develop other curriculum guides that will make use of the information contained in the resource guide.

The master plan

The chief purpose of the master plan is to put into perspective all of the elements that constitute the total health program of the school. Although content and format may vary from one situation to another, the master plan will always contain at least (1) a statement of the school's philosophy of health education, (2) the aim of the total health program, (3) the goals of health education, (4) the scope and sequence of health education, and (5) the overall evaluation program plans. Essentially it is an overview of the what, when, and why of the health program. Except in the statement of philosophy and evaluation program plans, the master plan tends to avoid detailed descriptions, leaving these for inclusion in the course of study guide.

Some school districts have developed what is called a curriculum guide. It is essentially a master plan but contains more details in regard to grade level offerings and other suggestions. The curriculum guide, for example, includes the master plan plus such things as resources available for each grade or developmental level, suggestions for use of the curriculum materials, specific objectives for each grade level, and so on. However, the usual procedure is to have these kinds of suggestions for inclusion in the course of study guides. The reader is referred to Figure 4–1 (on page 73), which diagrammatically provides the framework for curriculum development. The master plan, when carefully conceived, puts all elements of the health program into proper perspective and provides the blueprint for more detailed curriculum development and implementation. This blueprint is illustrated in Figure 11–2.

The course of study guide

The course of study is a detailed written guide for each grade or developmental level. Again, the specific design or format will vary, but certain essential elements are vital for its useability by the teacher. As such, the course of study guide contains at least the terminal and enabling objectives,* a wide variety of suggested learning experiences, suggested learning aids, evaluation procedures, and informational content.

The course of study must be carefully developed, since it is the document that provides teachers with all of the information and guidance necessary to implement the health education program for the learners. It is the document from which the teacher develops the daily lesson plan. Therefore, it must provide a wide variety of suggestions for learning experiences from which the teacher can choose, so that all learners will be motivated to learn and will have opportunities to proceed at their individual rates.

The course of study guide provides the teacher with sufficient information so as to minimize further research, but stimulates teacher creativity. Its design is extremely important and should be selected based upon its potential useability as a guide for teaching and learning. Specific suggestions along these lines are presented in the following section of this chapter.

---

* Many different terms are used to describe objectives. They may be called macro and micro objectives, goals and behavioral objectives, or terminal and enabling. Regardless of the label used, they should be carefully selected and precisely written. They are learner-centered rather than teacher or program-centered.

FIGURE 11–2   A Blueprint for Curriculum Development

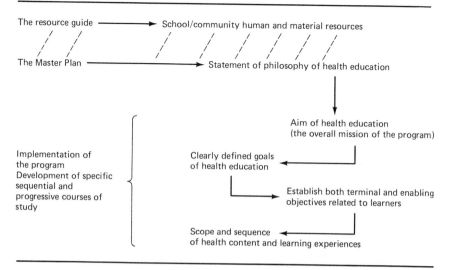

The lesson plan

There are nearly as many different kinds of lesson plans as there are teachers. Lesson plans by necessity must be tailored to the individual learners and qualities of the teacher. At any rate, the lesson plan is the culmination of all curriculum planning and development. It determines what will happen to the learners on a day to day basis.

Characteristics of lesson plans will vary considerably not only from teacher to teacher, but also with the same teacher on different occasions. However, it is generally agreed that lesson plans should contain, either overtly or by implication, at least four characteristics. First, they must be flexible and subject to adaptation to spontaneous circumstances that can arise on any particular day. Second, the objectives for the day should be clearly stated and understood by both the teacher and the learners. Objectives should be in behavioral, performance, or measurable form. Third, learning experiences should be learner-centered or experiential in nature and tailored to meet the varieties of individual learner needs, interests, motivational levels, and capabilities. They should be related to real life situations. Finally, each lesson should contain provisions for evaluation of the quality of learning taking place. Evaluation is always related to objective achievement.

CURRICULUM GUIDE DESIGN

Choosing the design

Choosing the design of the curriculum guide is one of the most important phases in planning the health education curriculum. The final format selected may very well determine the useability of the guide by the teacher. It is, therefore, essential that a variety of formats be considered. (Some suggestions regarding this are presented in the final discussions of this section.) Below is a list of criteria that should be used in the early stages of planning and development of the health education curriculum.

Criteria for curriculum development
1. Is the program justified?
2. Are the curriculum materials necessary for the success of the program?
3. Do the guides provide relevant suggestions for teaching strategies?
4. Are there a variety of learning activities?
5. Is the informational content meaningful, relevant, and important?
6. Are the learning experiences appropriate for the developmental levels of the learners?
7. Do the suggestions in the guides allow for learner variations?
8. Is the aim realistic and achievable?
9. Are the goals and objectives meaningful and achievable?
10. Do the goals and objectives point toward completion of the aim?
11. Is completion of the aim vital for promoting health and preventing disease, disability, and premature death?
12. Is the format of the guide functional?
13. Does the format and content of the guide expedite learning?
14. Is the content of the guide essentially positive?
15. Does the guide suggest a progression of learning?
16. Is there direct or implied evaluation of learner progress?
17. Does the content of the guides promote learner success? Is threat of failure avoided?
18. Do suggestions for learning include the development of the cognitive, affective, and psychomotor domains?
19. Are there opportunities for learner choices?
20. Do learner activities motivate the learner?
21. Does the guide provide the teacher with sufficient information regarding the topic?
22. Are suggested learning resources appropriate, accurate, timely, attractive, useable, available?
23. Do the activities encourage active, rather than passive, learning?
24. Do the suggestions promote student-centered learning rather than teacher-dominated teaching?
25. Do the learning experiences promote cooperative rather than competitive learning?
26. Is learning primarily inductive rather than deductive?
27. Do learning experiences promote comprehension rather than superficial memorization of facts?
28. Is the content of the curriculum guide consistent with present health education philosophy and practice?

29. Are the suggestions contained in the guide consistent with the principles of learning?
30. Is the guide based upon acceptable psychological and educational principles?

The curriculum developers should establish the most likely format to achieve the goals or purposes for which the curriculum materials are intended.

Determining the content and process

As stated above, the kind of content of any particular guide is dependent upon its purpose; that is, the purpose of the master plan is quite different from the purpose of the course of study guide. In this respect, it is necessary for the curriculum development committee to establish clearly the intent of each guide and to make certain that its content satisfies this intent.

Looking at the comprehensive health education curriculum as a whole, and the kinds of curriculum guides necessary, as described earlier, the guides in one way or another should achieve the following goals:

1. To provide teachers with a philosophical foundation for health education.
2. To provide teachers with the aim of health education.
3. To provide teachers with the goals of health education.
4. To provide teachers with in-depth factual information regarding pertinent health problems and issues.
5. To provide teachers with descriptions of the most effective methodologies to be used in health education.
6. To provide teachers with sources of the most current health research information available.
7. To provide teachers with suggested evaluative procedures and techniques to be used in determining the effectiveness of the program, methods, and learner progress.
8. To provide teachers with essential factual health information necessary to effectively help the learners achieve their objectives.
9. To provide teachers with a variety of suggested learner activities related to and directed toward the achievement of specific learner objectives.
10. To provide teachers with a variety of suggested educational aids related to enhancing learning experiences for learners to more effectively and efficiently achieve their objectives.
11. To provide teachers with ways in which learning aids can most effectively be used under a variety of circumstances.
12. To provide teachers with the most appropriate scope and sequence for health learning and the most efficient method for implementing the health education program.

13. To provide teachers with suggestions of how to use the curriculum materials most effectively.
14. To provide teachers with sources of assistance within the school.

Examples and comparisons of design

Functionalism is the key to curriculum design. Curriculum designers and developers should ask the following preliminary questions before deciding on the final format of the curriculum guides:

1. Is the design functional?
2. Will it be used by the teacher?
3. Does it reflect the school's overall philosophy of health education as well as education in general?
4. Is it experientially oriented? Does it provide for learner involvement?
5. Does the guide's format allow for progressive health learning?
6. Are learning experiences sequential and progressive? Are they appropriate and dynamic?
7. Does the design tend to put the elements of teaching and learning in perspective? Are objectives, informational content, learning experiences, and evaluation tied together throughout the guide?
8. Is the design such that the teacher and learners can make adaptations readily as occasions arise?
9. Is the format learner-centered?
10. Does the format reflect the school, the community, and the world as learning environments?

Over the years, many styles of curriculum design have evolved. The two most popular and general formats are the vertical and the horizontal. In the vertical format, which is the most traditional, the usual procedure is to (1) identify the specific topic to be covered, (2) identify the objectives for the topic, (3) outline the informational content, (4) list several learning or teacher activities, and (5) list several learning and teaching aids. Generally, the format of the vertical design would appear as follows:

1. Topic
2. Objectives
3. Content Outline
4. Activities
5. Resources

The advantage of the vertical format is its simplicity of development. However, it tends to be cognitively oriented, its parts are fragmented, making it difficult to conceptualize its elements, and it is difficult to use as an aid in planning lessons. It is a design that is being used less and less, since it fails to meet the functionalism criterion.

Over the past two or three decades, more curriculum developers have been using a variety of forms of the horizontal design. Its advantage rests primarily with its useability, since it shows progressive development of informational content and relationships between all of its elements at a glance. A popular variation of the horizontal format is shown in Table 11–1. A variation to this design is presented in Table 11–2. This latter variation, it will be noted, is more simplistic, flexible, and useable. It provides the teacher not only with suggestions for student learning, but also suggestions for carrying out these activities most effectively. The "Information for Teachers" includes factual information for dealing with anticipated questions, as well.

A final variation to the horizontal format is illustrated in Table 11–3 (on page 264). It provides for a conceptualization of topic, objectives, and related experiential learning strategies.

TRENDS IN CURRICULUM DEVELOPMENT

The informational approach

We have stressed the importance of accurate and relevant health information in several contextual frames of reference. At point for further clarification is in order as we continue our discussion of curriculum development. First, curriculum development is one of the most important steps taken for applying what is known about health and education to favorably influence each learner in all matters concerned with individual and societal health. As such, educators and curriculum developers must be clearly conscious of precisely what it is that they want to accomplish and the most effective and efficient approaches needed for this purpose. If cognitive or intellectual development is what is considered important, then the informational approach is justified.

However, we must also remember that intellectual development is expedited and enhanced when the learner is emotionally aroused. Emotional arousal is the result of motivation; motivation takes place when learners want to learn and perceive the importance of this learning. Affective-experiential learning is the most effective method of doing this. Therefore, curriculum development that emphasizes the informational approaches will need to take into account these basic philosophical and psychological principles.

The informational approaches to health learning are concerned with the acquisition of health knowledge and its comprehension and application to the health issue being explored. It is not necessary to create a totally new curriculum design that usually constitutes merely a rewriting of information that has already been done. The procedure usually used is to simply review the various textbooks and other printed matter already available and to select those parts that seem to best apply to local philosophy, goals, and practices. These are then arranged in a logical format and sequence as the curriculum guide.

TABLE 11-1 A Horizontal Design for Curriculum Development

Outline of Content	Major Understandings and Fundamental Concepts	Suggested Teacher Aids and Learning Activities	Supplementary Information for Teachers
This section provides an outline of content necessary to reach the objectives and to develop the basic concepts and understandings. The teacher should select those topics that are most appropriate to the students and the kinds of interests and needs they manifest. It is not always necessary to follow the sequence of the outline.	Included here are the major ideas that should be developed by the student or that should evolve as a result of their learning experiences and activities. Student evaluation should be based on the extent to which they understand these major concepts and how well they can relate these to reality. These concepts and understandings should develop as a result of the learning experiences.	These activities are suggested to assist the teacher in developing understandings of the basic content and to develop desirable attitudes and behavior. The teacher and students may find other more effective learning activities to supplement or supplant those listed. The more meaningful experiences students have, the more likely they are to develop the basic health concepts and attain the desired health objectives.	This section is also intended to assist the teacher in planning, conducting classes, and answering questions from students.

SOURCE: *Suggested Guidelines for the Development of Courses of Study in Health Education for Junior and Senior High Schools*, The University of New York, The State Education Department, 1970.

TABLE 11–2   A Variation in Horizontal Design for Curriculum Development

TOPIC
TERMINAL OBJECTIVE: (also called goal or macro-objective)
ENABLING OBJECTIVE: (also called behavioral, instructional)

Learning Experiences	Teacher Information
Describes the variations of learning experience that will contribute to the achievement of the objectives as listed above. Learning experiences should be listed in some logical order or sequence.	Provides the teacher with the most pertinent factual information needed to assist the learners, to answer questions, or to conduct discussions. In addition, the teacher may be provided with suggestions regarding the best ways to motivate learning or to conduct the learning experiences. Evaluation techniques may also be suggested.

The chief danger, however, is the tendency to clutter the guide with irrelevant information. Frequently, informational approaches tend toward teacher-dominated classes with the lecture approach being the only one that is used. It is essential to recognize that if health information is to be internalized it must be learned in such a way as to allow internalization to occur. Again, we return to experiential learning as the most valuable procedure for health learning.

The learner-centered guide

Throughout all of our discussions we have emphasized that schools and learning are for the learner. In developing curriculum, it is essential that we emphasize not what the teachers can do for learners, but what learners can do for themselves. In this regard, curriculum committees have been prone to include students as members of these committees. Such representation tends to focus attention more on what they, as learners, feel is important for their health promotion and survival. The curriculum committee acquires greater insight into the feelings of the learners and there is a tendency to make curriculum more relevant for them.

Learner-centered guides describe what learners will be doing to achieve their objectives rather than what teachers will be doing. They also demonstrate what the learner is thinking and feeling about health issues and how they can contribute to their solution. Finally, we have seen that curriculum development can possess many faces but in the final analysis, regardless of the form it may take, its purpose is to facilitate learning—learning that is permanent, positive, and useable for improving human effectiveness. The curriculum guide provides the direction for this.

The conceptual approach

We have discussed some of the basic factors related to conceptual development. But we would be remiss if we failed to describe the essential components of this in regard to curriculum design.

The result of the School Health Education Study have had more influence on this approach than any other single factor. The study was initiated in 1961, supported by grants from the Samuel Bronfman Foundation. These funds ran out in 1966, but further grants were awarded by the Minnesota Mining and Manufacturing Company (the 3–M Company) to continue its work in developing a national health education curriculum design. There evolved what is now known as the *conceptual* approach to curriculum design in health education.

The curriculum materials that eventually were formed were designed for teachers, not learners. The aim was to provide teachers with a document that would facilitate the teaching of health education at all grade levels. However, in the process, the curriculum design identified and stressed key learner characteristics and processes for learning consistent with these characteristics.

The conceptual approach is predicated upon three key concepts: (1) *growing and developing,* (2) *decision-making,* and (3) *interaction.* This approach introduced the "triad of health education" consisting of (1) health as a unity of physical, mental, and social well-being; (2) health behavior as knowledge, attitudes, and practices; and (3) a focus upon the health education of individual, family, and community.

The conceptual approach to health education encompasses ten major concepts related to the three key concepts:

1. Growth and development influences and is influenced by the structure and functioning of the individual.
2. Growing and developing follows a predictable sequence, yet is unique for each individual.
3. Protection and promotion of health is an individual, community, and international responsibility.
4. The potential for hazards and accidents exists, whatever the environment.
5. There are reciprocal relationships involving man, disease, and environment.
6. The family serves to perpetuate man and to fulfill certain health needs.
7. Personal health practices are affected by a complexity of forces, often conflicting.
8. Utilization of health information, products, and services is guided by values and perceptions.
9. Use of substances that modify mood and behavior arises from a variety of motivations.

10. Food selection and eating patterns are determined by physical, social, mental, economic, and cultural factors.[4]

These ten concepts were subdivided into thirty-one organizing elements. Although this approach emphasizes concept development, it does not ignore the importance of focusing on behavioral objectives as the stabilizing force for experiential learning to occur.

Table 11–3 provides a comprehensive listing of many of the key concepts that should be developed by elementary school pupils.

THE ELEMENTARY SCHOOL CURRICULUM

Major emphasis

Many of our serious health problems today are the result of individual living patterns that were established very early in life. These have come about because of many adverse factors, not the least of which is inadequate or erroneous health learning during the early, formative years. The fault lies with many of our social institutions, including the family and the educational community. However, they are not alone, for many other social influences have played significant roles in establishing faulty health attitudes and harmful living patterns. It probably does little good to place the blame without exploring ways in which these significant influences can be corrected so that the next generation has acquired more positive attitudes and more constructive modes of living. Willgoose established a perspective along these lines when he stated that "both formal and informal education must emphasize the maintenance and promotion of total health. This is especially true in the elementary school, and it is for this reason that the school health program exists."[5]

As with all health education, the curriculum design should be directed toward satisfying the health needs of children. This brings us to the most vital question: What are the needs of elementary school children? Nearly 25 years ago, the essential needs of elementary school children were listed in a document released by the New York State Education Department: 1. Interpersonal and intergroup relations, 2. Understanding of the world and people, 3. Self-development, 4. Control of the communicative arts and skills, 5. Moral and spiritual values.[6] If these are true and if they are all-inclusive, then the teacher needs to ask, "In what ways can the health education curriculum offerings assist each child to satisfy these needs?" The answer to this question will do two things: (1) it will establish the major emphasis for the elementary school health curriculum, and (2) it will provide guidance for the processes to be used at each progressive grade level as these needs are being developed.

TABLE 11–3 A Curriculum Design for Grades K–6 (A Sample)

Topic	Grades K–3 Concepts	Grades 4–6 Concepts
Mental, Social, and Family Health	1. Family members have specific responsibilities important to the unity of the total family. 2. Sharing responsibilities and activities with family and friends can make life more enjoyable. 3. Family members help each other in many ways. 4. Satisfaction and pleasure can be realized from helping each other. 5. Family members show consideration for each other. 6. It is important to respect others. 7. Cooperation in work and play is essential. 8. Babies need special care and attention. 9. Living things reproduce being like themselves. 10. Boys and girls are different. 11. It is good to be what you are—boy or girl. 12. There are special names for different parts of the body. 13. Plants come from parent plants; baby animals come from parent animals; human babies come from the mother's body. 14. Children come from many different kinds of families and homes.	1. The family unit is important to our society. 2. Parents may express affection differently to younger children than to older ones. 3. Communities should provide opportunities for constructive social and emotional outlets. 4. People express feelings and react differently to various situations. 5. Learning to deal with frustration, conflict, and stress are part of personality development. 6. Problems can arise which disrupt normal family living. 7. The problem-solving technique is helpful in making decisions. 8. It is fun to succeed. 9. Dependability, loyalty, and kindness are a few qualities which are essential to wholesome relationships. 10. Learning to lead and to follow is important to relationships with others. 11. Working independently and planning with others are essential ingredients for successful living. 12. Newborn babies need special care in the hospital and at home. 13. American family patterns have similarities to and differences from those in other parts of the world.

14. The development of self-control is essential to growth and maturity.
15. Some human emotions are fear, anger, and love.
16. Learning to accept disappointment helps to develop the habit of adjusting to things we cannot change.
17. A good sense of humor is a valuable asset throughout life.
18. Heredity is the process by which traits are passed from parents to children.
19. An appreciation of family traditions can enrich family life.
20. Environment influences behavior.
21. Assuming responsibility for one's own behavior increases with maturity.
22. People have basic psychological and physiological needs.
23. Human emotions affect performance, personality, and health.
24. Boys and girls mature at different rates.
25. Understanding menstruation and seminal emission are important to the development of mature attitudes.
26. Reliable sex information is available from parents, teachers, doctors, and nurses.
27. Accepting people of varied religious, social, economic, and racial backgrounds is a sign of social maturity.

TABLE 11-3 A Curriculum Design for Grades K-6 (A Sample) (continued)

Topic	Grades K-3 Concepts	Grades 4-6 Concepts
Nutrition	1. Food is necessary for growth. 2. Water is important to life. 3. Eating a variety of foods is important to health. 4. Eating new foods can be fun. 5. Many people help to grow and prepare foods. 6. Mealtime should be pleasant—family time. 7. Meals should be given an adequate amount of time. 8. It is important to eat a good breakfast, lunch, and dinner. 9. Between-meal snacks can be fun and important to good nutrition.	1. It is important to include food each day from the four basic food groups. 2. Milk is valuable to growing boys and girls. 3. Pasteurization helps to make milk safe. 4. Enriched and homogenized foods contribute to nutrition. 5. Milk is available in many forms. 6. Only safe water should be consumed. 7. Fruits, vegetables, whole grain products, and water help prevent constipation. 8. Attractive meals add to mealtime pleasure. 9. Refrigeration helps to preserve food. 10. Essential nutrients are part of an adequate diet. 11. It is important to distinguish between food facts and fads. 12. Sanitation is important to health. 13. Foods originate in many parts of the world. 14. All fruits and vegetables should be washed before eating. 15. Reliable sources of information about food should be known. 16. Eating patterns vary in different parts of the world. 17. Advertisements about food need to be evaluated.

Safety and First Aid

1. Play things should be carefully stored.
2. We need to know where safe places are.
3. It is important to share and cooperate with play-mates.
4. Boys and girls should use safe routes to school and home again.
5. Policemen help to make streets and roads safer.
6. Certain tools and toys must be used with special care.
7. Boys and girls need to know the differences between friends and strangers.
8. Everyone should know their name and their parents' name, as well as their address.
9. Fire drills in school are important.
10. Adults should be present when boys and girls are swimming.
11. Bicycles can be fun.
12. In case of injury or sudden illness, an adult should be notified.

1. Accident prevention is related to the development of responsible behavior.
2. Boys and girls can help to eliminate safety hazards in their homes and at school.
3. Bicycle riding requires knowing the rules of the road.
4. Fires can be prevented in many ways.
5. It is important to know what to do in case of an emergency.
6. Fire drills help people to know what to do in case of an emergency.
7. Boys and girls can help to make home and school safer places to work, play, and learn.
8. Accidental poisoning can be prevented.
9. Being safety minded is a sign of growing up.
10. Each family member should know where to get help in an emergency.
11. A number of professional organizations are concerned with the promotion of safety.
12. People should swim only in supervised areas.
13. Knowing how to prevent sunburn is important to health.
14. Keeping calm when faced with an emergency helps to keep the situation under control.
15. Knowing how to care for *minor* injuries is important.
16. Recognizing and avoiding poisonous plants can help to prevent much discomfort.

TABLE 11-3 A Curriculum Design for Grades K-6 (A Sample) (continued)

Topic	Grades K–3 Concepts	Grades 4–6 Concepts
		17. Laws and safety procedures pertaining to scuba diving and water skiing help to protect us.
		18. Injured persons must be kept warm and calm and left unmoved until a doctor or an adult arrives.
		19. Proper first aid may save lives and prevent further injury.
		20. First aid kits should be maintained and be available.
Medicines, Drugs, Alcohol and Tobacco	1. Milk and fruit juices are important at parties.	1. Skill in making decisions is important to healthful living.
	2. All medicines should be stored in safe, secure places or flushed down the toilet.	2. A good self-image helps to insulate the individual from improper use of alcohol and drugs.
	3. Accepting things from strangers can be dangerous.	3. Tea, coffee, and carbonated beverages contribute little toward good nutrition.
	4. Children should never take medicines without first asking parents.	4. Many people have played important roles in medical advances through the years.
	5. People should not experiment with drugs, tobacco, or alcohol.	5. Many medicines which promote health have been developed through medical research.
	6. Some medicines can be helpful if properly supervised by the family doctor.	6. Modern medicines assist the physician in preventing and treating diseases.
	7. Some medicines can be very dangerous.	7. Only a physician or certain others are qualified to prescribe medicines and instructions as to their use should be carefully followed.
	8. Children should know that medicines are not candy —even though they may taste good.	
	9. Children should know that medicines have a special purpose as medicines—not as candy.	

10. Alcohol and tobacco can be harmful, especially to young people.

Disease Prevention and Control

Public Health

1. Community health workers assist in providing clean, healthful, and sanitary communities.
2. The school nurse-teacher, dental health teacher, and school physician help pupils to stay healthy.
3. Children should stay home from school when they are sick because this helps to protect their friends and helps them to get well sooner.
4. Children should wash their hands thoroughly after going to the toilet.
5. Boys and girls should know how to use drinking fountains.
6. Children should know that it is important to tell an adult if they don't feel well.

8. Buying patent medicines without a prescription can perpetuate self-diagnosis and self-medication.
9. The sale of drugs is controlled by laws in order to prevent their misuse and abuse.
10. Alcoholic beverages contribute nothing essential to growth.
11. Alcoholic beverages affect body systems.
12. Research indicates that there is a relationship between cigarette smoking and lung cancer and heart disease.
13. There are many reasons why people start smoking.
14. Cigarette advertisements try to persuade people to smoke.
15. Smoking is an expensive practice.
16. The smoking habit is very difficult to break.

1. Hospitals help people to maintain and regain their health.
2. Periodic health examinations are important to health.
3. It is important to protect oneself and others from communicable diseases.
4. Each individual within a community has a responsibility for promoting cleanliness and sanitation.
5. Insect control is important to health.
6. Immunization can affect personal health.
7. Immunization can affect world health.
8. Water and air pollution are growing community health problems.

TABLE 11-3 A Curriculum Design for Grades K–6 (A Sample) (continued)

Topic	Grades K–3 Concepts	Grades 4–6 Concepts
Personal Health A. Dental Health	1. Clean teeth look and feel better. 2. We need to know how to clean our teeth to keep them healthy. 3. Teeth can be cleaned partially at school by eating an apple, celery, or rinsing the mouth with water. 4. The dentist and dental health teacher help people protect their teeth. 5. Teeth should be cleaned by the dentist at least twice a year. 6. Primary teeth are important even though we lose them later. 7. Some teeth that come in for the first time are permanent teeth. These should be given special care.	1. Proper care of teeth helps to prevent decay and injuries to tooth enamel. 2. Eating a variety of foods from the basic four groups promotes healthy teeth. 3. Teeth affect our health and appearance. 4. Criteria for the selection of toothbrushes is important. 5. A toothbrush needs special care. 6. Teeth are important to general health, for they aid in digestion and assist in articulation. 7. Permanent teeth should last a lifetime. 8. Certain types of teeth perform particular functions and all teeth have special parts. 9. Water fluoridation, topical applications of fluoride, and the ingestion of fluoride tablets have all proved helpful in preventing tooth decay. 10. Orthodontists often help people who are troubled with malocclusions.
		9. Safeguarding the community water supply is an ongoing process. 10. The programs of the World Health Organization influence world health. 11. Individuals have a responsibility for themselves and for the welfare of the community.

B. Conservation of Hearing and Vision

1. Eyes and ears are precious and need special care.
2. Eyes and ears need to be checked by the doctor to determine whether special care or correction is needed.
3. Objects should be kept away from eyes and ears.
4. Proper lighting helps to keep the eyes from getting tired.
5. Eye glasses should be protected and cared for.
6. Children should tell an adult if objects get into the eyes or ears.

1. Eyes and ears are delicate structures and need protection from injury and infection.
2. Vision and hearing tests differ from eye and ear examinations.
3. Eyes and ears enrich our lives through vision and hearing.
4. Older children can help younger children to protect their eyes and ears.
5. Looking directly at the sun may injure the eyes, even if smoked glasses or sunglasses are used.
6. Usually earaches should have the attention of a physician.
7. Contrasts in room lighting contribute to eye fatigue.
8. Changing eye tasks help to prevent eye fatigue.
9. Eyeglasses are corrective, not therapeutic.

C. Personal Appearance

1. Children should learn to become responsible for their appearance—clothes and cleanliness.
2. Boys and girls should dress appropriately for the occasion and weather.
3. Each person should have his own toilet articles.
4. Keeping clean is important to appearance and health.
5. Physical activities are good for a healthy body.
6. Rest is important.

1. Frequent baths help to promote general cleanliness.
2. Attractive and appropriate dress and styles of hair enhance personal appearance.
3. Regular and proper care of hair and skin is important to general health and appearance.
4. Good posture enhances personal appearance.

Consumer Health

1. Statements in advertisements may not be true.
2. Advertised products are not necessarily superior to unadvertised products.

TABLE 11-3   A Curriculum Design for Grades K-6 (A Sample) (continued)

Topic	Grades K-3 Concepts	Grades 4-6 Concepts
		3. Labels on products should be carefully read.
		4. Sound criteria should be used in the selection of health products.
		5. Factors that influence buying are: family customs, fads, and education.
		6. Laws help to protect the health of the consumer.
		7. Health information from mass media should be checked with health authorities.
		8. Reliable and accurate information is available locally from health departments, medical societies, and teachers.
		9. The Government tries to control the quality and sanitation of food and other products.
		10. The Food and Drug Administration, Federal Trade Commission, post office, World Health Organization, and health departments help to protect the health of the community.
		11. Health service organizations such as the American Medical Association, American Dental Association, and voluntary health agencies have an influence on the national health.
		12. The Better Business Bureau helps to protect the consumer from improper business transactions.
		13. Quackery is a serious health problem.

Primary grades: content

In a study conducted by the Connecticut State Board of Education, 5000 students from kindergarten through grade 12 were surveyed to determine those aspects of health about which they wanted to learn more. The following is a summary according to grades of these general health and health-related areas:

Kindergarten through grade 2[7]
- the body
- aches, pains, and diseases
- accidents
- hygiene and safety
- sex
- babies
- relations with parents and family
- relations with peers
- pets
- hospitals and doctors
- heart transplants

Grades 3 and 4[8]
- the body
- food and nutrition
- personal health and grooming
- exercise and physical education
- first aid and safety
- babies
- mental health
- disease and accidents
- drugs, smoking, and alcohol

Certainly, many of these topics are probably genuine student interests and concerns, but upon careful analysis one can also detect that pupils have learned that these areas are expectations of the teacher or others. In addition, we will find that they expressed concern about areas that were receiving wide media coverage for the times (for example, smoking, drugs, and heart transplants, which were news subjects during the late 1960s). However, their expression of concern can provide the teacher and curriculum developers with a point of departure for planning the primary grade health education program. Stone, et al. suggest that "results of the Connecticut survey of health interests provide clues to child responsiveness, rather than guidelines for curriculum development."[9] This is a rather astute observation, since curriculum development in health education—especially at the elementary school level—should be personalized for each group of learners rather than for a generalized national curriculum endeavor.

Regardless of the grade level or the locale, the development of curriculum will be based upon those fundamental principles we have discussed. The content of the curriculum refers to all of the elements to be included, not merely the informational content, as is widely assumed. Selection of the content for the intermediate grade learners must be predicated upon their general as well as specific characteristics—interests, readiness, and so on. Furthermore, what is to be included will also be influenced by the selection of the design of the written guides and the aspect of the program being emphasized. As with the primary grades, it is vital that the health curriculum for intermediate grade pupils stresses learner involvement, creativity, exploration, and inquiry. The curriculum should begin to take shape only after careful planning related to the nature of those learners who are going to be affected by it.

Standardized curricula (textbooks can be considered in this grouping) should be adapted to rather than being adopted for a local school situation. A noteworthy example of a standardized curriculum is the Berkeley Model Elementary Health Curriculum developed by the San Ramon Unified School District in California. It is a comprehensive health education program involving maximal integration into other basic curriculum areas of the elementary school program. This model emphasizes the development of an understanding and appreciation of the human body, prevention of disease, and making personal decisions regarding factors that adversely or favorably affect health. It stresses learner motivation, individual and group interaction, community and parental involvement.

Under a contract with the National Clearinghouse for Smoking and Health in 1968, the Berkeley Unified School District in California trained eight teams of educators from as many geographic areas in the United States. Each team consisted of two classroom teachers, their building principal, and one or two additional support personnel, usually the school nurse-teacher, a health educator, or a curriculum director. Two requirements were placed upon each team: (1) they were to implement the program in their home school classroom, and (2) they were to conduct similar training programs within their home district for other teachers and school personnel. This would result, eventually, in full implementation in all elementary schools within the geographic area.

Although specific evaluative data regarding the success of the model are lacking, general reactions are that it is one of the better elementary health education programs yet developed. This is supported by the pupils who have demonstrated overwhelming enthusiasm for the kinds of health learning experiences offered by the program. Probably the greatest criticism concerns the focus of the informational content, which consists of an in-depth study of one system of the body in each progressive grade level. Finally, some who have participated in the program indicate that an important factor for its success is the fact that the school administrators participate in the training program, providing them with a profound understanding of the program and support for its implementation; they develop a sense of "ownership."

Teacher-learner relations

In a paper presented at the 22nd annual conference of the Association for Supervision and Curriculum Development in 1967, Rogers[10] began by stating that "teaching, in my estimation, is a vastly overrated function." He emphasized that the "goal of education . . . is the *facilitation of change and learning*," and described facilitation of learning as the ability to "free curiosity."

This, in our judgment, is the fundamental relationship that should exist between teacher and learner. The teacher providing the opportunity for health learning to take place and the learner motivated to take advantage of this opportunity. Thus, the teacher and the learner become partners in education for health.

THE SECONDARY SCHOOL HEALTH CURRICULUM

Major emphasis

Health education at the secondary level is significant since this may be the final formal health education that many students will receive. Therefore, it should help each learner become self-sufficient, with the ability to recognize their capacity to contribute to their own health as well as that of society. The curriculum needs to focus on those health problems whose solutions are most likely to result from a more health informed generation of young people. This will prepare them to be directly influential in determining the health of still another generation of young people—their own children. In this regard, health education should place its major emphasis on self-understanding, interpersonal relations, community and political interaction, health decision-making regarding self, others, and society, continuing health awareness and education, analysis of health-related information from all sources, and synthesis of new health horizons for the future. To achieve this, the secondary health curriculum must enable learners to participate in the community's health affairs and must make all learning experientially oriented. Table 11–4 (p. 284) provides some suggestions in this regard. In addition, some urgent health issues that should be considered for all grade levels was suggested in Table 4–1 (p. 84). It might be well to review these in view of curriculum development and some of the general objectives which follow. These objectives are not intended to be all-inclusive; rather, they are suggestions for planning the secondary curriculum in health education. Each objective represents what the learner will be able to upon completion of the learning experiences for each topic listed.

Alcohol education

- to analyze the effects of the alcohol beverage industry on the American economy
- to describe the uses of alcohol
- to identify the possible physical effects of excessive use of alcohol over a long period of time
- to identify the factors that must be considered in deciding whether or not to drink alcohol
- to describe the attitudes regarding alcoholic beverages among various religious and ethnic groups
- to analyze the effects of alcohol abuse and alcoholism on the family unit
- to describe what the personal consequences of excessive periodic drinking can be
- to identify the ways that alcohol abuse affects communities
- to identify reliable resources of alcohol information
- to describe how excessive amounts of alcohol affects one's ability to function
- to explain the psychopharmacodynamics of alcohol abuse
- to discuss how one's environment can influence personal decisions regarding the use or nonuse of alcohol
- to demonstrate how responsible drinking is one alternative
- to identify the physical, social, and emotional risks involved in alcohol abuse
- to describe how one's peers can influence the choice to drink responsibly, not to drink, or to drink to excess
- to describe the varieties of approaches used to treat and rehabilitate the alcoholic
- to analyze the effects of advertising on one's choice to drink or not to drink
- to outline possible solutions to the alcohol abuse problem
- to identify the varieties of agencies dealing with the alcohol abuse problem
- to list the reasons why some people abuse alcohol
- to describe why viewing drunken behavior as humorous is counterproductive
- to analyze the effects of apathy, indifference, and ignorance on progress toward solving the alcohol abuse problem

Consumer health education

- to identify the criteria to be used in selecting and making use of the health services that are available
- to identify the psychological and sociological factors that influence self-medication

- to describe how the functions of various governmental agencies protect the consumer from unsafe or ineffective health products
- to distinguish between prescription and over-the-counter drugs
- to identify the characteristics of over-the-counter drugs
- to identify the chief medical and nonmedical health practitioners
- to compare the responsibilities of medical and nonmedical health practitioners
- to describe the characteristics of health quackery
- to analyze the influence of health advertising
- to identify the characteristics of misleading or false health advertising
- to develop criteria for evaluating the truth of advertised health products and services
- to describe the hazards inherent in the practice of health quackery
- to identify the reasons why some people make use of health quacks and nostrums
- to identify the motivational mechanisms that affect the behavior of the health consumer
- to identify reliable sources of health information
- to describe the various methods used for paying for health services and products
- to distinguish between voluntary and governmental health insurance programs

Dental health
- to describe how dental health can affect one's general health
- to describe the value of periodic professional dental care
- to identify ways in which the teeth and other oral structures can be protected from injury
- to analyze the effects of proper nutrition on oral health
- to demonstrate the continuous personal actions necessary for maintaining dental health
- to analyze the unique qualities of the oral structures
- to describe the value of flouridated water in maintaining the dental health of individuals and communities

Disease prevention and control
- to identify the fundamental principles of disease prevention and control
- to distinguish between communicable and noncommunicable diseases
- to analyze the historical efforts of people to understand and control diseases
- to analyze the significance of disease prevention and control as compared with treatment and rehabilitation
- to identify the chief causes of death from diseases
- to identify the chief degenerative diseases affecting people
- to identify ways in which individuals, communities, and governments can protect against contracting diseases

- to identify the physical, mental, and social consequences of disease
- to describe the value of research in the prevention and control of disease

Drug education
- to identify the various psychological and sociological causes of drug abuse
- to analyze the physical, psychological, and social effects of drug abuse
- to show how drug abuse affects the national economy
- to describe the relationship between drug abuse and crime
- to describe the various substances that modify mood and behavior
- to illustrate how family attitudes and practices regarding the use of drugs can influence one's own attitudes toward drug use
- to describe the influence of peers on decisions regarding drug use or nonuse
- to analyze the effectiveness of legal controls of drugs on preventing and decreasing the incidence of drug abuse
- to describe the role of drugs in the prevention and control of disease and pain
- to show how personal, social, family, and environmental forces can affect drug abuse or nonuse
- to describe the personal and social consequences of drug abuse
- to describe the physical, social, and emotional factors associated with drug dependence
- to show how drugs have contributed to the welfare of humanity
- to list the reasons why some people become drug users
- to develop realistic ways of preventing further increases in the incidence of drug abuse
- to show how attitudes regarding drug abuse vary among differing socioeconomic groups
- to define the various classes of drugs
- to describe the psychopharmacodynamics of drugs
- to compare the effects of short-term use of drugs with long-term behavioral changes
- to analyze the effectiveness of treatment programs for drug addicts
- to describe constructive alternatives to drug abuse
- to evaluate the effectiveness of current preventive practices and programs
- to become involved in programs designed to alleviate the drug problem
- to analyze the political implications of drug abuse

Ecology and epidemiology
- to describe the interrelationship between people and their environment
- to identify the ecological factors that influence health
- to describe the relationship between technological advances and the creation of new health problems

- to explain the epidemiological method
- to list the epidemiological factors affecting the health of people
- to describe the relationship between the etiological factors of disease

Public health
- to describe the nature of public health practice
- to list the major public health problems that exist today
- to describe the causes of the major public health problems and their solutions
- to explain why some health problems are the concern of the community while others are the concern of the individual
- to show how political action can have a definite beneficial effect in dealing with our public health problems
- to describe how the principles of epidemiology are applied to alleviate some public health problems
- to show how major improvements in the environment are necessary to alleviate some public health problems

First aid
- to identify the kinds of emergencies requiring first aid care that are most likely to occur
- to demonstrate proficiency in first aid procedures and the use of first aid equipment
- to categorize injuries according to the immediacy of treatment needed
- to describe the purpose of first aid care

Genetic health
- to analyze the significance of the numerous misconceptions regarding genetic health
- to describe the impact of personal and social stigmas on advances in genetic health technology
- to describe the importance of acquiring factual information on genetic health in favorably influencing one's own genetic decisions
- to distinguish between the various causes of genetic disorders
- to appreciate that certain groups or populations are more likely to transmit or acquire certain types of genetic diseases
- to describe the personal, social, and economic impact of genetic diseases
- to describe the psychosocial impact of genetic health issues
- to describe the various procedures being used to prevent some genetic diseases
- to describe the nature and kinds of rehabilitation programs that exist for those with genetic defects
- to describe the kinds of genetic research being conducted on selected genetic diseases
- to appreciate the significance of the various aspects of genetic health as a critical and urgent health matter

- to become motivated to be actively involved in the political ramifications of genetic health issues

Mental health education
- to describe the importance of communications as they relate to interpersonal relations
- to analyze the influence of persuasion on human behavior
- to analyze the relationship between perceptual ability and reality
- to describe the factors that may change the perception of reality
- to describe the importance of the self-concept to mental health
- to show how physiological and psychosocial need satisfaction affects behavior
- to explain how need satisfaction may vary as a result of cultural influences
- to describe the role that heredity plays in establishing basic human needs
- to show how attainable goals affect mental health and total behavior
- to describe how the decision-making process affects mental health
- to relate creativity to mental health
- to demonstrate how stress can affect decision-making as well as other behavioral outcomes
- to contrast impulsive behavior with rational behavior
- to describe how cultures can influence mental health status
- to describe the influence that the emotive force may have on behavior

Nutrition education
- to identify the varieties and sources of foods
- to relate food intake to the body's health and to growth and development
- to describe the importance of eating a variety of foods each day
- to show how food choices vary among families and cultures
- to develop valid criteria for food selection
- to describe how social and emotional factors influence nutritional behavior
- to describe the consequences of an inadequate diet
- to explain the relationship between adequate diet and achievement
- to describe the factors that influence individual preferences in food selection
- to show how individual differences influence individual daily nutritional requirements
- to describe the purposes that foods have in human life
- to relate nutrition to overall health
- to distinguish between food fadism and nutritional fact

Safety education
- to identify the characteristics of unsafe situations and ways to avoid them

- to describe the characteristics of a safe home, school, and community environment
- to explain the causes of accidents
- to demonstrate safe behavior
- to identify social and personal factors that contribute to safe living
- to analyze personal attitudes related to safe behavior
- to identify those factors that can prevent or reduce accidents

Sensory perception
- to describe the role of the sense organs in human perception
- to identify the characteristics of visual and aural acuity
- to describe the prevention, detection, and correction of common visual disorders
- to analyze perceptual ability and effective living
- to demonstrate the proper care of the sense organs
- to describe services available to alleviate the causes of perceptual disorders
- to identify health personnel available to assist individuals with perceptual problems

Smoking and health
- to identify ways that tobacco influences individuals and society
- to describe the immediate effects of tobacco smoke on the body
- to show how tobacco smoke affects performance
- to describe the relationship of tobacco smoke to health
- to explain how tobacco production affects the American economy
- to compare the attitudes of smokers, nonsmokers, and ex-smokers toward the use of tobacco
- to evaluate the effects of tobacco advertisements on smoking behavior
- to identify the forces that influence one's decision about whether or not to smoke
- to state reasons why cigarette smoking constitutes one of America's major health issues
- to justify the rights of nonsmokers to breathe unpolluted air

World health
- to describe the significance of world health problems on self and American society
- to analyze the effectiveness of worldwide programs dealing with world health problems
- to compare the kinds of health problems prevalent in developing countries with those of developed countries
- to analyze the international political implications of world health problems
- to describe the nature of cooperative research as it relates to international health problems
- to relate cultural differences to the nature and extent of health problems

- to identify some of the constraints obstructing international solutions to world health problems
- to describe the economic implications of some major world health problems
- to identify the chief world health agencies

As has been stressed earlier, the selection of objectives must be related to numerous factors other than just the health topic area. Therefore, it is not possible to present in a textbook exactly what each learner throughout the various geographic areas of the country should be achieving. In addition, the wording of objectives must be precise for the particular group of learners. Thus, the preceding discussions are intended to provide the reader with an example of the nature and scope that a comprehensive health education program at the secondary level can have and a beginning for curriculum development at the secondary level.

How much? When?

These questions have been partially answered in the earlier discussions. However, let us explore briefly what is generally taking place in many states throughout the country.

Children attend school for approximately 2,240 days from the time they enter kindergarten until graduation from high school. This is, of course, assuming that there are no absences during their entire school experience. During this time, the learner progresses through many learning stages acquiring knowledge, skills, attitudes, and behavioral expressions. Some are health-related; others are not. Many states require a minimum of one year of health education at the secondary level. Sometimes this is under a trained health educator and other times it may be a teacher trained in another discipline. At any rate, a learner will receive only about 2.8% of the total secondary school time for direct health education.

It is obvious that with such a short period of time devoted to direct health education, it is essential that all of it be used economically, and that all learning be important and relevant toward achieving carefully selected objectives.

Content and process

The scope of the informational content was discussed in Chapter 4. In addition, previous discussions in this chapter will provide further guidance in this regard. Generally, however, the scope of the informational content is limited only by the urgency of the health issues that exist, the interests and needs of the learner, the qualities of the teacher, and the philosophy and policies of local boards of education.

Since health education is directed toward improving the quality of life of each individual, society, and the world, it is vital that the processes being used will have the greatest influence on achieving these ends. In this regard, learning takes place best when the learner is experiencing directly and contributing to the improvement of health in this total context. Therefore, learning should be experientially oriented. An illustration of some of the kinds of experiences in which secondary school students can become involved are presented in Table 11–4 as they relate to alcohol education. Similar experiences are also appropriate for other critical health issues. You may want to compare the activities to the alcohol objectives presented earlier to determine whether or not the activities seem to achieve these.

THE ADULT HEALTH EDUCATION CURRICULUM

Organization

Adult health education should be an integral component of the comprehensive health education program of the school. Its basic organization should place it under the direction of the health education administrator, but it should be implemented in cooperation with the continuing education department of the school. In addition, the health education administrator should explore the possibilities of cooperating with community agencies in establishing community-based health education programs on a continuous basis. Again, goals of the adult health education program may vary from one community setting to another, but certain common goals will most likely prevail. These goals aim at having parents and other adults . . .

1. acquire an awareness of the kinds and extent of health problems that affect children and adults in the community.
2. acquire factual health information regarding key health issues.
3. bring adults together in a cooperative effort to deal adequately with the community's health problems.
4. be given opportunities to share experiences with each other regarding significant health issues.
5. find new and better ways of communicating with their children regarding their health concerns.
6. acquire ways in which they can assist the school in reinforcing the health learning of their children.
7. acquire a deeper understanding of and appreciation for the total health education program.
8. be given opportunities to share their knowledge and attitudes regarding health issues with their children and with school personnel.
9. have the opportunity to become more actively involved in finding solutions to the health problems of the community.

TABLE 11-4 Learning Experiences Related to Alcohol Education (A Sample)

Experientially-oriented activities for secondary school students

1. Have students interview an individual who works with people with an alcohol problem. Have them determine what their function is and report back to the class.
   The following is a suggested source list of such people.

   —physician
   —psychiatrist
   —psychologist
   —family and marriage counselor
   —judge
   —lawyer
   —police
   —Alcoholics Anonymous
   —Alanon

   —Alateen
   —mental health clinic
   —children and family service agency
   —alcohol information center
   —tavern owner
   —management of an industry
   —alcohol beverage industry
   —alcoholic beverage commission

2. Invite individuals from this list to speak to the class about their function and about their experiences with people with an alcohol problem. Divide the class into small groups with the guest speaker as a consultant. Have students discuss such problems as:
   1) What is the socioeconomic impact on the community as a result of alcohol abuse?
   2) What is the impact on family structure, children, spouse, etc.?
   3) What is the extent of the problem? Age groups, ethnic groups, sexes?
   4) What personnel and facilities are available to deal with the problem? How effective are they?
   5) What does the community need to do further to prevent, treat, rehabilitate? What would the cost be?
3. Visit an industry that manufactures alcoholic beverages—winery, brewery, or distillery. Determine the process, quantity produced, distribution, quality control, number employed, etc. What can be concluded about the industry in terms of contributions to society? To the economy?
4. Have a committee of students design a bulletin board or other display showing the uses of alcohol in industry, in medicine, and as a beverage. A self-test related to the display could be included; for example:
   1) Why is alcohol rather than water used in iodine?
   2) Why is alcohol used in the making of shellac or similar products?
   3) Why does beverage alcohol come in such a wide variety of forms?
5. Select a panel of students to prepare and deliver a presentation regarding how the excessive use of alcoholic beverages affects the user, other members of the family, employer, friends, and business associates.
   An expert consultant may be used to moderate the panel and summarize the presentations.
6. Divide the class into at least two small groups. One group is to write a story regarding a family whose attitudes toward drinking are liberal, while the second group writes a story about a family whose attitudes are conservative. The groups should consider justification for the attitudes they identify.

Experientially-oriented activities for secondary school students

    Have each group dramatize their views in role-playing situation wherein each attempts to convert the other to their way of thinking about alcohol.

7. Have students bring to class magazine and newspaper advertisements regarding various alcohol beverages.

    Analyze the contents of the ads. What is the central message of the ad? Identify misleading or false statements or illustrations. What needs are being appealed to?

    Have class identify other ways in which drinking is insidiously encouraged (e.g., heroes in movies who drink—cocktail parties, political toasts, etc.). What influence do these scenes have on young people's attitudes?

8. Have students identify the organs and systems of the body that are most significantly affected by the excessive use of alcohol.

    Describe how these organs and systems are affected and what it means to the overall health of the individual.

9. Collect labels (or containers) of products that contain alcohol.

    Determine the purpose of the alcohol as an ingredient.

10. Have a committee of students develop an alcohol attitude survey instrument. Survey the attitudes of the student body regarding alcohol use and abuse. Have the committee interpret the results and write an article for the school or local newspaper.

    The survey could also be given to the students' parents and these results compared with the students'.

11. Make a survey of the people and agencies in the community that are concerned with the alcohol problem. Determine the varieties of people and agencies and the aspect of the problem with which they are most concerned. Are their efforts coordinated? What is the cost to the citizens? Are there duplicated effects? Are there areas or aspects of the problem that are ignored?

12. Invite local or state legislators to class to discuss their views regarding the alcohol problem. What are the legislative controls? How effective are they? What further legislation is needed?

    Have a committee of students draft legislation that will help to solve the alcohol problem.

13. Survey tavern owners about their view of the problem of alcohol abuse. What are their responsibilities in this regard? What do they suggest as a possible solution to alcohol abuse? Who are the abusers?

14. Develop a class resource center on alcohol. Have pupils write to various agencies that produce educational materials for copies for the center. Have pupils evaluate the materials and catalogue them for the center.

15. Develop a class scrapbook on alcohol. Include newspaper clippings from local newspapers describing events related to alcohol. At the end of the year have a committee of students analyze and summarize the events. What can be concluded about the importance of alcohol use in the community?

To achieve these and other goals, the adult health education program should be organized formally within the continuing education department of the school. It should be planned and continuous with formal classes meeting regularly. Community-based programs can be formal or informal, or both. Formal programs should be planned with the voluntary and governmental health agencies in the form of a series of workshops, seminars, or lectures emanating from the community agencies. Informal programs may take the form of newsletters or other printed materials, use of the media, displays, health fairs, and the like. Incidentally, the school/community health education advisory committee should be actively assisting the health education administrator in initiating and implementing the adult health education program.

Content

As with all health education programs, the adult health education program's informational content is determined by the health issues deemed important and the needs and interests of the adult learners. Adult learners should be involved in planning the curriculum. This can be accomplished during the early class sessions. The first step should be to establish goals and objectives. This should be followed by discussions of ways in which these goals can best be achieved. Generally, the health concerns of children and youth are probably not much different from those of adults. Therefore, these health issues should be explored with the adults as a step toward ascertaining the content of the adult health education curriculum.

DEFINITIVE UNDERSTANDINGS

Health education is one of the most basic curricular offerings in the school's educational program. In a study conducted by the Connecticut State Board of Education, it was found that 87.2% of the respondents felt that the most important goal of education was for each student to learn to communicate effectively. This is also one of the chief goals of the health education program.

The health curriculum can be conceived of as any and all of the factors that influence health learning. In this regard, it may be planned or unplanned. Generally speaking, curriculum is defined as that aspect of teaching and administration that designedly, systematically, cooperatively, and continuously seeks to improve the teaching-learning process. Therefore, the health education curriculum should be planned for greatest effectiveness. Essentially, it is a continuous process that embraces initial design and construction, evaluation, reorganization, revision, experimentation, administration, and adaptability. As such, it reflects the importance of health learning from all segments of the learner's environment.

The principles of humanization of the educational programs apply directly to the development and implementation of the health education curriculum. Humanization is not only a process but a goal of health education and should be obvious in the design of the curriculum.

The chief purpose of the health education curriculum guide is to commit to writing the entire plan of action; it becomes the blueprint of learning and teaching, describing what, how, when, and by whom health learning and teaching will occur. It is in essence the culminating document of all evaluation and planning of the health education program.

Simply speaking, the development of the health curriculum will follow certain basic principles of curriculum construction. First, we need to ascertain a definite need for the educational offerings, plan its construction, implement it with procedures consistent with the school's general educational philosophy, and evaluate its effectiveness. In this sense, the curriculum guide should contain a statement of the aim of the program, the goals to be achieved, and the terminal and enabling objectives for the learner. These establish the boundaries of the program and suggest the approaches to be used. The curriculum guide, therefore, becomes an educational tool, with clearly stated purposes that are understood by those who will be using it. In this regard, curriculum developers need to ask certain preliminary questions prior to designing and constructing the guide.

Curriculum guides may take many forms and a variety of guides may be necessary for complete program development. The common guides being used today include:

1. The resource guide, which is essentially a listing of all of the material and human resources available in the school and community.
2. The master plan, whose purpose is to put into perspective all of the elements that make up the total health education program.
3. The curriculum guide, which is similar in content to the master plan, but which contains more detailed description of content and process.
4. The course of study, which is the most detailed curriculum guide. It is developed for each grade level and is the working document from which the teacher develops daily lesson plans. To be effective, the course of study should contain: terminal and enabling objectives; a variety of learning experiences; suggested learning aids; the informational content; and evaluation procedures.
5. The lesson plan technically is not a curriculum guide, but rather the results of the suggestions presented in the course of study guide. It is simply a document that describes what the teacher and learners intend to do on a daily basis.

The specific design that a particular guide takes will vary under different circumstances, as intended use varies, and with the quality of the teacher. With this in mind, it is well for the curriculum developers to establish basic criteria for curriculum design that will prove helpful in final determinations.

The content of the guides, along with the education processes to be used, should evolve from the goals, purposes, and other factors related to the health education program. Essentially, informational content should reflect relevant health issues, while the processes should be experientially oriented. It is important that guides be functional; criteria for their development should direct attention toward this goal. The two most widely used formats for achieving functionalism are the vertical and horizontal designs. For most, the horizontal design has distinct advantages over the vertical design.

There are currently three chief approaches to curriculum design: (1) the informational approach, (2) the learner-centered approach, and (3) the conceptual approach. The informational approach stresses the importance of intellectual development or the acquisition of accurate health knowledge. The learner-centered approach emphasizes the needs, interests, and developmental levels of the learners. The conceptual approach attempts to place health learning within a conceptual framework. Obviously, each of these approaches may include ingredients of the other two. No one approach is autonomous or isolated from all other approaches. Their distinction lies chiefly in their major emphasis.

Health education at the elementary school level is probably the most important for establishing constructive attitudes and practices. Many of our major health problems today stem from inappropriate health behavior acquired during the firset ten to twelve years of life. Therefore, health education at the elementary school level should place a major emphasis on continuous health guidance of children at this age and should be directed toward satisfying their health needs. It becomes obvious that the elementary school health education curriculum, in all of its segments, must focus on assisting all children in better understanding themselves and others and on ways of dealing adequately with the environment. A study conducted in Connecticut has provided us with some knowledge about what kind of health information elementary school children feel is important.

Finally, health learning at the elementary school level should emphasize creativity and opportunities to explore and express inquisitiveness. Learning should be concrete and experientially oriented. The Berkeley Model Elementary Curriculum is an example of a standardized curriculum that emphasizes these characteristics. However, it is not recommended that these kinds of programs be adopted without appropriate alterations for local implementation. In the end, the success of the elementary school health curriculum will be determined by, among many other things, the relationship between the learners and the teacher.

Health education at the secondary school level has a special significance since for many students this may be their final formal health education experience. Therefore, it should provide them with the skills and knowledge for becoming health educated. That is to say, emphasis should be placed on self-understanding, interpersonal relations, and community and political interaction. Decision-making skills should be developed so that these students will be able to deal effectively with future health issues as they arise. There are at least sixteen broad health areas that should be included in the secondary school health education program. The specific objectives should reflect achievement of the aims described above. However, since the amount of time allocated for health education in most schools is extremely short objectives must be carefully selected and clearly stated so that maximum achievement is possible. In addition, it may be necessary to limit the scope of the program to the most urgent health issues.

Adult health education should be an integral component of the comprehensive health education program of the school. It should consist of two major thrusts: (1) a planned program within the continuing education department, and (2) a community-based program in conjunction and cooperation with the various community health agencies.

PROBLEMS
FOR DISCUSSION

1. Describe the philosophical foundations of the health education curriculum.
2. Outline the chief components of a written curriculum guide.
3. Detail the specific purposes of both the health curriculum and the written course of study.
4. Develop a written guide for the elementary school health education program and justify the format being used.
5. Develop a written guide for the secondary school health education program and justify the format being used.
6. Distinguish between a resource guide and a course of study guide.
7. Compare the advantages and disadvantages of a vertical and horizonal format for a written course of study.
8. Describe why the identification of goals and objectives is important for curriculum construction.
9. Distinguish between curriculum guides that emphasize the informational, learner-centered and conceptual approaches.
10. Why should adult health education be an integral component of the total health education program?
11. Develop criteria for evaluating the effectiveness of the curriculum design.
12. Develop a master plan for a comprehensive health education program for learners from kindergarten level through adulthood.
13. Describe the factors that determine the content and process of the health education curriculum.
14. What are the chief purposes of a written curriculum guide in health education?
15. Develop a lesson plan for a hypothetical class in health education.
16. Should the major emphasis in health education be for secondary school students? Justify your response.

REFERENCES

1. Koopman, G. Robert, *Curriculum Development*, The Center for Applied Research in Education, Inc., New York, 1966, p. 9.
2. Wilhelms, Fred T., "Humanizing Via the Curriculum," *Humanizing Education: The Person in the Process*, Robert R. Geeper, ed., Association for Supervision and Curriculum Development, NEA, Washington, 1967, p. 21.
3. Saylor, J. Galen, and William M. Alexander, *Curriculum Planning for Modern Schools*, Holt, Rinehart and Winston, Inc., New York, 1966, p. 6.
4. School Health Education Study, *Health Education: A Conceptual Approach to Curriculum Design*, Minnesota Mining and Manufacturing Company, St. Paul, 1967, p. 20.
5. Willgoose, Carl E., *Health Education in the Elementary School*, 3rd edition, W. B. Saunders Company, Philadelphia, 1969, p. 27.
6. The Bureau of Elementary Curriculum Development, *The Elementary School Curriculum*, The University of the State of New York, The State Education Department, Albany, 1954, p. 13.
7. Byler, Ruth V., Gertrude M. Lewis, and Ruth J. Totman, *Teach Us What We Want to Know*, Connecticut State Board of Education, Mental Health Materials Center, Inc., New York, 1969, chap. 1.
8. Ibid., chap. 2.
9. Stone, Donald B., Lawrence B. O'Reilly, and James D. Brown, *Elementary School Health Education: Ecological Perspectives*, William C. Brown Company, Dubuque, 1976, p. 198.
10. Rogers, Carl R., "The Interpersonal Relationship in the Facilitation of Learning," *Humanizing Education: The Person in the Process*, Association for Supervision and Curriculum Development, NEA, Washington, 1967, pp. 1–2.

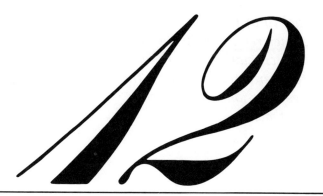

Health
Education
Methodology /
Theory
and Practice

*It is the quality of the
teacher-learner relationship that is
crucial. More crucial, in fact, than
what the teacher is teaching, how the
teacher does it, or whom the teacher
is trying to teach.*

Thomas Gordon

No one can tell another how to
teach, only how others have taught.
Would-be health educators must
first become people, and only then
can they become teachers.

AEB
DAB

INTRODUCTION: INFORMATION THEORY

Description

In Chapter 7, we discussed the fundamental principles that help to explain learning and thinking in humans. Methodology in health education can be viewed as the science (and art) of altering the environment for maximum learning to result. Learning is influenced by a kind of stimulus contact with the environment; it is, in essence, the result of a form of communications. Communications is an interchange of thoughts, ideas, or opinions through definite channels or network. Without communications there is no learning. The field of study of communication systems is called *information theory*. It is concerned with the principles governing understanding, control, and predictability in communications.

Information theory is related to and explains the transmission of information from a source to a final destination. It has five essential elements:

1. The *source* of the message, which can have a variety of origins (e.g., the physical environment, learning resources, teacher, or the individual's thought processes).
2. The *transmitter* changes the information into a form that can be easily conveyed from the source to the destination. This conversion is called encoding and can take the form of the spoken word, for example, or may be in the form of visual or other sensory symbols or stimuli.
3. The *communication channel* is the mechanism that carries the information. In the case of the spoken word, the communication channel would be the air. The stimuli of symbols passing through the channel are called the coded message. Language is thus a coded message that must be decoded for communications to take place.
4. The *receiver* decodes the coded message; that is, the spoken word, in this example, is interpreted by the individual receiving the information for use at its final destination.
5. The *destination* of the information is the point at which it results in some form of reaction. For instance, the coded message is decoded to alter in some way the learning of the individual, who then reacts accordingly.

Figure 12–1 illustrates the application of the information theory to health education methodology.

Communications may be interrupted or interfered with by extraneous disturbances in the learning environment. In the communication model, these disturbances are called *noise*.

As we have seen, humans are inherently goal-seeking organisms. As such, they can be compared to servomechanisms that have been devel-

Two-way verbal and/or nonverbal feedback is essential for successful communications to take place.

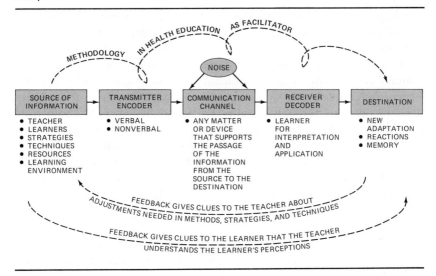

oped with intrinsic goal-seeking devices; that is, they are sensitive to certain external stimuli and respond accordingly until the programmed goal is reached. The stimuli are called feedback, which directs the servomechanism in its course. The servomechanism adapts to the feedback until the goal is reached. An example of this type of servomechanism is a ground-to-air missile. The feedback from the target is essential for its success. The science that studies the relationship of computer engineering and human neurology is called cybernetics.

The methodology chosen for health education should be sensitive to the principles of the information theory and flexible enough to make appropriate adjustments based upon feedback from the learner. In this regard, the teacher must constantly evaluate the effectiveness of the communications as methods are being applied to the learning process. Methods must allow for and encourage feedback. The feedback may be either verbal or nonverbal in nature but either way it must provide the essential information (i.e., changes in the learner) for directing the source of learning to its final destination.

Communications: verbal and nonverbal

Communication is a two-way phenomenon. Effective communications can not take place unless the person originating the message is aware of the degree to which the receiver understands the information being transmitted. Feedback may take the form of verbal or nonverbal energy.

The learner may receive the coded message through the use of one or more sense organs: hearing, seeing, feeling, tasting, smelling, or a combination of these. The use of a sound film, for example, makes use of both seeing and hearing. Such a technique can profoundly stimulate the learner's perceptual and interpretive abilities, increasing the possibilities of accurate communications occurring. Follow-up discussions of the film's content can provide the teacher with an indication of the accuracy of the learner's comprehension of the information presented. This is an example of verbal communication in the form of feedback.

During the showing of the film, the teacher can observe learner reactions—facial expressions, for instance—and acquire some indications of whether or not the film's message is being received. This is an example of nonverbal communications. The teacher, however, must also learn to decode the coded messages being transmitted by the learner in this way. To fail to do so can result in misunderstandings and serious communications breakdowns between the learner and the teacher. Breakdowns, like communications, are two-way phenomena. Gordon suggests that "the most effective method for preventing such breakdowns in communications is active listening that all but insures understanding what students communicate. Active listening, as opposed to passive listening (silence), involves interaction with the student, and it also provides the student with proof (feedback) of the teacher's understanding."[1] Accordingly, feedback is a symptom of active listening and, as such, is also a two-way phenomenon, as illustrated in Figure 12–1.

Learning strategies

Methodology is a term encompassing a broad spectrum of planned and orderly processes designed to make health learning as simple as possible to insure accuracy of learning. It can be expressed either as teaching methods or learning methods. In either case, the focus is upon the learner rather than the teacher.

Teaching methods are those planned approaches or procedures that the teacher employs to most effectively influence students' comprehension of a new situation or to further influence their comprehension of a familiar situation. *Learning methods* are those procedures that the learner uses (and that may be directed by the teaching methods) to acquire greater insight into a new or familiar situation. Specific methods will be discussed later.

Methods are composed of teaching/learning techniques and strategies. These imply specific skills needed to effectively carry out the method to its completion. For example, a person using the lecture method effectively must possess unusual skills in verbal communications. A teaching (or learning) *technique* is essentially the manner in which the method is performed. A *strategy*, on the other hand, implies techniques of maneuvering the learner into a position in which learning will occur more readily. Motivational techniques may be used as a strategy, for example, within the boundaries of the planned method. However, Stone, et al.[2] equate strategies with methods: "Teaching strategies or methods are the tools an educator utilizes for the development of health attitudes, knowledge, and behavior." He suggests that the term strategy "denote[s] a broader concept of teaching tools." Regardless of definition, it is generally agreed that *methodology in health education is the chief facilitator of communication and of learning.* And it is its application in this regard that is of utmost importance.

Finally, teaching methods, techniques and startegies are designed to influence learning, and as such, they become learning strategies when properly applied. *Learning strategies* are the skills that learners use to facilitate learning and are generally energized by the strategies used by the teacher. Russell[3] supports this contention, stating that teaching and learning "are not antithetical." He goes on to explain that "in one strategy the one who knows, tells. In the other, the one who knows would rather learners developed other ways of knowing rather than simply listening to him/her."

Methods related to curriculum

As we discussed earlier, curriculum has many faces. Some curricula possess the "face" of a textbook while others are designed by the health educator for a specific group of learners. The textbook curriculum is usually less effective, since it does not take into account specific methods, strategies, and techniques designed for the characteristics of the individual teacher or the specific group of learners. Instead, it should be used as a guide or strategy within the curriculum that is developed by the teacher and learners. Its use therefore, becomes a method, a tool—as it should be.

As we will see, methods are specific for learners and teachers. They become a basic and inherent component of a specific curriculum design based upon teacher and learner characteristics and a philosophy of health education consistent with these and other factors. Methods must be planned and implemented in this context to be maximally effective. They may, however, be motivated and expanded ideas that others have developed.

BASIS FOR METHOD SELECTION

Characteristics of the learner

We have stressed the importance of all health education efforts being geared toward learner characteristics—physical, psychological, and sociological developmental levels. This becomes especially significant in planning the methods to be used to achieve goals and objectives for health, since these are the vehicles that will be used for this purpose.

The characteristics of each individual must be appraised, and learning experiences selected and provided, in accordance with these findings. Sweeping generalities regarding typical characteristics of people in a given age group simply will not do. *Learning, as with growth and development in other human dimensions, is a very personal process and must be treated as such.* Every teacher that has completed a teacher education course of study in an accredited institution has studied at length the psychology of childhood and adolescence. These principles are important as a foundation for an understanding of the nature of children and youth in general terms. But when time comes to apply these principles to the teaching-learning situation, it is vital that learners be viewed as individuals rather than as norms. (Some procedures for assessing individual learners will be discussed in Chapter 13.)

In addition to the existing developmental characteristics of the learner, their momentary attitudes, desires, and motivation play a part in method selection. In one instance, a particular learner may simply not be motivated, and although the method being used is appropriate in other respects, it may fail to achieve the desired learning. For efficient learning to occur, the method being used must sustain motivation as well as direct learning. Finally, regardless of all that has been said about similarities between the sexes, there are some significant differences that need to be considered when selecting methodologies. Boys and girls at various developmental levels (although chronological ages may be identical) view certain phenomena in their lives differently. Their interests and abilities will vary and consequently, learning experiences appropriate for one sex may be inappropriate for the other.

One might then ask, "But what are the general characteristics of children and youth at various age levels? What can one expect to find? What criteria can be established with which intelligent judgments can be made for selecting the best method of learning?" Health learning begins at birth with the first breath and continues through the last. The teacher must be concerned with the development of the child in the past, the present, and the future. The first formal health education with which schools deal usually begins in kindergarten and it must be built upon those experiences and developments with which the child enters school.

Maturation includes both the biological (physical) changes taking place in the cells, tissues, organs, and systems (growth) and the improvement in their functioning. The rate of maturation for each child is unique, and this uniqueness must be considered by the teacher; but there is also a general pattern which a group of children of the same chronological age manifest. The maturation process is influenced by such factors as genetic potentials, nutrition, rest, recreation, or other activities and the richness of the culture or other stimuli that affect personality, emotional and social growth, and intellectual development. Since these differences exist, children develop at their own rate, and these individual rates together form a norm of maturation for the age group. *It is this norm that determines the method of education that is appropriate, while the individual differences determine the techniques and strategies to be used for individualized instruction.*

Characteristics of the teacher

There is no single method that is considered the best to use with a particular group of learners. Selection of methods depends in part upon the depth and breadth of teacher competency. A teacher should: (1) feel comfortable with the method selected; (2) have the training needed to properly implement it; (3) recognize its limitations and impact upon the learners; and (4) know its value for motivating learning and guiding the learner toward goal achievement. In this regard, teachers must know the extent of their abilities and experience in making the method as effective as possible. The importance of the teacher in health education (as in all education) was emphasized by Dewey when he stated that "everything the teacher does, as well as the manner in which he does it, incites the child to respond in some way or another and each response tends to set the child's attitude in some way or another."[4]

The characteristics of the teacher, therefore, become critical considerations when the health education plan of action is being formulated. Inappropriate approaches may very well resent effective education, while appropriate approaches can guarantee a high quality of education. This was exemplified in the case of Maryland Association for Retarded Children versus Maryland in 1974 when it was stated that education is "any plan or structured program administered by competent persons that is designed to help individuals achieve their full potential."[5] The competency of the teacher is deliberately emphasized. From this viewpoint, one may ask whether the method or the teacher is the chief factor influencing learning. The answer is obviously that it is not a question of either/or; the two must be compatible with each other.

Health science or health education?

A teacher must not only be highly trained in the health sciences, but also highly skilled in the procedures for educatiing others. We have defined both health and education elsewhere, but when the term "science" is added (which is in vogue these days), a new dimension is implicated. Science is described as a "possession of knowledge attained through study or practice." Science, essentially, "seeks to establish general laws connecting a number of particular facts."[6] However, when health, science, and education are combined into a single term, a new meaning that is quite different from that of each term individually results. Health science education is much narrower in its meaning than health education, since it refers basically to the acquisition of health facts, their relation to each other, and how these relationships can establish health principles or laws. If, however, the term "applied science" is added, still another dimension is implicated. Applied science is "concerned with the application of discovered laws to the matters of everyday living."[7]

The point of this discussion is that teacher characteristics generally include training and experience in the health sciences, education, health (and disease), and the applied sciences. These factors are essential for health learning to occur with a high degree of effectiveness and efficiency. The quality of the teacher (hence, the quality of the approaches being used) are inseparably intertwined with the quality of the training received in these areas. *Methodology in health education is therefore an application of the principles of the health sciences by use of the educational process by a competent individual.* In this regard, health education must be considered a "multidimensional process."[8]

Availability of learning resources

Learning resources may be either materials, such as films, books, posters, etc., or people. They are generally used as a technique or strategy in conjunction with a particular approach to enhance learning by adding new sensory dimensions to the method being used. As with other phases of the program, learning aids should be used only after careful evaluation and determination of their useability, quality, and appropriateness. Chapter 13 provides some suggestions along these lines.

Once material resources have been selected, they should be made available to the learner. One technique is to establish a learning resource center convenient for learners and available to them for such activities as independent study and research, as well as being used for large and small group discussions and analyses. A well stocked and up to date resource center can add much to the learning environment and to the motivation of learning.

Most communities have a wide variety of agencies whose personnel possess special expertise in particular areas of health. Many are anxious to work with children and youth and to share their knowledge and experiences with them. Resource people can be used in a variety of ways, but they appear to be most effective when they are acting as consultants in small group discussions and research, rather than merely as speakers. The following is a list of general sources* of resource people:

1. The local or state health department
2. The local or state mental health department
3. The local or state social services department
4. The council of churches
5. The parent-teacher association
6. The professional societies (medical, dental, psychological, pharmaceutical, etc.)

---

* An extensive listing of organizations at the national level is included in Appendix B. They can provide names and addresses of local affiliates.

7. The varieties of voluntary health agencies (Lung Association, Heart Association, etc.)
8. Hospitals, clinics, nursing homes
9. Research centers

Many communities have available a directory of agencies and people concerned with various health matters. Like material resources, human resources should be evaluated prior to their use. (A suggested procedure is presented in Chapter 13.)

In 1946, Dale[9] introduced his "cone of experiences" which categorized learning on a continuum from abstract to concrete experiences as "doing," "observing," and "symbolizing." "Doing" is labelled today as learner-centered experiences and characterized by direct and purposeful learning, contrived experiences, and dramatic participation, all of which were described by Dale. "Observing" is described below as learner-observational and includes those experiences that students see others doing. "Symbolizing" is usually referred to today as teacher-centered methods. The less mature learners are and the fewer past experiences they have had, the more important it is that concrete (learner-centered) learning experiences be used. For example, teacher-centered approaches are more likely to be more effective in college settings than in elementary school settings. However, it is important to recognize that teacher-centered approaches under ordinary circumstances are never as effective as learner-centered approaches.

TRADITIONAL METHODS

Advantages and disadvantages

Simply because a method may be traditional does not necessarily mean that it is ineffective. Although there has been a move in recent years to discover new and more effective approaches to health teaching and learning, a careful analysis of many of these will reveal that they are essentially modifications of approaches that have been in use for decades. Some old ways of doing things are still the best; however, admittedly, some should be discarded and replaced with other proven ways of teaching. For example, one of the major movements underlying educational progress has been in the direction of making education more humanistic by giving greater attention to the individual student as the basic unit of value in the total learning process. Education in a democratic society should seek to maximize the sense of personal worth of the learner. With appropriate alterations in some of the traditional approaches, this goal can be achieved. Some of the so-called traditional methods are: (1) the lecture method, (2) the textbook method, (3) the recitation and rote method, (4) the discussion method, (5) the question and answer method, (6) the demonstration method, (7) the problem-solving method, (8) the project method, (9) the dramatization and role-playing method, (10) the unit method, (11) the media-oriented method, (12) the laboratory method, and (13) the oral report method.

Some of the more popular approaches used in the past are briefly described below. With some alterations, many of these can be adapted to conform with current philosophical thinking and practice. As a matter of fact, many of the so-called current or even experimental methods which we will discuss later are in reality adaptations from traditional methods, applications of philosophical thought of many decades ago, or both.

Teacher-centered approaches

These methods originate with the teachers and remain within their control throughout the learning period. There may from time to time be some learner participation, but generally this is controlled by the teacher and held to a minimum. Some of the methods that possess these characteristics are:

1. *The lecture method,* which is one of the oldest methods used in formal health education. It continues to be popular among college and secondary school health educators. It is characterized by the presentation by the teacher of a body of facts through verbal (and usually one-way) communication. It has the advantage of facilitating the coverage of a large amount of information in a short period of time. However, it defeats its own purpose, since very little learning usually takes place during the lecture period. It tends to bore students, discourage critical thinking, remove interest, and lessen motivation.

   The lecture method should be used rarely, if at all, at the elementary school level. It may be effective if used sparingly at the secondary school level in conjunction with other modified methods (e.g., questions from students, use of visual aids, and general discussions following the presentation). Even then, the lecture should be used only with information that students can not obtain in other more effective ways. For example, there is no valid reason for the teacher to lecture about information contained in the textbooks or other printed sources available to the student. Also, the content of many lectures can be reproduced for students who can then read the material and critically analyze it for discussion later.

2. *The textbook method* may appear in several variations. For instance, oral reading, where a learner reads a portion, then another, and so on, until the topic has been covered; or silent reading, related to a specific assignment. These approaches have proved to be nearly completely ineffective in bringing about any significant learning.

   Textbooks should be used as reference materials related to acquiring factual information and/or seeing a variety of opinions of authorities regarding a particular health issue or problem. The use of textbooks and the lecture methods are probably among the most abused approaches to learning being used in health education. However, reading, if purposeful, can be a valuable aid to learning.

3. *The recitation method* implies memorization of health information which is then recited during class time. It has very little value as an indication of what the learner understands about what is being recited; it tends to remove individuality and creativeness, while emphasizing rote learning and indoctrination. It is used frequently in relation to memorization of health vocabulary without a comprehension of significances and applications.

4. *The question and answer method* could be either teacher– or learner-centered, depending upon who is in control of the questioning. If the questions originate with the teacher, it is teacher-centered. This approach can be modified to stimulate in-depth learning and debate whether teacher- or learner-controlled. It is especially valuable for motivating two-way communication and important feedback. Questions should be formulated to direct discussion toward specific conclusions about the health issue.

Learner observational

This includes a wide variety of methods that provide the learner with the opportunity to observe others who are actively engaged in some sort of activity, or to observe the operation of machinery or other mechanical devices. Although this approach is generally passive learning in that the learner does not actively participate in the activity, it may bring about an emotional participation. It can bring into play several of the other senses besides sight, for example, smelling the cooking of foods, tasting, and feeling the texture of foods. The most frequently used examples of this approach are the demonstration, the field trip, and the use of media resources.

The *demonstration method* is usually teacher-centered or conducted by a visiting authority in some aspect of health. The method can become more effective if the learners are involved in the planning and conducting phases. Student participation should be considered, especially at the secondary school level, but many kinds of demonstrations can also be done by elementary school pupils. Demonstrations should allow for learner questions and follow-up discussion. They are most effective when kept short and focus on a particular health concept.

Field trips provide learners with experiences beyond their normal environmental contacts; they can broaden the learners' view of the community and the world in general and develop an appreciation for the work of others and an understanding of some of the problems encountered in business, industry, and the health professions. Field trips should be carefully planned by both the teacher and the learners. Specific things or events to observe should be anticipated, and opportunities for students to ask questions during the trip should be provided. In addition, there should be an opportunity for students to share their experiences upon return to class.

The use of media resources has long been an integral part of most health education programs. The media available for this method include sensory stimulators; for example, textbooks, pamphlets, and other literature, workbooks, scrapbooks, chalkboard, bulletin board, flannel or magnetic boards, slides, photographs or other still pictures, the diorama, posters, charts, models, radio, videotapes, audio tapes, films, filmstrips, and the use of numerous projective devices, such as the opaque projector and overhead projector. Media resources are generally more effective when used in conjunction with other teaching/learning approaches. They can provide a variety of dimensions for learning and enhance the effectiveness of other approaches such as the lecture method. Media can also be used in a variety of ways to motivate learning or as a substitute for field trips when they are not practical. The use of media can become even more valuable when the learner is involved in the selection or actual creation of the device. For example, learners could plan, write, perform, and produce a videotape or movie which could then be shared with other classes, the faculty, or parent groups.

Learner-centered approaches

Motivation for learning is more likely to occur when the learner is actively engaged in all phases of the learning process: planning, selection of objectives, the learning experiences, and self-evaluation. As we will see later on in this chapter, methods currently used by many health educators and those still in the experimental stages of development concentrate on student involvement in their own learning. This has also been true with some traditional methods that have been developed over the past few decades. They include such approaches as problem-solving, creative activities, decision-making, research, debates and discussions, and fieldwork experiences.

The *problem-solving method* is characterized by a series of discoveries by learners as they proceed to solve the health problem. This method may use a variety of other methods in the process, such as research to gather pertinent information necessary to arrive at a solution. It also involves several principles of learning: trial and error, inductive thinking, decision-making, experimentation, and the like. Essentially, this method entails learners identifying the problem, obtaining information (usually from many sources), confirming the accuracy of the information, interpreting it, deciding on the alternative solutions, and selecting the best solution. The culminating experience is the application of the solution selected to the problem and observing the consequences. Health education authorities have long recognized the value of this approach in favorably influencing health attitudes and behavior of students as well as in encouraging the acquisition of in-depth knowledge related to the health problem. It tends to be a lasting experience for the learner. Moreover, the problem-solving approach can be adapted to every developmental level of learners.

Creative activities provide ways in which the learners can acquire insight into the health problem or ways they can assist others to understand the problem. This approach gives opportunities to learners to become expressive and individual in demonstrating their knowledge of a particular health matter. It is a most effective method for use with elementary school children.

The *decision-making method* is usually an outcome of other approaches such as the problem-solving method. Essentially, the learner is given several alternatives and can then discover the consequences of each upon which a decision for personal action is based. As a result, learners learn to make judgments about their analysis of the health information available. Such learning can have valuable long-term implications when learners are faced with health decisions in the future.

The *research method* affords learners an opportunity to develop a research design and carry it through to a conclusion. During the process, they will acquire knowledge about the health issue, a sense of objectivity, and the ability to make a contribution to the learning of others or perhaps to society. As an example, a learner may conduct a survey of a community health problem (such as water pollution), discover why it exists or who is responsible, suggest a solution, and present it to the media or responsible community leaders for consideration. This method is applicable to an individual learner or to a small group of learners.

Debates and discussions have long been popular with health educators as a method to motivate both intellectual and emotional exchange among learners. It is an effective method for developing a respect for the ideas and opinions of others as well as for acquiring insight into a particular health problem. This method needs to be carefully planned (as do all of them), and it should be moderated by a person that the class respects. Another important outcome of this method is that students learn to listen, communicate, and analyze what is being said.

Fieldwork experiences for elementary and secondary school pupils is a relatively new approach to health learning that has shown great promise for success especially in achieving the goal of attitude development. Essentially, students spend a part of their day actually working in a health-related community agency. They have an opportunity to work in close association with experts in the health area. As a result, learners will develop an appreciation for the occupation, increase their knowledge of the health problem and the ways in which it is handled, and, most important, they will be providing a community service. The experiential approach requires careful planning, coordination, and supervision. The personnel of the community health agency must be aware that the student is there to learn and to work, not merely to observe or to do menial tasks.

CURRENT METHODS FOR HEALTH LEARNING

Introduction: learning or teaching?

Many of the traditional methods we have been discussing are currently in use on a wide scale. There has been, however, a major trend toward modifying some of these approaches or combining effective aspects of several of them to form what appears to be a completely new and different way of teaching about health. This is exemplified in the emphasis on learner-centered philosophy over teacher-centered philosophy of just a few years ago. For instance, instead of the teacher leading class discussions, there is now a tendency to provide learners with the opportunity to direct their own discussions either in large or small group arrangements. Such a move places greater emphasis on the learning process than on the teaching process. As a result, the teacher takes the role of a catalyst for learning rather than a giver of information. This is a procedure that is vital for the success of current effective approaches, as well as the experimental methods discussed later. Such an approach stresses the application of the principles of group dynamics.

In all fairness, however, it is important to recognize that the bulk of methods used through the 1960s and early 1970s placed major emphasis on teaching rather than on the learning process. And, in practice, teachers generally conducted health education classes with a focus on passive rather than active learning. The teacher with authoritarian inclinations is more likely to feel comfortable with teacher-dominated approaches, while the secure and open-minded teacher will feel comfortable with learner-centered approaches that stress cooperative rather than competitive learning. On the one hand, we have teacher-centered classes with active learning and the teacher taking a passive, catalytic role, while on the other hand, we have teacher-centered classes with the teacher taking a dominating role, resulting in passive learning. Learner-centered classes always require that the teacher facilitates active learning. Figure 12–2 illustrates this relationship between teacher and learner.

Inductive and deductive learning?

Discovery is learning; it is the fundamental principle underlying inductive thinking. The inductive method, introduced by Francis Bacon in the 1600s, became the forerunner of modern scientific methodology. Prior to the Renaissance, demonology dominated the thinking of people as they attempted to explain natural phenomena. During these times, conclusions were deduced from historical premises, most of which evolved from beliefs that spirits (or demons) were responsible for the fate of humanity.

The inductive method begins with a question (or hypothesis), followed by an accumulation of empirical evidence (discoveries). Con-

FIGURE 12–2 Teacher-Centered Approaches vs Learner-Centered Approaches
Active learning is most desirable, permanent, and applicable to improved health behavior.
Learner-centered approaches are more apt to result in active learning than are teacher-
centered approaches.

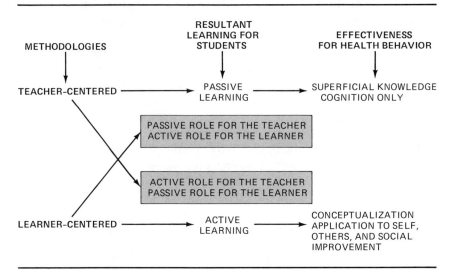

clusions are then formed from the evidence. The deductive method
assumes certain facts and premises to be accurate, with a conclusion
based upon these "known" truths.

Deductive reasoning is akin to syllogistic reasoning. That is, conclusions necessarily follow the premise. For example, three plus three
is necessarily six. In health education, this kind of learning is exemplified
by rote memorization of certain health facts and its result. In simplistic
terms, if one does not brush one's teeth, tooth decay will result. In this
approach, the learner acquires a body of health information with the
hope that certain results will occur. For instance, it was thought by
health educators at the turn of the century that if students memorized
the structure and function of the body they would by necessity respect
and take better care of their bodies. Finally, deductive reasoning is
characterized by moving from a general premise to a specific conclusion.
The real problem with this method is that as students are memorizing
certain facts, they are unaware of the reasons for it. Consequently, the
information is perceived as irrelevant and is soon forgotten, frequently
before conclusions can be made. In addition, this approach tends to
limit learning to the facts at hand; it generally limits creativity and the
discovery of new knowledge and encourages indoctrination.

In contrast, *inductive reasoning* encourages discovery and creativity
and discourages indoctrination. This approach is characterized by an
understanding by the learner of the nature of the health issue followed

by techniques to acquire evidence or other information to explain it. It tends to open new doors to learning; new discoveries are made, and new issues arise. The inductive method tends to initiate and perpetuate motivation and learning. Its principles are the basis for problem-solving and the scientific method. Figure 12–3 compares inductive and deductive learning.

Individualized learning

Individualized learning means many things to many people. It may mean, for example, grouping learners according to certain kinds of abilities or talents; differentiating the curriculum; meeting the learning needs of individuals on an individual, one-on-one basis, and the like. Health educators generally perceive individualized learning as a means of arranging the learning environment so that all learners have the opportunity to satisfy their health needs and interests according to personal capabilities and at times and in ways that best suit their motivation and speed of learning. Individualized learning can occur whether the learners are in large groups, small groups, one-on-one, or working independently. Essentially, it all depends upon the goals, the point of learning for each individual, and the approaches being used. *If each*

FIGURE 12–3   Inductive and Deductive Learning

Inductive learning is more effective for developing decision-making skills and for solving health problems than deductive learning. Deductive learning tends to limit creativity, exploration, and comprehension.

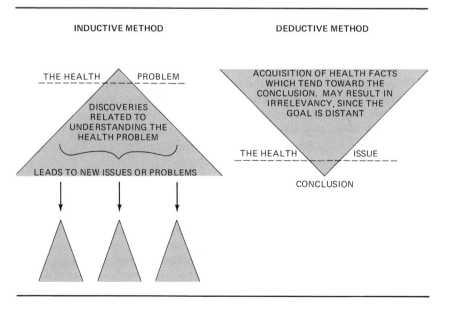

learner is learning according to anticipated levels of achievement, it is individualized learning. Individualized learning is determined by whether or not each individual is in fact learning.

Of course, this is an oversimplification of what frequently is a complex problem, since it is not always possible, or even desirable, to select approaches that will affect learning equally among all learners. Therefore, it becomes necessary to ascertain what needs to be done with some learners and to arrange the learning environment and techniques accordingly. The use, for example, of programmed .materials, a variety of visual and other resources, peer teaching, independent study and research, and variations in strategies may be necessary. In any event, there should be opportunities for slower learners to proceed at their own pace and for faster learners to be allowed to exceed general expectations. Nearly any effective method can be adapted to achieve these ends.

Self-directed learning

The term self-directed learning is probably a misnomer. It is more accurately described as directed learning, a procedure that became popular during the middle to late 1960s. It is very closely associated with individualized learning, since its characteristics include many of those in this area and its primary purpose is not only to provide a means for learners to proceed at their individual pace, but also to offer a variety of learning options under the direction of a teacher. One such program* was developed in health education and implemented in 1969.

INNOVATIVE HEALTH EDUCATION   (A sample)
(Secondary Level)

Introduction
This developmental program in health education utilized three basic approaches to teaching and learning; (1) traditional organization and methodology in a modified form, (2) some aspects of team teaching, and (3) independent and self-directed study and research.

Secondary school principals continued to provide health education time, personnel, and scheduling in the traditional patterns. However, the secondary health education department planned who, what, and how the program would be implemented. This gave teachers a direct, professional role in decision-making regarding health content and methodology. It used the specific expertise of each teacher more effectively. The result was that students benefited more directly from teachers and their learning became greater. Obviously, this required that health educators take an active part in planning, that they cooperate with each other in a total team effort, and that departmental efforts become highly coordinated.

---

* "Innovative Health Education" was developed and implemented by Albert E. Bedworth in 1969 in the Ithaca City School District (New York).

Although teachers were assigned to a building and scheduled traditionally, their expertise was used at any level or in any building. This greater use of individual talents was decided by the department. This approach used professional staff most effectively and tended to decrease loss of continuity and learning for students in the event of teacher absence or turnover.

It was essential to emphasize the need for the health education department to function as a team in planning and developing materials and procedures for the most effective educational experiences for the student. This required weekly department meetings to discuss the next one or two week's work in relation to the students and teachers. Further, it was important that the health department continuously evaluate the effectiveness and success of the program as it developed.

The function of the teachers was necessarily changed from that of dominating the learning situation to the role of counselor, consultant, motivator, and organizer of learning experiences. Teachers needed to prepare better—more thoroughly—and to improve self-evaluation and student evaluation, arrange for continuous self-improvement, learn new teaching methods, and concentrate more on student motivation and inspiration. Students, on the other hand, needed to be given the opportunity to evaluate themselves, become involved in decision-making regarding what and how they should learn, and be given time and assistance for self-directed study.

Purpose of this Health Education Reorganization
1. To provide students with greater motivation to learn.
2. To provide students with more relevant health information.
3. To provide students with opportunities to accept responsibilities for their own learning.
4. To provide students with opportunities to investigate and discuss health content and problems in greater depth through large group discussions, small group discussions, and self-directed study.
5. To provide students with more direct contact with teachers and others who could share their expertise with them.
6. To provide more direct learning guidance for students.
7. To use teacher time and professional competence most effectively as they related to the learning of students.

Independent Study
Students were given greater opportunity to investigate, either superficially or in detail, health areas in which they had the greatest interest and need. Time during the week was provided for this. Students were provided with specific guidelines, suggested activities, goals, and self-testing materials to assist them in the learning of basic information. Also, there was always available at least one teacher aide, and frequently a professional teacher to provide the students with guidance and direction in self-learning. This provision for independent study . . .
1. Allowed students to investigate those areas of health content in which they needed to obtain more basic information and greater understanding, or in which they had a special interest and wished to investigate in depth.

2. Provided students with more opportunities to learn greater amounts of materials covering a broader scope.
3. Eliminated almost completely "busy work" wherein all students did the same things regardless of their individual needs and desires.
4. Provided students with more valuable learning experiences and greater opportunity to make choices about their learning.

Further, this organization provided teachers with time to work more directly with the students, to develop more effective curriculum materials, and to plan more meaningful class discussions. Independent study was neither homework nor required written work.

Peer approaches

Lawler stated that "many approaches to solving the drug problem are being tried. The main advantages of the peer group approach is that we are involving students to help us with a mutual problem. The realization that students are an untapped resource to help society influence others is the hope of the seventies."[10]

It was the drug crisis of the late 1960s that gave birth to the peer approach to solving health problems. Peer approaches were varied; some were characterized by rap sessions by students and others by students becoming trained in working with other students. Even training sessions were quite varied. Some involved merely an orientation, while others involved extensive workships conducted by highly trained, skilled instructors. Finally, some peer approaches consisted of high school students attempting to teach elementary school pupils. Some have experienced a degree of success while others were tragedies.

Experience has told us that for the peer approach to be successful the peer teachers must be trained as any teacher would be. The advantage, apparently, to this approach is that students are sometimes able to relate more specifically to other students. But upon close examination, the peer approach is nothing more than an educational environment that encourages a free interchange between the learners. It is our contention that unskilled and untrained students are not a substitute for an understanding, skilled, and open-minded teacher. The peer approach, therefore, is essentially a label.

EXPERIMENTAL APPROACHES

What is an experimental approach?

As we have seen, health education methodologies have evolved from greater understanding of the principles of learning and their application to health learning. Many of these have established themselves as effective ways of assisting the learner in comprehending the nature and ramifications of societal and personal health issues, at least with some learners under certain kinds of circumstances. Experimental approaches are those that have not as yet proved themselves as effective or as more effective than those presently being used. They are generally based upon sound logic and application of research findings, but still need to be used in a variety of situations with a variety of learners to ascertain their actual worth. However, some approaches that have been tried in recent years have their roots primarily in a philosophical rather than a scientific base. Examples of experimental approaches that have received varying amounts of popularity include values clarification, transactional analysis, transcendental meditation, and computerized learning. Transactional analysis and transcendental meditation remain as very controversial, unproven methods, and are shunned by most health educators. Values clarification and computerized learning have received widespread popularity and for this reason we shall discuss only these methods, since they have shown the greatest promise for success for future generations of learners.

Values clarification

The essential elements of this approach originated with John Dewey in the early part of this century. In his book, *How We Think*, Dewey laid down principles that gave impetus to problem-solving and other methodologies. During the 1960s, Raths, Hochbaum, Simon, and others contributed to the development of values clarification as a vital methodology for health learning. Its application has become widespread in the ensuing decade and a half.

Values clarification approaches contain two essential elements: (1) strategies for identifying areas for value judgments to take place, and (2) making personal decisions regarding one's own values. This approach emphasizes the processes used by learners to arrive at a value judgment consistent with their own intellectual, moral, and social structure. It is not concerned with what the value judgment is or with whether or not it is right or wrong. Its purpose is to assist learners in clarifying their moral, ethical, and social relationships, resulting in self-understanding.

Simon, et al[11] emphasize that success in this method is more likely to occur if the strategies used are based upon a value grid approach. Briefly, this grid requires learners to indicate whether or not they chose the belief freely, considered alternatives, considered any consequences from the choice; whether or not they prized or cherished the choice, affirmed the choice to others, acted on the choice; and whether the choice was repeated to become incorporated into their life-style.

Stone, et al[12] suggest the use of the following strategies for formulating one's value judgments: rank order, wherein the learner chooses among alternatives; voting techniques on health issues; a values continuum; a values whip that forces learners to state how they arrived at their decision; interview techniques to acquire opinions of others; open-ended statements; the use of the "devil's advocate" role play; the use of the Likert scales; role play techniques; autobiographical sketches;

the use of appreciation activities that assist learners in developing a positive self-image; and the use of a variety of communications activities.

This methodology is intended to assist learners to identify and clarify their thinking regarding vital health issues and to understand (clarify) their values. It is not intended to force the values of others upon them. It is completely void of any attempts at indoctrination. The method, when used appropriately, results in a learner-centered atmosphere with the teacher's role being one of a facilitator and catalyst.

Computerized learning

Originally conceived by Harnack in the early 1960s, the development of computer-based resource units (CBRU) forged the trail for a whole new process of learning. Although CBRUs were initially intended "to encourage and to aid individualized instruction by providing instructors [not students] with pre-planning suggestions,"[13] they have been used by teachers as a technique to involve learners in their own learning. This is accomplished by learners selecting their own objectives and identifying their own characteristics, which are then entered into the computer, providing suggested learning experiences that learners can pursue to achieve their objectives.

The use of computers continues to make great strides forward as a method for assisting learners in solving a wide variety of health problems. Computers have the potential for making readily available to the learner an enormous amount of current information almost instantly. There have been attempts at using the computer in conjunction with video equipment that makes it possible for learners to communicate directly with the computer. We can anticipate more widespread use of this approach in the coming years, especially in view of some of the educational constraints that have been developing recently, not the least of which is the economics of educating children and youth through conventional channels. However, computerized learning, as with all methods, should be perceived as an additional tool to aid both the teacher and the learner in educational pursuits.

Experiential strategies

The foregoing discussions emphasize the basic concept that there are numerous methods, strategies, and techniques available to teachers and learners alike. New ones are developing almost daily. In the final analysis, the effectiveness of health learning will depend upon the skill, creativity, understanding, and compassion of the teacher. *No one can direct the teacher to the best approaches that must be used with specific groups of learners.* At best, we can only explore what is known and share experiences with each other. The experiential strategies are offered as a starting point only; they are not intended as a recipe for teaching and learning about health.

These strategies exemplify the close relationship between curriculum design and its application to methodology and ultimately to the health learning of students. It is suggested that the reader return to Chapter 11 and *analyze* the strategies presented in light of our discussion of methodology.

The suggestions are categorized according to some of the major health issues already discussed; broad objectives are also given with the intent that the successful application of the strategies will affect achievement of objectives for most learners. Neither the objectives nor the strategies are presented in any progressive order or priority. It must be left to the teacher to make relevant choices regarding this matter.

DEFINITIVE UNDERSTANDINGS

The basis for learning is effective communications. Communications take place when there is an interchange of ideas, thoughts, and opinions between individuals or between a person and the environment. The science of the study of communications systems is called information theory. There are five elements of information theory: (1) the source of the information, (2) the transmitter, (3) the communication channel, (4) the receiver, and (5) the destination.

People are goal-seeking organisms that can be compared to servo-mechanisms. These are devices that have built-in mechanisms that direct the object to a predetermined target or goal. The target provides feedback to the servomechanism which guides it to its destination. Learning also follows a similar pattern when teachers are aware of the learners' reactions to the learning experiences and when they respond to this feedback by achieving the goal. The science that is concerned with computer engineering and human neurology is called cybernetics.

Methods of health learning should be selected on the basis of their effectiveness for communicating adequately with the learners and for helping them achieve their objective. In this regard, communication is the most fundamental consideration in method selection; it is a two-way process. Feedback is a two-way process characterized as verbal and/or nonverbal. Feedback, therefore, determines the effectiveness of the communication process as well as the appropriateness of the methodology.

Methodology is the broad process that motivates learning. It consists of techniques and strategies that are planned and organized in such a way as to guide the learner through experiences vital to achieving the objectives. Methods may be either learner– or teacher-centered, but when appropriate and effective, either approach ultimately affects learning. Teaching methods should influence the quality of learning methods. They essentially originate with the learner but their purpose is to facilitate learning. With this in mind, methods must take into account the characteristics of the learner as well as those of the teacher and the learning environment. Such an accounting tends to increase the likelihood that learning will be individualized. Teachers should avoid approaches with which they feel uncomfortable or about which they lack adequate knowledge regarding their implementation. Methods being used should always be dynamic, creating an atmosphere that results in learner enthusiasm. However, it is important to recognize certain factors may preclude the use of even an excellent method at any particular time. Moreover, some learners may not be prepared for learning in some instances, regardless of the care taken in selecting a method. It is also vital that new learning be built upon existing readiness patterns. Readiness will vary from learner to learner because of different rates of maturation, past experiences, and present circumstances that may interfere with learning motivation. As a result, techniques and strategies may need to be used with individuals to overcome these differences.

Health education is essentially an applied science. It differs from health science, which is narrower in view and practice. Science is concerned chiefly with the acquisition of knowledge, while health education is concerned with application of knowledge to favorably influence one's life. The health educator must be trained in the health sciences, education, health, and the applied sciences. Therefore, health education is a multidimensional process.

Learning resources are valuable as techniques within the perimeters of a method. They are used to enhance the learning experience, to add a new dimension to the process. Learning resources may take the form of materials or people. In either case, they should be carefully evaluated and selected as an adjunct to the learning experience.

Learning experiences range from those that are abstract to those that are concrete. Abstract experiences are chiefly characterized by passive learning, while concrete ones are characterized by active learning. The more mature the learners are, and the richer their past experiences have been, the more likely that abstract methods will be effective. However, under no set of circumstances are abstract methods more effective than concrete and direct experiences, all other things being equal.

Traditional methods of health education are those that have been used for many years, many of which have proved themselves to be effective. However, many of those methods were introduced during times when teacher-dominated classes were popular. With the introduction of the humanization of education, teacher-centered approaches are gradually being discarded and replaced by learner-centered approaches. Some of the teacher-centered approaches are the lecture, textbook, recitation, or rote. Learner-centered methods include problem-solving, creative activities, research, independent study, debates, and fieldwork experiences.

Current methods stress the importance of the learning process without ignoring the importance of the teaching process for bringing about learning. The teacher is more and more being conceived of as a facilitator of learning and as a catalyst for learning. This is exemplified by the use of such methods as inductive learning, individualized learning, learner-controlled discussions, small group work, self-directed learning, peer approaches, values clarification, and computerized learning.

PROBLEMS
FOR DISCUSSION

1. Select a traditional, teacher-centered method and alter it to make it learner-centered.
2. Describe ways that the teacher can identify significant nonverbal feedback from the learners. Describe the characteristics of nonverbal feedback. What are some strategies that a teacher can use to motivate feedback?
3. Distinguish between method, technique, and strategy.
4. Develop a lesson plan. Include learner objectives, methods, techniques, and strategies to be used. Describe the pertinent characteristics of the learners and why you think the approach selected will be effective. Roll-play the lesson plan and have the class evaluate its effectiveness.
5. Identify some of your strong qualities as a potential teacher. Describe why you feel you possess these qualities and how they will make you a better teacher.
6. Effectiveness of teaching is dependent to a great extent upon the relationships established between the learners and the teacher and among the learners themselves. Explain why this is so, if you believe it is or why it is not so, if you do not agree. How do relationships affect learning?
7. Describe at least five ways that material and/or human resources can be used most effectively to influence learning. Try one with your classmates.
8. Describe in detail five experiential strategies that can be used with a variety of learners. For example, "Have learners develop a survey instrument to determine the community's attitudes toward alcohol use (abuse). Conduct the survey, organize the data, interpret them and draw conclusions." Describe the teacher's role regarding each of the five strategies described.
9. Suppose that you wanted to use the peer approach with a group of senior high school students. Describe what you would do to implement the approach and to evaluate its effectiveness.

REFERENCES

1. Gordon, Thomas, T.E.T.: Teacher Effectiveness Training, Peter H. Wyden, Publisher, New York, 1974, p. 66.
2. Stone, Donald, et al., Elementary School Health Education: Ecological Perspectives, William C. Brown Company, Publishers, Dubuque, 1976, p. 255.
3. Russell, Robert D., Health Education, Joint Committee on Health Problems of the National Education Association and the American Medical Association, Washington, D.C., 1975, p. 171.
4. Dewey, John, How We Think, D. C. Heath and Company, Boston, 1933, p. 9.
5. Bersoff, Donald N., "Child Advocacy: The Next Step," New York University Education Quarterly, New York University Press, 1976, p. 12.
6. Dorland's Illustrated Medical Dictionary, 24th ed., W. B. Saunders Company, Philadelphia, 1965.

7. Ibid.
8. Stone, et al., op. cit., p. 133.
9. Dale, Edgar, *Audiovisual Methods in Teaching,* Holt, Rinehart and Winston, Inc., New York, 1946.
10. Lawler, John T., "Peer Group Approach to Drug Education," *Journal of Drug Education,* 1(1), 1971, p. 63.
11. Simon, Sidney B., Leland Howe, and Howard Kirschbaum, *Values-Clarification: A Handbook of Practical Strategies for Teachers and Students,* Hart Publishing Company, New York, 1972.
12. Stone, et al., op. cit., pp. 277–279.
13. Center for Curriculum Planning, *Computer-Based Curriculum Planning,* State University of New York at Buffalo, 1974, p. 1.

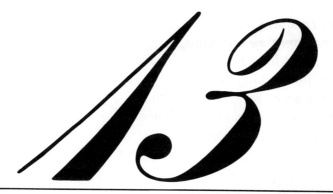

Evaluation in Health Education

*We can encourage professional
excellence only by redefining
academic excellence . . . which may
well include looking for the ways in
which learners are excellent rather
than merely measuring how they are
not by limited, traditional
evaluation modes.*

Robert D. Russell

Health educators do not seek an easy
life for self or others, but do seek
to make people stronger. They do
not seek tasks equal to their
strengths, but do seek strength equal
to their tasks.

AEB
DAB

PRINCIPLES OF EVALUATION

Our discussions of evaluation will include those principles and procedures that can be adapted by the school, community, and patient health educator. Because of the variations in learning environments and the nature of the learners in each (some are well, some are sick, some are children, some are adults), it would be impossible to describe specifically evaluation techniques for each. Therefore, we will concentrate chiefly on school health education evaluation. However, the general principles of evaluation apply to all health education programs. Decisions regarding what techniques should be used and when they should be used must be left to the judgment of the individual evaluator. Finally, although this section deals with the principles of evaluation, discussions of principles will appear throughout the chapter.

Definitions

We need to begin by eliminating the misconceptions that measurement and evaluation are synonymous, that evaluation techniques can be either objective or subjective (all contain some degree of both), and that attitudes can not be ascertained. (We will see that some attitudes can be determined with a high degree of accuracy.)

Anderson states that "evaluation may be considered an appraisal, assessment, or measurement in the *broadest* and most complete sense."[1] Evaluation may be described by the use of such terms as estimation, calculation, determination, approximation, worth, or even opinion. The use of such synonyms, however, fails to recognize that evaluation is a process as well. Bedworth and D'Elia define evaluation as "a complex process of measurement and judgment which includes *gathering, organizing and interpreting* information."[2]

The extent of complexity of evaluation is influenced by the nature of what is being evaluated. For example, it is relatively simple to gather accurate data regarding the increased acquisition of learner health facts. Test instruments can be developed or existing standardized ones may be used for this purpose. The chief quality of standardized tests is that they are generally developed by authorities and as such, each test item is most likely to be carefully written, decreasing the possibility of ambiguity. The items, therefore, are apt to possess a high degree of validity. The chief weakness, however, is that they are developed with general objectives in mind for the entire (or at least large) learning population rather than being geared to the specific group of learners. Therefore, they can not be used to determine the degree to which local teacher and learner objectives have been achieved.

Gathering information about changes in health attitudes or behavior is much more difficult, since we are dealing with less concrete, extremely complex results of learning. This is especially true in the measurement of health attitudes. Standardized tests are also available to evaluate health attitudes and behavior; however, many are obsolete. Standardized tests may be used to verify strengths and weaknesses and to justify what is being done. They may be useful for comparing the class of learners with statistical norms as well.

Objectivity and subjectivity of an evaluation instrument refers to scoring consistency. An objective instrument is one that reflects a high degree of scoring consistency regardless of who is doing the scoring. Little if any judgment is needed by the scorer. A subjective instrument is one that requires the scorer to be trained, experienced, and skilled in interpreting the responses obtained with the instrument. The scorer must possess skills in judgment. As a result, two or more persons may arrive at quite different scores from the same instrument. This is due simply to the fact that one person may place a greater (or lesser) value on a response than another person. Both objective and subjective instruments are valuable devices for evaluating specific objective achievement for a specific learner or group of learners by a specific health educator. Subjective instruments become less valid and reliable with larger populations whose objectives and learning approaches may be quite varied.

There are two chief faults with an objective instrument: (1) they measure simple recall or recognition of health facts and are limited in measuring comprehension, and (2) the instrument is subjectively developed, since the test items and their design are selected (valued) by the person developing the instrument. Another person, for example, may judge the items and/or design as unimportant. Therefore, an objective test is one that is designed in such a way that it is likely to yield objective results.

A valid instrument is one that measures what it is intended to measure. For example, a tape measure or ruler are valid instruments for measuring short, linear distances. A reliable instrument is one that yields consistent results each time it is used. A valid instrument is always reliable, but a reliable instrument may not always be valid. For instance, an automobile odometer is valid for measuring relatively long, linear distances and will produce the same approximate results each time it is used.

The validity and reliability of a measuring device can be determined by the use of rather complex mathematical procedures. However, such procedures are unnecessary for teacher-made instruments, since they are intended for use with a specific group of learners providing care is taken to establish at least a face validity. *Face validity* simply means that the instrument, in the judgment of experts (and a health educator is an expert in this case), will evaluate what it is purported to. That is to say, the test is obviously designed to elicit certain kinds of data.

It is clear that although some methods used to evaluate program effectiveness can be highly objective, the final results of evaluation are always subjective. The very nature of evaluation requires judgment on the part of the individual making the interpretations. Interpretations, however, can become more accurate if care has been taken in planning the evaluation program, developing the measuring devices so that complete and accurate information is obtained, and organizing the data in the most useful way.

What should be evaluated?

The economics of education has generated unprecedented interest in accountability in education in recent years. This is especially true in regards to those areas of the curriculum that deviate from the basic disciplines that have established themselves over the decades, Specifically, such areas of the curriculum as reading, writing, and arithmetic are generally understood areas and are subject to scrutiny only when test scores indicate that learners in a particular school appear to fall below certain state or national norms. Curriculum areas that have been introduced into the schools in relatively recent years, or those that are not understood by the community, school administrators, legislators, and others, are subject to reduction or elimination in times of economic crisis. The school health program is an example of just such an area. It is therefore imperative that those responsible for the health program develop and implement an evaluation program that will yield concrete data about its effectiveness. This will demonstrate to concerned persons how it can contribute to the education of children and youth and the reduction of both the prevalence and incidence of current critical health problems.

The first step in planning an evaluation program is to decide specifically what should be evaluated. This will be determined primarily by the goals and objectives of the health program. Generally, the broad areas to consider are: (1) the health education program through all of its progressive phases, (2) the health services program, both school- and community-based (in Chapter 2 we outlined some basic criteria regarding this important aspect of the health program), and (3) the environment in which people must live, work, learn, and so on.

Each of these general areas takes on different evaluative dimensions when we begin to consider the varieties of settings in which they may occur. Health education, as we have seen, can occur in three forms: school, community, and patient. The same is true with health services and healthful environments. And, as we discussed in Chapter 2, the primary goals for people in the three levels of health are necessarily different; therefore, what to evaluate will also be necessarily different. For example, school health education, broadly speaking, is concerned with keeping well people well and providing them with the intellectual essentials for improving their health status. The patient health educator is concerned with returning individuals to society as contributing members. The public health educator is chiefly concerned with health education directed toward the proper utilization of community health personnel and facilities. The degree to which these primary goals, as well as more specific ones, are achieved should be the focus of the evaluation program.

Purpose of evaluation

The overall purpose of evaluation is adequately described by Stone, et al. as "useful in determining the needs, assessing the strengths and weaknesses, and improving various areas that comprise the total health program."[3] Evaluation is positive and purposeful; it is conducted to determine the following:

- The value of learning experiences, past and present.
- The value of learning aids and the ways in which they have been used or are being used.
- The effectiveness of methods, techniques, and strategies.
- The effectiveness of program planning, organization, and implementation.
- The speed at which learning is taking place.
- The quality of learning for each individual as well as for the group.
- The consistencies or inconsistencies that may exist between goals and processes.
- The changes that must be made in any element of the program (goals, objectives, processes, etc.).

Evaluation not only indicates what is right or wrong with what is being done, it provides a procedure to question certain aspects of the program. *Evaluation is a cyclic and continuous process developed and implemented as an integral component of any educational effort.* It should provide information regarding the impact that the educational program is having on the learner. Evaluation should begin, be accomplished, be finished, and provide a basis for beginning again. It should not be a hit or miss, sporadic, crisis-motivated process. In this sense, the evaluation program is diagnostic as well as prognostic, indicating what changes are needed.

No element of the evaluation should ever be used for disciplinary purposes. Grades should inform the teacher, the parent, and the learner about the degree to which the objectives are being achieved. They are essentially a progress report. They tend to act as a barometer of the learning that is occurring. Oberteuffer states: "When evaluation procedures are used as a threat, they can have negative results not only on learning but on the students themselves as well as their perception of the course and the learning process."[4]

Qualitative and quantitative evaluation

Information obtained from testing techniques may become more meaningful if grouped according to some common characteristics. The usual practice is to categorize the data either qualitatively or quantitatively, even though there is a rather fine distinction between the two.

Qualitative information is grouped according to similar characteristics or qualities; for example, boys or girls, youth or adults, teachers or parents, smokers or nonsmokers, and so on. As a result, comparisons can be made and information interpreted more readily. Quantitative information, on the other hand, has a measurable dimension that can be given a numerical value (e.g., the number of students who do or do not smoke cigarettes). Obviously, the accuracy and meaningfulness of the interpretation of the information is dependent not only upon the quality of the instrument being used but upon the care taken to organize the data appropriately.

DEVELOPING EVALUATIVE CRITERIA

Evaluation related to objectives

In Chapter 4 we discussed the importance of identifying realistic and achievable goals and stating objectives precisely and in measurable terms. Objectives must convey specifically what is to be measured and they may indicate directly or indirectly how the measurement is to be accomplished. In this regard, the objectives establish the criteria upon which measurement and ultimately evaluation will be based. Finally, the way in which objectives are stated will influence the validity of evaluation. Oberteuffer, et al.[5] emphasized this point when they stated that "specification of instructional objectives in behavioral terms not only facilitates but assumes the validity of related evaluation procedures. . . . Objectives provide a blueprint for what is to be evaluated and how it might be done." Figure 13–1 put this concept into perspective.

Once objectives have been identified, teaching strategies must be determined. These influence the quality of learning experiences that will take place. Evaluation approaches are selected to assess the degree to which these objectives have been achieved. They provide information regarding the effectiveness of the teaching/learning strategies as well.

Dependent and independent variables

Although evaluation in health education does not need to be so highly structured as to incorporate all the elements of the experimental method, it is important to understand some of its basic principles. Objectives of health education can be equated with the hypothesis of an experi-

FIGURE 13–1 Objectives as Evaluative Criteria
The results of comprehensive evaluation techniques provide clues for changes in the elements affecting health learning. These changes can be inferred from the degree to which learners are achieving their objectives (learner progress).

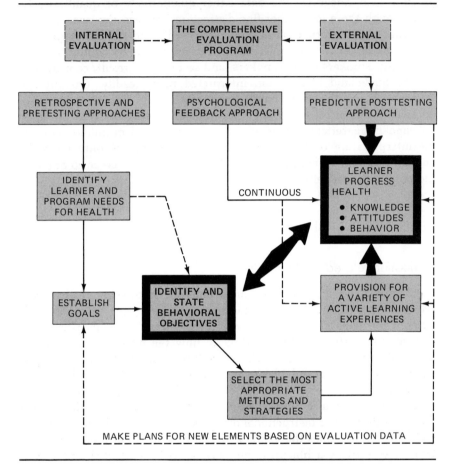

mental design, for example, since it is the factor that is being tested (evaluated). The *independent variable* is the factor whose effects are being evaluated. In health education we are concerned with the effectiveness of the teaching/learning strategies as the independent variable. The *dependent variable* is the factor that is expected to change as a result of the action of the independent variable. The dependent variables in health education are health knowledge, attitudes, and behavior.

One of the difficulties associated with evaluation of health education is the complexity of controlling all the relevant variables. As a consequence, interpretation of evaluative data may be biased by the existence of these variables, or may not be taken into account sufficiently. The relevant variables would include such factors as the learning environment, learner motivation, existing attitudes toward the learning experience, and the learner capabilities and past experiences. With these influences on both learning and evaluation in mind, it is essential to take great care in selecting the type of evaluation to be used and the development of the instruments for obtaining the desired information.

Instrument construction

For evaluation to be most effective, the instruments to be used must be well constructed. The quality of information is dependent entirely upon the quality of the instrument or other techniques used to obtain it. The same high standards of construction of standardized tests should be employed when developing teacher-made tests. However, as Tinkelman points out, "Constructing a good test is always a demanding task, challenging the best creative effort and professional judgment of the teacher."[7] These are the principles of instrument construction:

- The instrument should constitute a fair and representative sample of questions.
- The teacher should clearly identify the purpose of the test, what skills and information are to be measured, what the priority areas are, and the relative weight each will receive on the test.
- An instrument blueprint should be formulated indicating the objectives to be measured, an outline of the nature of topics, their weight allocation on the test, and the types of items that will best meet the purposes of evaluation.
- Regardless of the types of objective items that are to be used, each question should be written so that there is only one correct response possible. Ambiguity should be eliminated.
- Evaluation instruments are intended to provide the teacher with accurate and objective information. Therefore, a test should never be constructed for the purpose of tricking the learner.
- Objective items may take the form of true-false, completion, multiple-choice, or matching.
- Care should be taken in designing the format of the test; items should be numbered, and all items should appear in their entirety on one page. There should be a generally equal distribution of correct replies, ease in scoring, indicated credits for items, clear directions for answering, and the instrument should be typed or printed for ease in reading.

In addition, there are many basic principles that will be helpful in writing the test items themselves. Tinkelman[8] offers the following suggestions:

Essay questions
- Use the essay question to measure objectives that cannot be measured as well with other question types.
- Limit and define the freedom of learner responses to essay questions.

- Use many brief essays rather than one or two extended essays.
- Indicate clearly in each question the desired extent and depth of the answer.

Completion items
- Avoid the loose, ambiguous item that does not tie down the answer to one or two specific words or phrases.
- Do not require more than one or two completions to be made in any one item.
- In general, place the blank near or at the end of the statement.
- Avoid extraneous clues to the correct answer.
- In general, do not use the completion form when no recall is involved.
- In computation problems, specify the degree of precision expected.

True-false items
- Avoid loosely worded and ambiguous statements.
- Base true-false items upon statements that are absolutely true or false, without qualification or exceptions.
- Highlight the central point of the question by placing it in prominent position in the statement.
- Avoid double-barreled and multi-barreled statements that are partly true and partly false.
- Avoid the use of long and involved statements with any qualifying clauses.
- Avoid trick questions.
- Avoid "window dressing" that may serve to confuse the learner.
- Avoid negative questions wherever possible, and double-negatives in any case.
- Avoid extraneous clues in the form of specific determiners (e.g., always, never, usually, etc.).
- In modified true-false type of items, indicate the word or words that should be corrected.

Multiple-choice items
- Use either a direct question or an incomplete statement as the item stem, whichever seems more appropriate to effective presentation of the item.
- Items should be written in clear and simple language, with vocabulary kept as simple as possible.
- Each item should have one and only one correct answer.
- Base each item on a single central problem.
- State the central problem of the item clearly and completely in the stem.
- In general, include in the stem any words that must otherwise be repeated in each response.
- Avoid negative statements.

- Avoid excessive "window dressing."
- Place the choices at the end of the incomplete statement.
- Make responses grammatically consistent with the stem and parallel with one another in form.
- Make all responses plausible and attractive to pupils who lack the information or ability tested by the item.
- Arrange the responses in logical order, if one exists.
- Make the responses independent and mutually exclusive.
- Avoid extraneous clues.
- Use the "none-of-these" options with caution.

Matching items
- Group only homogeneous premises and homogeneous responses in a single matching item.
- Keep the lists of premises and responses relatively short.
- Arrange the lists of premises and responses for maximum clarity and convenience to the learner.
- Explain clearly in the directions the basis upon which items are to be matched and the procedure to be followed.
- Avoid extraneous clues.
- Provide for extra responses to reduce guessing.

Examples

The previous discussions provide us with some concrete examples of subjective and objective instruments that can be developed for evaluation at any or all of the four levels of evaluation. (These levels will be described later in this chapter.) Other examples of subjective techniques include observations, interviews, questionnaires, surveys, checklists, anecdotal records, and self-inventories.

- *Observations* may be structured or unstructured. Structured observations require the use of a criteria checklist. The checklist contains items that the teacher feels are important in noting any change in the learner's attitude or behavior. It is limited to determining present behavior as it occurs. The teacher simply records (or checks) behavior of the learner that is actually observed.
- *Questionnaires, surveys,* and *checklists* have several features in common. They can provide a wide range of information in a very short period of time (although they are more effective when their scope of information is kept to a limited body of facts). The shotgun approach is likely to yield faulty information as well as a variety of data that are difficult to organize and interpret. A serious drawback is the fact that the learner may not choose to provide completely honest responses to the items. Also, learners may not be aware of their true feelings regarding the question being asked.

- *Anecdotal records* on the behavior of learners under a variety of circumstances may be kept by the teacher. This technique is closely related to the observation methods mentioned above. The chief difference is that the teacher records what is observed in a brief, objective manner. This approach is time-consuming for the teacher and is often done only sporadically. It is also difficult to use this method with all learners at one time. Anecdotal records may reflect positive and/or negative behavior. They are probably best used for a specific purpose and time period.
- *Self-inventories* are instruments designed to require learners to provide information about themselves. Obviously, the information depends on how individuals perceive themselves. This may or may not be accurate. Items, therefore, should be carefully selected and worded so that only simple responses are required.

AREAS TO BE EVALUATED

Introduction

It is obvious that there are a variety of specific as well as general techniques available for obtaining relevant data upon which to base certain interpretations associated with health learning. We also know that health learning takes place in numerous ways and in many different environmental settings. An evaluation program, therefore, should be directed toward obtaining the information necessary for ascertaining what learning has taken place, what the learner's present health knowledge, attitudes, and behavior are, what needs to be done, how best to do it, and whether or not it was done. Accordingly, there are five general objectives of evaluation of health education that should be considered:

1. To ascertain the quality and speed of learner progress, past and present.
2. To make judgments regarding the effectiveness of teaching/learning methods and strategies being used as they relate to learner progress.
3. To ascertain the effectiveness of teaching/learning aids being used to enhance methodologies and learning.
4. To determine the value and relevance of the informational content in affecting the learner's health comprehension, attitudinal status, and behavioral reactions.
5. To appraise the effectiveness of the overall program including organization, administration, and cost-effectiveness.

Learner progress

There are four levels of evaluation that apply to health education; these are illustrated in Figure 13–2. The approach to evaluation—retrospective,

FIGURE 13–2 Levels of Evaluation in Health Education
The level, kind, and techniques of evaluation are determined by the kind of information needed.

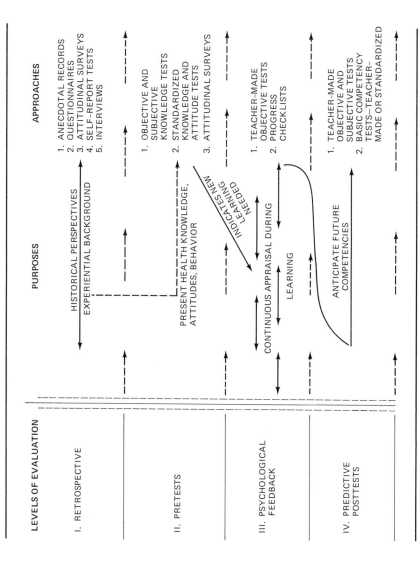

pretest, psychological feedback, or predictive posttest—will be dependent upon the level of evaluation selected. The level of evaluation is determined by the kind of information desired. In all cases, both subjective and objective techniques as well as standardized or teacher-made instruments may be used.

A *retrospective approach* is used to assess what learning has taken place and what experiences have been significant in establishing the individual's present health behavior. In essence, it provides information for judging a historical learning perspective. Such techniques as anecdotal records, surveys, questionnaires, self-reports, checklists, and interviews will provide the data desired. The use of the information acquired can be directed toward new learning experiences designed to build upon past successful experiences.

Psychological feedback approaches are valuable for both the health educator and the learner. The health educator will be kept continuously informed as to the effectiveness of the methodologies being used, while the learners receive periodic and continuous feedback regarding their learning progress. As mentioned in Chapter 8, psychological feedback can be valuable in sustaining learning motivation. Because of the purpose of this approach, it is essential that techniques are teacher-made (not standardized tests) and related to the immediate learning situation.

Pretests are best used to determine specific health knowledge, attitudes, and behavior that the learner can demonstrate at the moment. The health knowledge, attitudes, and behavior reflect the quality of previous learning and are therefore an indication of earlier health education whether or not it was direct or incidental. The results of pretesting provide base-line data that are valuable for ascertaining the effectiveness of new learning experiences and the progress the learner is making. Subjective or objective techniques may be used for this purpose.

Weekly, unit, or final health examinations are common practice. They are frequently called *posttests* and provide the health educator with data that are interpreted in terms of the learning that has taken place for a given period of time. Scores are usually used to record report card grades. In actuality, the scores from posttests can be interpreted in more empirical terms since they suggest that the learners have achieved a level of learning that is satisfactory (or unsatisfactory) for them to behave healthfully in the future. In this respect, we can coin the term "predictive posttest" since the results may anticipate future learner competencies. When posttest scores are compared with pretest scores, a relatively accurate measure of learning progress can be ascertained. Basic competency scores imply, at best, a minimal level of achievement. The following is an example of one attempt at such an endeavor.

In March, 1976, the Board of Regents of the New York State Education Department adopted a proposal advocating basic competency tests as a requirement for high school graduation. In regards to health education, the State Education Department, as of this writing, is in the process of developing a competency test in "the practical sciences, including health and drug education." In the official publication of the New York State Education Department the following description of these tests is given: "The basic competency tests have been described as 'criterion referenced tests' or tests which are designed to measure mastery of specific skills. As such, they are developed independently of norms or grade levels. A student who passes the tests could be expected to handle most of the normal adult activities required in each of the subject areas."[9]

The "practical science" test is designed to contain 50 multiple-choice items, only 13 of which will be related to measuring adult health competencies. Obviously, predictive evaluation is most difficult, since final results can lie at some future date. In the above example, 14 or 15 year old students who take the test and pass it are *presumed* to be able to deal with complex (or perhaps basic) health problems which will occur in adult life. To determine validity, it will be necessary for the New York State Education Department to conduct follow-up studies of these students for at least ten years into the adule life of those who have taken the test. However, there is no mention in the proposal of any such follow-up evaluation.

Effectiveness of methods

If methods have been selected on the basis of learner outcomes and teacher competencies, if learner outcomes are related to needs and learner capabilities, and if evaluation of learner progress demonstrates the ability to apply knowledge, to analyze health problems, and to exhibit positive health attitudes and behavior, one can conclude that the methods being used are effective. Ways should then be sought to incorporate into the learning process even more effective methods. If, on the other hand, the evaluation indicates that learner progress is not as thorough or rapid as desired, steps should be taken to determine why. The use of the following criteria will be valuable in finding the strengths and weaknesses in the approaches being used:

1. Are approaches primarily learner-centered rather than teacher-centered?
2. Are learners genuinely motivated?
3. Are objectives real and attainable?
4. Have a variety of methods and techniques been used?
5. Do methods stimulate learner involvement?
6. Do approaches build upon learner experiences and capabilities?
7. Do methods allow for learner field experiences?
8. Do methods stimulate inductive learning?
9. Do methods extend beyond the school environment?
10. Do methods allow for independent study and motivate learner exploration and discovery?

11. Are the learners involved in planning and method selection?
12. Do methods include the use of team teaching, team learning, and the use of expert consultants?
13. Do methods motivate cooperative rather than competitive learning?
14. Do approaches relate learning to real-life situations?
15. Are affective learning approaches used?
16. Are opportunities provided for learners to discuss, analyze, and synthesize?
17. Are there opportunities for the learner to be expressive and creative?
18. Do methods allow for learners to clarify their own health values?
19. Is the learner provided with continuous psychological feedback?

Effectiveness of learning aids

In recent years, governmental and voluntary health agencies as well as commercial producers have developed a wide variety of printed, audio, and visual learning aids. These will range from very effective to worthless, from innovative to conventional, from scientifically accurate to inaccurate, and from stimulating to boring. With such a diversity of materials available, it is imperative that selection and use with the learner be based upon a careful evaluation by the health educator beforehand. Evaluation is also important to insure the selection of the best aid available to enhance the learning experience and to assist the learner in achieving the predetermined objectives.

In addition to the increased use of material aids in health education, teachers have been making greater use of community resource people. Again, some can provide learning experiences that can not be acquired in any other way. However, prior to the selection and use of these human resources, they too should be carefully evaluated. Below are two suggested checklists to assist in this important task. (In addition, listing of sources of materials will be found in Appendix B.)

Criteria for evaluating material resources
1. Are the materials authored or developed by recognized authorities?
2. Do the materials contain undesirable innuendoes?
3. Are products advertised in or on the learning aid?
4. Is the content of the material scientifically accurate?
5. Is emotionalism avoided?
6. Are there hidden moralistic values or views present in or on the materials?
7. Are the materials appropriate for the developmental level of the learner?
8. Do they appear to have sufficient value in contributing to learner goal achievement?
9. Will the materials enhance learning and motivate learner action?
10. Are the materials attractive in appearance?

11. Are the materials appropriate for classroom use?
12. Do the materials seem to possess the potential for stimulating learner discussion, analysis, and synthesis?
13. Will the use of the materials be more effective than some other technique?
14. Does the cost and apparent value of the materials seem justified?
15. Is the content and presentation consistent with the school's overall educational philosophy?
16. Are the materials' content and presentation consistent with the general standards of the community?
17. Is the content of the materials and their presentation positive and obviously geared toward realistic outcomes?
18. Is there a minimum of morbid or pathological content present in the materials?

Criteria for evaluating human resources
1. Is the person a recognized authority in the subject area?
2. Is the person's presentation more than just a lecture?
3. Does the person provide a learning experience that can not be obtained more readily and effectively in some other way?
4. Has the person a reputation for planning for the presentation?
5. Does the person possess credentials for the subject area?
6. Will the person relate positively with the learners?
7. Is there a cost factor (honorarium) for the person's services? Is it justified?
8. Does the presentation allow for learner interaction?
9. Is the person willing to reappear for a follow-up discussion?
10. Have others made use of the person? What are their reactions to the person's presentation?
11. Does the person use material aids during the presentation? Have they been previewed by you?
12. Has the use of the person been approved by the school administration?
13. Does the school district have a written policy regarding the use of resource people? Does the person meet the standards of the policy?

Value of informational content

We have discussed in detail the value of the informational content of the health education program. It is important to reemphasize that health education is much more than health information, the memorization of health facts, and the recall of these facts for testing or grading purposes. Learners should be able to demonstrate their knowledge of health issues, health maintenance, and health care. The components of evaluation should be designed to measure the learners' problem-solving and decision-making skills and their relationship with their health attitudes and behavior, even though the acquisition of health knowledge does not guarantee their favorable development. Nevertheless, the relationship of health knowledge to health attitudes and behavior is undeniable.

However, one might ask if the quality of health knowledge affects the quality of health attitudes, which in turn, affects the quality of health behavior, how can we explain the health behavior, for example, of cigarette smokers who continue to smoke, knowing the health hazards of smoking and even believing that these hazards apply to them. The answer obviously lies in exploring other significant variables. Health behavior is seldom simply explained as $A + B = C$. We must also recognize the presence and influence of possible intervening variables. In this case, for instance, the addicting nature of the chemicals found in tobacco smoke, or the possibility of emotional factors that reinforce the smoking behavior may be significant intervening variables. Smoking may be perceived by the individual as satisfying some emotional need. Emotional factors may dominate intellectual factors. We can evaluate the intellectual factors quite accurately, but the emotional and behavioral factors may require the use of rather sophisticated psychological procedures. The results of knowledge tests could be correlated with the results of psychological tests and begin to provide us with some clues regarding the success of the health education program.

Health knowledge tests can provide evidence as to how much accurate health information learners have acquired and some indications regarding how well they understand the significance and relationships of this information. This can further provide the health educator with evidence of the kinds of attitudes the learner has developed either as a result of the health learning experiences or from other sources. However, we can not conclude that health knowledge, attitudes, and behavior will necessarily be developed to the same degree. Nor can we infer that the measurement of one, such as health knowledge, is a measure of the other two. We can only assume that with an increase in accurate health knowledge, there is more likelihood that one *will* behave more favorably. If evaluation is valid, we may be able to conclude that people *can* behave more favorably although they may not choose to do so.

One weakness in evaluating health is the result of expecting too much from health education programs. We must recognize that there are many factors influencing life and therefore evaluation must be limited only to the extent that the health experiences have favorably influenced behavior. Finally, evaluation needs to be geared to measuring either the health-related or health-directed behavior. This is determined by the goals and the objectives of the program. If the purpose is to help the learners direct their behavior to more desirable ends, then we are evaluating health-directed behavior. On the other hand, if the purpose of the program is to provide the learners with general information for use in improving their life-style, then we are evaluating health-related behavior. Techniques can be devised to accurately measure health knowledge, attitudes, and behavior, but the question remains as to how well we do it. This is dependent upon how extensive we feel the evaluation must be to provide us with the data necessary to support contentions regarding the effectiveness of the total health education program.

Effectiveness of the program

Program effectiveness is reflected in the results of learner achievements. Assuming that the predetermined goals and objectives are accurate and the learner achieves these in the anticipated time, it is possible to conclude that the overall program is effective. However, it should be an integral component of the total evaluation program and given periodic scrutiny as with other elements, since it is possible that goals and objectives may be too simplistic or may contain other faults. Evaluation of the program is usually directed toward identifying inherent strengths and weaknesses. The following outline lists some of the areas of the program to be evaluated and provides some criteria for conducting such an evaluation.

Goals
1. Are the goals realistic and consistent with current health education philosophy and practice?
2. Are the goals clearly stated and measurable?
3. Are the goals related to learner health needs and those of the community?
4. Are the goals consistent with general educational philosophy and practice?
5. Are the goals achievable?

Objectives
1. Are the objectives obtainable?
2. Are the objectives measurable?
3. Will achievement of an objective satisfy some learner health need or needs?
4. Are objectives related to goal achievement?
5. Are the objectives consistent with the developmental characteristics of the learners?
6. Do objectives allow for individualized learning?
7. Are the learners aware of their objectives?
8. Have the learners been involved in identifying the objectives?

Organization and administration
1. Is the health program an integral and recognized component of the total educational program?
2. Is the program sequential and progressive through developmental levels of the learner?

3. Is the program under the direction and coordination of a qualified health educator?
4. Does the program have priority in the school's educational program?
5. Are adequate time, funds, facilities, resources, and personnel provided for the health education program?
6. Does the health education program have the active support of the administration and the community?
7. Is the health education program comprehensive?
8. Are there provisions in the organizational structure of the health education program for parent and community involvement?
9. Are adequate learning resources made availabe?
10. Are teachers adequately prepared to assume the responsibilities of teaching about health?
11. Is provision made for interdisciplinary approaches?
12. Is there a comprehensive and continuous evaluation component?

HOW TO EVALUATE

Teacher-made tests

The principles of test construction discussed previously should be applied to the development of teacher-made tests. Here we will explore the purpose and value of teacher-made tests and other instruments to be used to evaluate specific aspects of the health education program.

Evaluation instruments, their design, and the amounts to be used should be constructed in conjunction with the development of the overall plans of the health curriculum. As the curriculum guides begin to take shape, methods for evaluating various aspects should be established. For example, following identification of learner objectives, the teacher should construct test items related to measuring achievement of each objective. Careful consideration should be given to the best way of ascertaining the extent to which each objective is achieved by each learner or by the group. Furthermore, the teacher should decide whether the learner achievement evaluation is related to learner motivation, effort, or capability; or to the effectiveness of methodologies, techniques, strategies, resources, and learning environments. Finally, consideration should be given to the extent that all elements of the program influence each other and whether or not the evaluation should be designed to indicate any correlations between them.

In essence, teacher-made evaluation instruments have the important purpose of providing information about the quality of plans and effectiveness of carrying them to completion. These measuring devices, therefore, have the inherent purpose of measuring periodic but continuous effectiveness of the program as it progresses through its various phases. As such, they are much more valuable for evaluating health education programs than are the standardized instruments that are available.

Standardized tests

Over the years, numerous standardized tests in health education have been developed and made available. There are tests to evaluate health knowledge, attitudes, and behavior as well as specialized areas of the health curriculum.* The most complete listing of these tests was published by the American Association for Health, Physical Education and Recreation in 1969.[10] The general topic areas included instruments for testing at the elementary school, junior high school, senior high school, and college levels. They are objective instruments for evaluating health knowledge, but there are also instruments for evaluating health attitudes.

The use of standardized tests has very little value in evaluating current health education programs. They should be used with extreme caution (if used at all). They are not designed to provide information about the effectiveness of a specific health education program. For the most part, their value is that of satisfying one's curiosity as to how well a particular group of learners compares with the norm. But even this can be misleading, since the purpose of a given health education program may be quite different from the purpose perceived by the author of the standardized test.

Why evaluate?

Evaluation provides the vehicle for gathering pertinent information that, when properly organized, can be interpreted accurately and used to modify the health program to make it more effective in the future. Evaluation guarantees that health programs will stay alive and continue to grow and improve. Evaluation also helps the health educator to define more precisely what health education is all about. With each modification incorporated into the program we come one step closer to providing this generation of youth with a process that will improve their effectiveness as members of society.

DEFINITIVE UNDERSTANDINGS

The general principles of evaluation apply to the school, the community, and the patient health educator. However, specific techniques will vary.

Evaluation can be defined in a variety of ways, but will always include techniques or measurement to gather information, organize it into meaningful categories, and interpret its meaning in regard to the program being evaluated. Specifically, evaluation is a process requiring judgments on the part of the evaluator.

An evaluation instrument may be either objective or subjective in

---

* For an interesting discussion of health education evaluation, see Pigg, R. Morgan, Jr., "A History of School Health Program Evaluation in the United States," *The Journal of School Health*, XLVI (10), 1976.

its design. An objective test is one that yields consistent scores each time it is used, regardless of who is doing the scoring. A subjective test is one that requires judgment on the part of the one who is doing the scoring. Objective tests are limited primarily to testing recall or recognition of health facts. Subjective tests provide the one being evaluated with some freedom of expression in answering the test items.

A valid instrument is one that measures what it is supposed to measure. Validity can be determined by a rather complex mathematical procedure whose use is important for establishing standardized tests. However, for teacher-made tests, such a precise determination of validity is not necessary as long as the instrument possesses at least a face validity. Valid instruments are always reliable, but a reliable instrument may not always be valid. Reliability refers to the consistency of results each time the test is used. It too can be determined by mathematical means.

Evaluation of the health program should take into consideration health education, health services, and the learning environment. Pressures by society for accountability in education have made it imperative that more precise approaches be used to determine the effectiveness of all phases of the health program.

The primary purpose of evaluation is to determine individual and group needs, assess the strengths and weaknesses of the program, determine learner progress, and modify the program in accordance with evaluation information received. In this sense, evaluation is a cyclic and continuous process, planned and implemented as an integral component of the entire health program. Evaluation, therefore, should always be usd for positive reasons, never for threatening or punishment.

The results of evaluation should provide an abundance of data upon which to base certain judgments regarding the quality of the program. To assist in the interpretation, information is usually classified in accordance with certain characteristics that can be compared. The data that can be expressed in numerical terms are quantitatively classified, while the data that are similar or comparable in certain qualities are classified qualitatively.

In health education, evaluation is always associated with objective achievements. Since all other aspects of the program are related to the objectives, evaluation of the extent to which learners have achieved them provides evidence for making certain inferences about, for instance, the effectiveness of the teaching and learning strategies.

Evaluation in health education can be compared to the experimental method. The objectives are, in essence, the hypothesis. Teaching strategies and learning experiences are the independent variables, and changes expected in health knowledge, attitudes, and behavior are the dependent variables. However, we must also be conscious of the other relevant variables which can have an influence on final evaluation judgments.

Instruments to be used in the evaluation program should be developed as an integral component of the total health program at the time the health program is being planned and formulated. Great care should be exercised in instrument construction because the quality of data received is entirely dependent upon the quality of the instruments being used. Therefore, the same principles governing the construction of standardized instruments should govern the development of teacher-made tests. Test items, for instance, should be representative, purposeful, weighted, fair, objective, in logical sequence, and readable. These principles generally hold whether essay or objective test items are to be used.

An evaluation program can be expanded to incorporate the use of such devices as observations, questionnaires, surveys, checklists, anecdotal records, and self-inventories. This is especially important when attempting to ascertain changes in health attitudes and behavior.

There are five general objectives of evaluation. They are associated with the speed of learning, the effectiveness of teacher/learner methods, the effectiveness of learning aids, the importance of health information, and the way the total health program is organized and administered. Evaluation of the effects learning experiences have on the learner takes place at four levels: (1) retrospective, (2) pretesting, (3) psychological feedback, and (4) predictive posttesting. These determine what has happened to the learners, their present status, how well learning is progressing, and how well the learners will be able to apply the new learning to future encounters. Basic competency tests are examples of predictive posttesting in that they indicate the extent to which the learner has acquired basic skills necessary for dealing with life's problems.

How effective the methods being used are can be inferred from the speed and progress of learning. Speed and progress are also associated with complexity of learner objectives. Methods can be evaluated by the application of direct techniques as well. Criteria used to make specific judgments regarding certain aspects of the methods as they relate to influencing the learner can be established. Criteria can also be established to evaluate the other influencers of learning (e.g., material and human resources, program planning, organization, and administration).

Health education is much more than the acquisition of health information. It is also concerned with problem-solving and decision-making. As such, the relationship between health knowledge, attitudes, and behavior is unquestionable, even though changes in the three areas may not take place equally. By ascertaining the comprehension of the informational content, we can be quite certain of what the learner's health behavior can be, even though we will be uncertain of what it will be.

The use of teacher-made tests or other evaluative devices is the best approach in evaluating a specific program. However, one should be cautioned against overinterpretation or underinterpretation of results, since there may be present other intervening variables which could bias judgments by the health educator. Standardized tests should also be used

discriminately since they are constructed for large general learner populations and are based upon general objectives of the test author rather
than any particular health program.

PROBLEMS
FOR DISCUSSION

1. Show how evaluative principles are adaptable for evaluating health education within the three spheres—school, community, and patient—according to measurement, test construction, organizing data, and interpreting
   data.
2. Distinguish between measurement and evaluation.
3. Explain why evaluation is always subjective to some extent.
4. Give reasons why even an objective instrument is subjective in some
   respects.
5. What are the chief faults of objective tests?
6. Distinguish between valid and reliable evaluative devices. Discuss why
   validity and reliability are important in gathering data for evaluating any
   aspect of the health program.
7. List the general areas of the health program that should be evaluated. List
   those that should be evaluated in regards to health education.
8. Describe why evaluation is and should be cyclic and continuous.
9. Distinguish between quantitative and qualitative evaluation.
10. Why should objectives always be stated precisely?
11. Show the relationship between learner progress and the other elements of
    the health education program.
12. Distinguish between the four levels of learner evaluation.
13. Using Figure 13–1 as a guide, develop an evaluation program for one health
    education topic or issue.
14. Show how evaluation in health education is comparable to the use of the
    principles of the experimental method.
15. Develop a health knowledge test that complies with the principles of test
    construction. State the objectives to be measured and develop appropriate
    test items.
16. Develop a health attitude instrument. What is the validity of the test in
    your judgment? Support your contention. Have others review the test
    and obtain their judgment. Give reasons why attitude scales may be weak
    in ascertaining the true attitudes of the learner.
17. What are the chief faults of basic competency tests? How can some of the
    weaknesses be overcome?
18. Analyze the various criteria lists presented in this chapter. How can they
    be improved to yield more specific and usable information?
19. Secure some material resources in health education. Evaluate each, using
    either your own criteria or those presented in the chapter.
20. Compare the values of using teacher-made tests with the use of standard-
    ized tests.
21. Develop a philosophy of evaluation in health education. Include purposes,
    goals, objectives, values, uses, areas to be evaluated, reasons, and how the
    evaluation will take place.
22. Obtain copies of final examinations being used in a local school district.

Review them, using the principles of test construction presented in the chapter. Are the instruments valid? Do they appear to measure student progress or achievement? Do they contain items to measure attitudes and behavior as well as knowledge?

REFERENCES

1. Anderson, C. L., *School Health Practice*, C. V. Mosby Company, St. Louis, 1968, p. 371.
2. Bedworth, Albert E., and Joseph A. D'Elia, *Basics of Drug Education*, Baywood Publishing Company, Inc., Farmingdale, N.Y., 1973, p. 228.
3. Stone, Donald, et al., *Elementary School Health Education: Ecological Perspectives*, William C. Brown Company, Publishers, Dubuque, 1976, p. 372.
4. Oberteuffer, Delbert, et al., *School Health Education*, 5th ed., Harper & Row, Publishers, New York, 1972, p. 179.
5. Ibid., p. 168.
6. Ibid., p. 169.
7. Tinkelman, Sherman N., *Improving the Classroom Test: A Manual of Test Construction Procedures for the Classroom Teacher*, The University of the State of New York. The State Education Department, Bureau of Elementary and Secondary Testing, Albany, 1976.
8. Ibid., chap. III.
9. *Inside Education*, 62 (8), The University of the State of New York, The State Education Department, Albany, April, 1976.
10. Solleder, Marian K., *Evaluation Instruments in Health Education*, The American Association for Health, Physical Education and Recreation, Washington, D.C., 1969.

Appendix A

Glossary

Ability. A pattern of behavioral tendencies responsible for skillful performance in a variety of related tasks. Ability may be expressed in health terms as the capacity for self-sufficiency.

Achievement test. An examination that measures the degree of proficiency already attained in some specific skill or ability. Such a measure may be directed toward ascertaining intellectual, social, or physical skills.

Accommodation. The adaptation by the individual to the assimilated experience.

Adaptation. Adjustment to physical and social environmental conditions as well as internal stimuli. Essentially, the process of homeostasis. (See also *homeostasis.*)

Adjustment. A general term that refers to the ability to meet the demands of society and satisfy drives. (See also *adaptation.*)

Affective domain. That aspect of health learning that involves one's interests, attitudes, and values, and the development of appreciations and adequate adjustment.

Aim. A term used to describe the mission of the accumulated learning experiences achieved through accomplishing goals, which act as intermediary guideposts.

Amniocentesis. A process of withdrawing amniotic fluid during the fourteenth to eighteenth weeks of pregnancy for the purpose of monitoring the growth of the fetus. Also, a process of determining the genetic makeup of the fetus to evaluate the potentials for abnormality after birth.

Anecdotal record. Utilized by the teacher in the observation of behavior of the learner. It may reflect both positive and negative behavior during a specific period of time.

Applied science. Having to do with the application of discovered laws to the matters of everyday living.

Aptitude. An ability that is potentially related to the skillful performance of some task.

Aptitude test. An evaluation instrument designed to measure potentials to perform or to learn.

Assimilation. The process of internalizing the learning experience as a part of self. Fitting an experience into one's existing cognitive structure.

Associationist. The school of thought that maintains that learning is determined by a link which is created between a stimulus and a response through action on the part of the learner (i.e., learning is a process of developing associative connections or bonds).

Attitude. A tendency to respond in a characteristic way to some social stimulus. A predisposition or set to respond in some consistent way toward an exogenous stimulus.

Authority structure. Those elected officials of a community who are mandated to make decisions on behalf of the people.

Basic need. An inborn drive. Basic needs are classed as biological (i.e., the need for food, water, etc.) or psychological (psychosocial) (i.e., security, love, etc.).

Behavior. Any internal or external, observable or nonobservable response of a person to a stimulus or stimuli. Internal responses such as thinking or feeling may be inferred from observable behavior. (See also *health behavior.*)

Behavioral objective. A statement describing precisely what the learner will be doing as a result of a learning experience. A behavioral objective is expressed in measurable terms. Also called performance or instructional objective. (See also *objective.*)

Biogenic motive. A drive or biological need; motivation originating from the need for biological survival.

Board of education. The legally constituted body for the establishment of educational policies governing a school district.

Bureau of Health Education. Component of the Center for Disease Control of the United States Public Health Service within the Department of Health, Education, and Welfare. It provides for prevention of disease, disability, premature deaths, etc., on a national basis.

Classical conditioning theory. A subschool of the associationist school of thought. The theory holds that learning occurs as a result of a link established between a stimulus and a response through the use of rewards.

Coded message. A component of information theory. The stimuli of symbols passing through the communication channel.

Cognitive domain. That aspect of learning that involves the recall or recognition of knowledge and the development of intellectual abilities and skills.

Cognitive learning theory. The theory that one's characteristics must be taken into account in addition to the various stimuli and responses when explaining learning. A theory which views learning as a process of intellectual development resulting in new insights, discriminations, and associations.

Communication channel. The mechanism which carries information from its source to its destination. A component of information theory.

Community health education. All of the methods, techniques, and strategies used by the community health educator to improve the health knowledge, attitudes, and behavior of members of the defined community.

Community health organizations. The voluntary, governmental, and professional agencies and associations concerned with certain aspects of health.

Community health program. Includes all functions directed toward improving the health of individuals within the community and the health of the community as a whole. Its components are fundamentally the same as those for the school health program; namely, health education, medical and health services, and a healthful environment in which to live.

Competency-based teacher education (CBTE). A system of teacher training in which students are required to demonstrate particular competencies in order to qualify for graduation and/or certification, rather than mere minimum grade point averages or a minimum number of credit hours. A student must demonstrate certain predetermined basic skills.

Components of the total health program. The health education program and all of its elements; the medical or health services and all of its functions and the quality of the school/community environment.

Comprehensive health program. Includes two broad areas: (1) the community health program, and (2) the school health program, which are made up of school/community environment, health education, and health services.

Computerized learning. Method of individualizing learning. This is accomplished by having the learners select their own objectives and identifying their own characteristics, which are then entered into the computer and, in turn, provide suggested learning experiences that can be pursued by the learners to assist them in achieving their objectives.

Concept formation. The process of categorizing learning experiences in a meaningful way, enabling the learner to appropriately communicate with others. It implies a generalized comprehension as a result of specific learning experiences. Significances and relationships of basic factual information result as concepts are formed.

Conceptual approach to curriculum design. This focuses upon the attainment of three principles: (1) growing and developing, (2) decision-making, and (3) interaction. Learning experiences are directed toward each individual developing health concepts which can be applied to improved daily living.

Conditioned response. The response which is evoked by the conditioned stimulus after conditioning has taken place.

Conditioned stimulus. The stimulus that is paired with the unconditioned stimulus and subsequently acquires the capacity to evoke a response similar to the one made to the unconditioned stimulus.

Coping mechanisms. A variety of complex, usually unconscious devices used to handle frustration or ego threats.

Correlated health experiences. Health learning within the health education program that is associated with learning taking place within another curricular discipline.

Course of study. A detailed written guide for each grade or developmental level. Such a guide contains all of the essential information and components for developing the lesson plan.

Creative activities. Learner-centered methods by which the learners can acquire insight into the health problem or ways they can assist others to understand the problem. Creative activities are designed to elicit individual potentials for learning.

Critical Health Problems Act (1967). Chapter 787 of the Laws of 1967 of the State of New York which provided for the first mandated comprehensive school health education program in the United States. Served as the model for corresponding legislation in other states.

Cue function. An environmental condition that provides the individual with an indication of the direction a behavioral response should take.

Curriculum. Any and all things which influence in any way the learning of the individual.

Curriculum development. A continuous process embracing initial construction, evaluation, reorganization, revision, experimentation, administration, and all other elements of the school and community that influence the quality of learning and teaching.

Curriculum guide. A written plan containing detailed information regarding grade level offerings and other suggestions for the health education program of the school district. It differs from the course of study chiefly in the lack of grade or developmental level details. The curriculum guide describes overall goals, philosophy, scope, and sequence of the health education program.

Cybernetics. The science which studies the relationship of computer engineering and human neurology.

Debates. Learner-centered method typically used to motivate both intellectual and emotional exchange among the learners. Through the use of this method, students learn to listen, communicate, and analyze what is being said. It encourages objective thinking and listening.

Decision-making method. A learner-centered method in which the learner is given several alternatives and allowed to discover the consequences of each, resulting in the best decision for personal action.

Deductive learning. Assumes certain health facts and premises to be accurate with a conclusion based upon "known truths". It is characterized chiefly by memorization of certain health facts presumed to lead to a change in health behavior. (See also *inductive learning.*)

Demonstration method. A learner observational method that is usually teacher-centered or authority-centered. May be effective if students are involved in the planning and conducting phases. It is most effective when the demonstration focuses upon a particular health issue.

Dental hygiene teacher. (Also a dental health teacher.) A person trained in oral health who is a member of the health services team.

Dependent variable. The factor expected to change as a result of the action of the independent variable. In health education, the learner is the dependent variable while the learning experiences are the independent variables. (See also *independent variable.*)

Destination of message. The point at which information results in some form of reaction; one of the components of the information theory.

Developmental tasks. Achievements necessary for development at various stages of maturity.

Dimensions of health. The interrelated factors of the physical, emotional, mental, and social aspects of each individual.

Direct health experiences. Planned and deliberate health education under the guidance of a trained health educator.

Disability. Any temporary or permanent condition of the body or mind which reduces the individual's ability to function at a higher level of effectiveness.

Disease. Any condition of the body or mind, acute or chronic, which interferes with the individual's ability to function effectively under ordinary environmental circumstances. Literally, a lack of ease of functioning. A disease may be either organic, functional, or both.

Drive. A condition or state of the individual which activates or directs behavior; hunger, thirst, etc. Drives are powerful motivational forces.

Education. A complex process of experiences that influences the way that we perceive ourselves in relation to the social and physical environments. It is a purposeful process for expediting learning, although it does take place in other contexts.

Enabling goal (objective). The achievements necessary for the learner to achieve the terminal goal or objective.

Encoding. The conversion of information from its transmitted form to a form which can be interpreted. In information theory, the encoded message is the thought or idea converted into speech, for example.

Endogenous. Factors originating or produced within the individual; intrinsic. (See also *exogenous.*)

Environment. The physical, social, effective, and noneffective influencers of human functioning.

Exogenous. Factors originating or produced by the social or physical environments. (See also *endogenous.*)

Feedback. Verbal or nonverbal responses of a learner that may be interpreted by the teacher and utilized to guide learning. Feedback may also originate with the teacher in verbal or nonverbal form, providing the learner with knowledge that the teacher is aware of the learner's coded messages.

Field trips. May be used to broaden the learner's view of the community and world in general. They should be planned by the teacher and learner together with an opportunity for students to share their experiences upon return to class. A field trip is basically a learner observational method.

Fieldwork experiences. A learner-centered method in which students spend a part of their day working in a health-related community agency. The experience should result in students developing an appreciation for the health occupation; increasing their knowledge of the health problem(s), and the ways they are handled by the agency. Most importantly, students provide a community service by contributing to the functions of the community health agency.

Genetic health. The quality of functioning as determined by inherited potentials.
Genotype. The combination of genes that determines genetic potentials.
Goal. A commodity or condition capable of reducing or eliminating a drive; an incentive; the end toward which the learner strives.
Governmental health agency. A health agency supported chiefly by tax revenues and under the authority of the government.

Health. The quality of physical, psychological, and sociological functioning that enables us to deal adequately with self and others in a variety of situations. It is related to self-sufficiency and effectiveness; a dynamic and relative state of functioning.
Health attitudes. The predisposition to behave in a particular way regarding health matters. They are characterized by health beliefs or feelings.
Health behavior. Actions and reactions one makes to promote personal and social health, maintain health, or restore health. Health behavior may be either health-related or health-directed.
Health care system. All of the facilities, people, and functions directed toward promoting, maintaining, and restoring health.
Health curriculum. All of the planned and unplanned learning experiences that affect health learning. Usually, it is the term used to describe the planned health education program within the school.
Health-directed behavior. The actions one takes to promote health, prevent the onset of disease or disability, maintain present health status, restore health that has failed, or solve a specific health problem. (See also *health-related behavior.*)
Health education. All of those experiences—planned or unplanned, direct or indirect—that influence the way learners think, feel, and act in regard to their own health as well as that of the community in which they live. It is a process affecting intellectual, psychological, and social dimensions that increase our capability to make informed health decisions affecting self, family, and community well-being. It is one of several processes for improving human effectiveness.
Health education administrator. An individual trained in health education and administration who provides direction and coordination so that programmatic goals are achieved with a maximum amount of efficiency and a minimum expenditure of human energy. Functioning categories include planning, structuring, administering, communicating, and evaluating.
Health education center. A focal point for the health education efforts of a geographic region comprised of five components: (1) research and evaluation, (2) personnel development, (3) community service, (4) communication and media development, and (5) program development.
Health education curriculum guide. The culminating document of evaluation and planning related to the health education needs of the learner. A tool to help teachers and learners systematically achieve health goals through predetermined processes. (See also *curriculum guide.*)
Health education methodology. The science and art of altering the environment for maximum learning to result. It consists of approaches which include teaching/learning techniques and strategies.

Health education movement. The events that have contributed to the progress of health education.

Health education practices. The application of theory to health learning. They include teacher education, organization and administration, curriculum development, methodology, and evaluation.

Health education program and curriculum committee. This consists of representatives from health educators, elementary school teachers, school administrators, medical and psychological services, and students. This committee establishes the basis for curriculum development.

Health education resources. These are the materials such as films, printed materials, posters, etc., and people which contribute to the health learning of pupils.

Health educator. A highly trained individual who attempts to improve the health of others through the use of the educational process. The health educator may function within school, community, and/or clinical settings.

Health and medical services. This is a component of the health program comprised of medical and dental services and psychological services. It provides for the treatment and intervention programs as well as educational functions within the health education program.

Health goal. (See *goal.*)

Health guidance. A broad term which implies a variety of counseling techniques used to provide individuals or groups with insight into personal health problems.

Health information. Facts related to the quality of individual and societal physical, psychological, and sociological effectiveness.

Health instruction. An obsolete term used in the past to describe direct and indirect health learning. Essentially, health teaching. More recently, health professionals have replaced this term with the broader one of health education, which implies a focus on learning rather than on teaching.

Health knowledge. The acquisition of health information which is assimilated and accomodated by the individual. It is health facts that become a functional and integral part of the individual in making health decisions.

Health learning. Any of a variety of experiences which change the way the individual responds to health-related aspects of the environment. Health learning can be either health-related or health-directed.

Health maintenance. The actions one takes to preclude the onset of disease, disability, or premature death, including health-related and health-directed behavior.

Health professions. Numerous occupations that are concerned with one or more aspects of human health.

Health promotion. A complex process of providing an environment conducive to optimal development of the individual and/or providing the necessary individual qualities for one to overcome obstacles standing in the way of growth and development.

Health-related behavior. All behavior, since all behavior is influenced by health and health influences all behavior. (See also *health-directed behavior.*)

Health restoration. The actions one takes to overcome a disease or disability.

Health science education. This refers basically to the acquisition of health facts, their relation to each other, and how these relationships can establish health principles or laws.

Health services. The medical and health-related functions found within the school and community which direct their attention toward promotion of health, prevention of disease, disability, and premature death, and restoration of health.

Health status. The level of functioning of the individual at any given moment in time.

Homeostasis. The tendency of an organism to maintain physiological equilibrium. It is also used to describe the tendency to maintain emotional and social equilibrium. (See also *adaptation.*)

Horizontal curriculum format. More simplistic, flexible, and useable than the vertical format. Provides teachers with suggestions for student learning, information, and methodology. (See also *vertical curriculum format.*)

Idiographic. The qualities possessed by individuals that make them different from all others.

Incentive. A commodity or condition capable of reducing or eliminating a drive or goal. It is an extrinsic motivational device and may take the form of reward or punishment.

Incidental health experience. Health learning that is unplanned and indirect and that results from daily activities.

Independent variable. The factor whose effects are being evaluated. In health education the independent variable is the method, technique, or strategy. (See also *dependent variable.*)

Individualized learning. A means of arranging the learning environment so that all learners have the opportunity to satisfy their health needs and interests according to their personal capabilities at times and in ways that best suit their motivation and speed of learning. It is the use of methods, techniques, or strategies that influence the learning of each individual most effectively.

Inductive learning. A methodology which begins with a health problem or issue followed by an accumulation of empirical evidence. This method tends to expose new health issues, resulting in broadened learning. Inductive reasoning is essentially the scientific method. (See also *deductive learning* and *problem-solving method.*)

Informational approach to curriculum development. Concerned with the acquisition of health knowledge and its comprehension and with application to the health issues being explored. This approach places emphasis on the acquisition of health facts.

Information theory. The field of study of communications systems which is concerned with the principles governing understanding, control, and predictability in communications.

Integrated health experiences. Health learning that is a component of another curricular discipline.

Intelligence. The term that refers to intellectual ability; an ability or pattern of abilities influencing intellectual functioning. It is related to learning, memorization, reasoning, comprehension, conceptualization, wisdom, etc.

Learner-centered curriculum guide. Describes what learners will be doing to achieve their objectives, rather than what teachers will be doing. (See also *teacher-centered curriculum guide.*)

Learner-centered methods. Includes a variety of approaches based upon the premise that learning is most effective when the learner is actively involved in all phases of the learning process: planning, selection of objectives, selecting the learning processes, and self-evaluation. These methods emphasize learning as opposed to teaching.

Learner observational methods. These include a wide variety of methods that provide the learner with the opportunity to observe others who are actively engaged in some sort of health activity. The field trip and demonstration methods are examples.

Learning. A change in behavior resulting from the individual's participation in various experiences or interactions with the environment. Positive learning results in improved adaptation to the environment. (See also *health learning.*)

Learning methods. Those procedures that the learner uses to acquire insight into a new or familiar situation. They may originate from the teacher, from other outside sources, or from the learner. (See also *teaching methods.*)

Learning resources. Used as techniques or strategies to enhance learning. They may be either materials or people.

Learning resources and evaluation committee. Functions to review, evaluate, and make recommendations regarding the varieties of learning resources available; makes recommendations regarding policies for the selection and use of material and human resources and assists in the development of the evaluation program.

Learning strategies. The skills used by the learner to facilitate learning that are generally energized by the strategies used by the teacher. (See also *teaching strategies.*)

Lecture method. A traditional teacher-centered approach to learning. It is characterized by one-way communication resulting in very little learning. May be used to cover a large body of information in a short period of time.

Lesson plan. The functional culmination of all curriculum planning and development. It describes what will happen to the learner on a day-to-day basis.

Master plan. Describes the elements that constitute the total health program of the school; it is a statement of the school's philosophy of health education, the aim of the total health program, the goals of health education, the scope and sequence of health education, and the overall evaluation program plans. It is characterized chiefly by its lack of detail. (See also *curriculum guide.*)

Maturation. The biological changes taking place in the cells, tissues, organs, and systems and the improvement in their functioning. It is influenced by such factors as genetic potentials, nutrition, rest, recreation, and the richness of the culture or other environmental stimuli that affect personality, emotional, and social growth, and intellectual development.

Media resources. These include any sensory stimuli that enhance learning when used in conjunction with other methods.

Methodology. (See *health education methodology.*)

Misconception (health). The erroneous acquisition of health information. A misconception may also influence the development of erroneous health attitudes resulting in unhealthful behavior.

Need. A variety of felt urgencies related to existence, continuation, maintenance of life, and enhancement of living. Biological and psychosocial needs are interrelated.

Noise. Extraneous disturbances in the learning environment that may interrupt or interfere with communications.

Nomothetic. The characteristics possessed by individuals that make them similar.

Nonobservable health behavior. Those instances in which an individual is functioning outside of the educational setting. It may also include those feelings and thoughts occurring within the individual. Health attitudes, a form of nonobservable behavior, may be inferred from observable health behavior.

Nonsense syllable. A combination of letters, usually consisting of two consonants with a vowel in between, that do not form a word in the langauge of the person using it. Used by Ebbinghaus in experiments investigating memory.

Objective. A statement that describes the outcome of teaching or learning. Objectives may be classified as teacher, learner, or method. Learner objectives are expressed in behavioral terms and fall within the cognitive, affective, or psychomotor domains. An objective states precisely what the learner will be doing as a result of the learning experience. (See also *behavioral objective.*)

Objective test instrument. One that reflects a high degree of scoring consistency regardless of who is doing the scoring. Little, if any, judgment is needed by the scorer.

Observable health behavior. Behavior which can be evaluated during or immediately after the learning experience; or when the learner utilizes what is learned in a later life situation. It is the overt behavior of the individual towards various aspects of the environment that affect health.

Operant (instrumental) conditioning. The process adhered to by one subschool of the associationist school of thought; rewarding or punishing an organism's emitted behavior.

Optimal health. The highest level of functioning the individual is capable of under the existing environmental constraints.

Patient health education. All of the methods, techniques, and strategies used by the patient health educator to favorably influence the health knowledge, attitudes, and especially the behavior of patients recovering from a disease or injury.

Peer approaches. Methods which provide an educational environment which encourages a free interchange among learners.

Perception. An intellectual process of becoming aware of exogenous events that stimulate the sense organs and of interpreting their relationships.

Phenotype. The expression of inherited traits.

Philosophy. A comprehension of the principles of reality; a body of knowledge that defines the perimeters of life and living.

Philosophy of health education. The beliefs, concepts, attitudes, and theory of individual health educators and the profession in general. It sets the boundaries of practice, clarifying the areas of professional concentration. It ties together theory and practice.

P-I-S-A. The process of internalization, where P equals perception; I equals interest; S equals significance, and A equals application. Internalization is incomplete unless the learner goes through each phase.

Posttest. An evaluation instrument that provides the educator with data that are interpreted in terms of the learning that has taken place over a given period of time. Measures learning progress over a given period of time.

Power structure. A group of people in a community whose power often supercedes that of the authority structure and that usually functions for the satisfaction of its own interests. The influential segment of the community.

Predictive posttest. Evaluation instrument used to anticipate future learner competencies.

Proactive facilitation. This occurs when past learning allows future learning to become easier.

Proactive inhibition. This occurs when one learning experience causes later ones to be inefficient.

Problem-solving method. A learner-centered method characterized by a series of discoveries by the learners as they proceed to solve a particular health problem. (See also *inductive learning*.)

Processes (health education). Methodologies, techniques, and strategies used to influence teaching and learning that are consistent with known learning principles.

Professionalism. The methods, manner, or spirit of a profession.

Program aim. The overall mission of the health program.

Psychological feedback. Evaluation procedure used to keep the educator continuously informed as to the effectiveness of the methodologies being used. It provides knowledge of results of communications.

Psychomotor domain. This includes those aspects of learning through which accumulated knowledge and attitudes are applied to particular life situations. It implies skill development.

Public relations. An enterprise designed to promote positive attitudes toward particular organizations, individuals, or ideas. It is a form of communications with the community.

Question-and-answer method. A teacher or learner-centered method depending upon who is in control of the questioning. It can be a valuable method of motivating two-way communications and important feedback.

Recitation method. A teacher-centered approach that requires the learner to memorize health facts that are recited to the rest of the class. It has very little value in indicating student comprehension.

Rehabilitation. The restoration to constructive functioning of one who has suffered a disability.

Reliability. The term used to describe a testing instrument that yields consistent results each time it is used.

Research method. A learner-centered method that affords the learner an opportunity to develop a research design and to carry it through to a conclusion.

Resource guide. A listing of all the human and material resources available within the school or community that can be used as aids in implementing the program once it is developed.

Retention. The amount of previously learned material that is remembered.

Retroactive facilitation. The review of material or the discovery of new explicit relationships resulting in greater retention of a previous experience.

Retroactive inhibition. The interfering effect present learning can have upon the retention of previously learned material.

Retrospective evaluation. This is used to assess how much learning has taken place and what experiences have been significant in establishing the individual's present health behavior. It provides information for judging a historical learning perspective.

School/community communications. This is a continuous process of informational exchange and direct interaction among all those concerned with health. It may take the form of locality development, social planning, and/or social action.

School/community health education advisory committee. This is comprised of representatives from governmental and voluntary health agencies, civic and service groups, professional health associations, parent groups, and clergy. The committee identifies health needs of the community, anticipates areas of possible concern in the future, coordinates the health activities of both the community and school, and establishes a system of effective communications.

School dentist. A licensed dentist who supervises the school dental health program; a member of the health services team.

School health education. All of the planned or unplanned methods, techniques, and strategies used by teachers and health educators to favorably influence the health knowledge, attitudes, and behavior of learners. Its elements include programs for elementary and secondary pupils, teachers and other school personnel, and adults.

School Health Education Study. Directed by Elena Sliepcevich in 1961. It resulted in the conceptual approach to curriculum design.

School health program. (See *comprehensive health program.*)

School nurse. A person trained and certified as a nurse but who functions within the school health services. Generally, this person does not function in an educational capacity within the school.

School-nurse-teacher. An individual who is trained in both nursing and education and who functions in both health services activities and educational endeavors.

School physician. A medical doctor who usually functions within the school health services component of the school health program. This person may be employed by the school on a full-time or part-time basis.

Science. Seeking to establish general laws connecting a number of facts resulting in a possession of knowledge attained through study or practice.

Self-directed learning. A method closely akin to individualized learning in some respects. Its primary purpose is to provide a means for learners not only to proceed at their individual pace, but to offer a variety of learning options under the guidance of a teacher. It is a learner-centered approach.

Self-inventories. Instruments designed to require the learners to provide information about themselves.

Self-sufficiency. The capability of meeting one's needs within the contex of existing environmental circumstances. The quality of one's health influences self-sufficiency.

Social stimulus value. The characteristics that influence the way others respond to us.

Sociogenic motive. A motive originating from social expectations or social aspirations.

Source of message. The place from which communications originate. It may originate from the physical environment, learning resources, the teacher, or the individual's thought processes. It is a component of information theory.

Standardized test. This is based upon the norms of a large population. It is best utilized to verify strengths and weaknesses of a program and to justify what is being done.

Strategy. This implies techniques used to maneuver the learner into a position in which learning will occur more readily. It is a component of methodology.

Subjective test. An instrument that requires the scorer to be trained, experienced, and skilled in the responses expected from the use of the instrument. Scoring is based upon judgments of the scorer.

Subliminal. A stimulus too weak to produce a response; below the normal threshold of consciousness.

Teacher-centered curriculum guide. Describes what teachers will be doing to affect learning.

Teacher-centered methods. Teacher-dominated approaches to teaching/learning. (See also *learner-centered methods.*)

Teaching/learning teams. A group of teachers and/or learners which implements the health education program with learners. Such groups also coordinate an interdisciplinary approach to health education.

Teaching methods. Those planned approaches or procedures that the teacher intends to employ to most effectively influence the learners by favorably affecting their comprehension of a new situation or influencing further their comprehension of a familiar situation. (See also *learning methods.*)

Teaching strategies. Techniques used by the teacher to motivate or manipulate learning. (See also *learning strategies.*)

Technique. The manner in which a teaching or learning method is performed.

Terminal goal (objective). The ultimate end result of the learning process. When all terminal goals have been achieved, the aim of health education has been accomplished.

Textbook method. A teacher-centered approach in which the student reads aloud or silently a specific assignment.

Transfer or learning. The influence the learning of one task has upon the learning or performance of another task.

Transmitter of message. Changes information into a form that can be easily conveyed from the source to the destination. A component of information theory.

Unconditioned response. The response that is made to the unconditioned stimulus in classical conditioning. An example of this is an inborn reflex.

Unconditioned stimulus. The stimulus that elicits the unconditioned response in classical conditioning.

Validity. The term applied to a test that measures what it is intended to measure.

Values clarification. The method dealing with techniques that help learners clarify their moral, ethical, and social relationships.

Vertical curriculum format. The most conventional format. Basically, it is composed of topic, objective, content outline, activities, and resources. (See also *horizontal curriculum format.*)

Voluntary health agency. A health agency, usually specializing in a particular health issue, that receives its financial support from donations or sources other than tax revenues.

Appendix B

Sources
of Learning
Aids

- Associations and Societies
- Commercial Sources
- Governmental Agencies
- Insurance Companies
- Voluntary Health-Related Agencies

ASSOCIATIONS AND SOCIETIES

Alcohol and Drug Problems Association
of North America
  3500 North Logon Street
  Lansing, Michigan 48914
American Academy of Pediatrics
  1801 Hinman Avenue
  Evanston, Illinois 60204
American Alliance of Health, Physical
Education and Recreation
  1201 Sixteenth Street, N.W.
  Washington, D.C. 20036
American Association for the Advance-
ment of Science
  1515 Massachusetts Avenue, N.W.
  Washington, D.C. 20005
American Association of Marriage and
Family Counselors
  225 Yale Avenue
  Claremont, California 91711
American Association of Motor Vehicle
Administrators
  839 Seventeenth Street, N.W.
  Washington, D.C. 20036
American Association of Ophthalmology
  1100 Seventeenth Street, N.W.
  Washington, D.C. 20036
American Association of Sex Educators
and Counselors
  815 Fifteenth Street, N.W.
  Washington, D.C. 20005

American Chemical Society
  1155 Sixteenth Street, N.W.
  Washington, D.C. 20036
American Dairy Association
  20 North Wacker Drive
  Chicago, Illinois 60607
American Dental Association
  Bureau of Dental Health Education
  211 East Chicago Avenue
  Chicago, Illinois 60611
American Dietetic Association
  1 West 48th Street
  New York, New York 10020
American Dry Milk Institute, Inc.
  130 North Franklin Street
  Chicago, Illinois 60606
American Educational Research
Association
  1126 Sixteenth Street, N.W.
  Washington, D.C. 20036
American Home Economics Association
  1600 Twentieth Street, N.W.
  Washington, D.C. 20036
American Hospital Association
  840 North Lake Shore Drive
  Chicago, Illinois 60611
American Medical Association
  Bureau of Health Education
  535 North Dearborn Street
  Chicago, Illinois 60610

American Nurses' Association
2 Park Avenue
New York, New York 10000
American Occupational Therapy
Association
250 West 57th Street
New York, New York 10000
American Optometric Association
Public Information Division
700 Chippewa Street
St. Louis, Missouri 63119
American Osteopathic Association
212 East Ohio Street
Chicago, Illinois 60611
American Physical Therapy Association
1790 Broadway
New York, New York 10019
American Podiatry Association
20 Chevy Chase Circle, N.W.
Washington, D.C. 20010
American Psychological Association
Task Force on Psychology, Family
Planning and Population Policy
1200 Seventeenth Street, N.W.
Washington, D.C. 20036
American Public Health Association
1015 Eighteenth Street, N.W.
Washington, D.C. 20036
American School Health Association
Kent, Ohio 44240
Child Study Association of America
50 Madison Avenue
New York, New York 10010
Evaporated Milk Association
910 Seventeenth Street, N.W.
Washington, D.C. 20036
Family Service Association of America
44 East 23d Street
New York, New York 10010
Institute of Makers of Explosives
420 Lexington Avenue
New York, New York 10017
International Apple Association
1302 Eighteenth Street, N.W.
Washington, D.C. 20036
National Academy of Sciences
Food and Nutrition Board
2101 Constitution Avenue, N.W.
Washington, D.C. 20418
National Apple Institute
Suite 410
2000 P Street, N.W.
Washington, D.C. 20037
National Association for Mental Health
Director of Education and Program
Services

43 West 61st Street
New York, New York 10019
National Better Business Bureau, Inc.
230 Park Avenue
New York, New York 10017
National Commission on Safety
Education
National Education Association
1201 Sixteenth Street, N.W.
Washington, D.C. 20036
National Congress of Parents and
Teachers
700 North Rush Street
Chicago, Illinois 60611
National Dairy Council
111 North Canal Street
Chicago, Illinois 60606
National Education Association
1201 Sixteenth Street, N.W.
Washington, D.C. 20036
National Fire Protection Association
470 Atlantic Avenue
Boston, Massachusetts 02210
National League for Nursing, Inc.
2 Park Avenue
New York, New York 10016
National Livestock and Meat Board
Nutritional Department
407 South Dearborn Street
Chicago, Illinois 60605
National Nutrition Education
Clearinghouse
Society for Nutrition Education
Suite 1110
2140 Shattuck Avenue
Berkeley, California 94704
National Recreation and Park
Association
1700 Pennsylvania Avenue, N.W.
Washington, D.C. 20006
National Rifle Association of America
1600 Rhode Island Avenue, N.W.
Washington, D.C. 20000
Pharmaceuticals Manufacturers
Association
Public Relations Division
1155 Fifteenth Street, N.W.
Washington, D.C. 20005
Society for Public Health Education, Inc.
655 Sutter Street
San Francisco, California 94102
The Tea Council of the United States of
America
16 East 56th Street
New York, New York 10022

United Fresh Fruit and Vegetable
Association
77 Fourteenth Street, N.W.
Washington, D.C. 20250

COMMERCIAL SOURCES

Abbott Laboratories
Department 33
Abbott Park
North Chicago, Illinois 60064
American Can Company
Home Economics Section
100 Park Avenue
New York, New York 10017
American Institute of Baking
Consumer Service Department
400 East Ontario Street
Chicago, Illinois 60611
American Meat Institute
59 East Van Buren Street
Chicago, Illinois 60605
American Visuals Corporation
381 Park Avenue South
New York, New York 10000
Amurol Products Company
Naperville, Illinois 60540
Armour and Company
Public Relations Department
401 North Wabash Street
Chicago, Illinois 60690
Automotive Industries
Highway Safety Committee
200 K Street, N.W.
Washington, D.C. 20015
B.F. Goodrich Company
500 South Main Street
Akron, Ohio 44318
Block Drug Company
Py-Co-Pay Division
105 Academy Street
Jersey City, New Jersey 07302
The Borden Company
Consumer Services
350 Madison Avenue
New York, New York 10011
Bristol-Myers Products Company
Educational Service Department
45 Rockefeller Plaza
New York, New York 10000
Carnation Milk Company
Home Service Department
5045 Wilshire Boulevard
Los Angeles, California 90036

Cereal Institute, Inc.
Home Economics Department
135 South LaSalle Street
Chicago, Illinois 60603
Ciba Pharmaceutical Products, Inc.
Division of Ciba-Geigy Corporation
556 Morris Avenue
Summit, New Jersey 07901
Colgate-Palmolive Company
300 Park Avenue
New York, New York 10010
DCA Educational Products, Inc.
4865 Stenton Avenue
Philadelphia, Pennsylvania 19114
Food Wonders of the World
P.O. Box 773
Detroit, Michigan 48232
Ford Motor Company
Research and Information
Department
The American Road
Dearborn, Michigan 48127
General Biological Supply House
Chicago, Illinois 60601
General Foods Corporation
General Foods Kitchens
250 North Street
White Plains, New York 10625
General Mills, Inc.
Public Relations Department
9200 Wayzata Boulevard
Minneapolis, Minnesota 55440
General Motors Education Aids
General Motors Building
Detroit, Michigan 48202
Goodyear Tire and Rubber Company
Public Relations Department
1144 East Market Street
Akron, Ohio 44316
H.J. Heinz Company
P.O. Box 57
Pittsburgh, Pennsylvania 15230
International Cellucotton Products
Company
919 North Michigan Avenue
Chicago, Illinois 60611
International Harvester Company
180 North Michigan Avenue
Chicago, Illinois 60601
Johnson and Johnson
c/o Director, Consumer Relations
501 George Street
New Brunswick, New Jersey 08901
Kellogg Company
Home Economics Service
Battle Creek, Michigan 49016

Kimberly-Clark Corporation
Life Cycle Center
P.O. Box 20001
Neenah, Wisconsin 54956
Lactona Products
Warner-Lambert Pharmaceutical
Company
201 Tabor Road
Morris Plains, New Jersey 07950
Lederle Laboratories Division
American Cyanimid Company
Public Relations Department
Pearl River, New York 10965
Lever Brothers Company
Public Relations Division
Consumer Education Department
390 Park Avenue
New York, New York 10022
Licensed Beverage Industries, Inc.
Division of Educational Studies
485 Lexington Avenue
New York, New York 10017
Mental Health Materials Center
419 Park Avenue South
New York, New York 10016
Minnesota Mining and Manufacturing
Company
2501 Hudson Road
St. Paul, Minnesota 55119
Pepsodent
Division of Lever Brothers Company
390 Park Avenue
New York, New York 10022
Personal Products Corporation
c/o Association Sterling, Inc.
P.O. Box 117
Ridgefield, New Jersey 07657
Pet Milk Company
Director of Home Economics
1401 Arcade Building
St. Louis, Missouri 63101
Proctor and Gamble
P.O. Box 599
Cincinnati, Ohio 45201
Public Affairs Committee, Inc.
381 Park Avenue South
New York, New York 10016
Ralston Purina Company
Checkerboard Square
St. Louis, Missouri 63199
Smith, Kline and French Laboratories
1530 Spring Garden Street
Philadelphia, Pennsylvania 19130
Sunkist Growers
Consumer Services Division
Box 2706 Terminal Annex
Los Angeles, California 90054

Swift and Company
Agricultural Research Department
115 West Jackson Boulevard
Chicago, Illinois 60604
Tampax Inc.
Department HL
Educational Director
5 Dakota Drive
Lake Success, New York 11040
United Fruit Company
Education Department
30 Saint James Avenue
Boston, Massachusetts 02100
The Upjohn Company
Trade and Guest Relations Department
Kalamazoo, Michigan 49001
Wheat Flour Institute
14 East Jackson Boulevard
Chicago, Illinois 60604
Whitehall Laboratories, Inc.
685 Third Avenue
New York, New York 10022

GOVERNMENTAL AGENCIES

Atomic Energy Commission
P.O. Box 62
Oakridge, Tennessee 37830
Bureau of Commercial Fisheries
Department of the Interior
Washington, D.C. 20025
Bureau of Education for the Handicapped
Office of Education
Seventh and D Streets, S.W.
Washington, D.C. 20202
Chief Postal Inspector
United States Post Office Department
Washington, D.C. 20260
Children's Bureau
U.S. Department of Health, Education
and Welfare
330 Independence Avenue, S.W.
Washington, D.C. 20201
Division for the Blind and Physically
Handicapped
Library of Congress
1291 Taylor Street, N.W.
Washington, D.C. 20542
Division of Drug Education, Nutrition
and Health Programs
Bureau of School Systems
400 Maryland Avenue, S.W.
Washington, D.C. 20202
Florida Citrus Commission
Production Department
Lakeland, Florida 33801

Heart Information Center
National Heart Institute
U.S. Public Health Service
Bethesda, Maryland 20014
National Center for Chronic Disease Control
Office of Information
4040 North Fairfax Drive
Arlington, Virginia 22203
National Center for Disease Control
1600 Clifton Road, N.E.
Atlanta, Georgia 30333
National Center for Family Planning Services
5600 Fishers Lane
Rockville, Maryland 20852
National Clearinghouse for Drug Abuse Information
P.O. Box 1635
Rockville, Maryland 20850
National Clearinghouse for Smoking and Health
U.S. Public Health Service
5600 Fishers Lane
Rockville, Maryland 20852
National Heart Institute
U.S. Public Health Service
9000 Rockville Pike
Bethesda, Maryland 20014
National Institute on Alcohol Abuse and Alcoholism
5600 Fishers Lane
Rockville, Maryland 20852
National Institute of Allergy and Infectious Diseases
Office of Information
Bethesda, Maryland 20014
National Institute of Child Health and Human Development
Office of Information
U.S. Public Health Service
9000 Rockville Pike
Bethesda, Maryland 20014
National Institute of Dental Research
Information Office
U.S. Public Health Service
Bethesda, Maryland 20014
National Institute on Drug Abuse
11400 Rockville Pike
Rockeville, Maryland 20852
National Institutes of Health
Department of Health, Education and Welfare
Bethesda, Maryland 20014
National Institute of Mental Health
5600 Fishers Lane
Rockville, Maryland 20852

Office of Civil Defense
Secretary of the Army, Pentagon
Washington, D.C. 20310
Office of Environmental Education
Bureau of School Systems
400 Maryland Avenue, S.W.
Washington, D.C. 20202
President's Committee on Mental Retardation
GSA Building
Seventh and D Streets, S.W.
Washington, D.C. 20202
President's Council on Physical Fitness
Superintendent of Documents
Government Printing Office
Washington, D.C. 20402
Public Health Service
Environmental Health Service
U.S. Department of Health, Education and Welfare
Rockville, Maryland 20852
Superintendent of Documents
U.S. Government Printing Office
Washington, D.C. 20025
U.S. Consumer Product Safety Commission
Bureau of Information and Education
Washington, D.C. 20207
U.S. Department of Agriculture
Agriculture Research Administration
Washington, D.C. 20250
U.S. Department of Agriculture
Consumer and Food Economics Institute
Washington, D.C. 20250
U.S. Department of Agriculture
Nutrition and Technical Services
Food and Nutrition Service
Washington, D.C. 20250
U.S. Department of Commerce
National Industrial Pollution Control Council
Fourteenth Street and Constitution Avenue, N.W.
Washington, D.C. 20230
U.S. Department of Health, Education and Welfare
Center for Disease Control
Bureau of State Services
Atlanta, Georgia 30333
U.S. Department of Health, Education and Welfare
Food and Drug Administration
5600 Fishers Lane
Rockville, Maryland 20852

U.S. Department of Transportation
National Highway Traffic Safety
Administration
Washington, D.C. 20590

Water Pollution Control Federation
3900 Wisconsin Avenue, N.W.
Washington, D.C. 20016

World Health Organization
Office of Public Information
1501 New Hampshire Avenue, N.W.
Washington, D.C. 20006

INSURANCE COMPANIES

Aetna Life Affiliated Companies
Information and Education
Department
151 Farmington Avenue
Hartford, Connecticut 06115

Allstate Insurance Company
Accident Prevention Department
Allstate Plaza
Northbrook, Illinois 60062

American Fire Insurance Companies
Engineering Department
80 Maiden Lane
New York, New York 10007

American Insurance Association
85 John Street
New York, New York 10038

Association of Casualty and Surety
Companies
Accident Prevention Department
Publication Division
60 John Street
New York, New York 10038

Connecticut General Life Insurance
Company
Advertising and Public Relations
Hartford, Connecticut 06115

Employers Mutual of Wausau
Safety Engineering Department
407 Grant Street
Wausau, Wisconsin 55402

Equitable Life Assurance Society of the
United States
Bureau of Public Health
1285 Avenue of the Americas
New York, New York 10019

Health Insurance Institute
277 Park Avenue
New York, New York 10017

Institute for Safer Living
American Mutual Liability Insurance
Company
Wakefield, Massachusetts 01880

Insurance Institute for Highway Safety
1710 H Street, N.W.
Washington, D.C. 20037

John Hancock Mutual Life Insurance
Company
Health Education Service
200 Berkeley Street
Boston, Massachusetts 02117

Kemper Insurance Company
Advertising and Public Relations
Department
110 Tenth Avenue
Fulton, Illinois 61252

Liberty Mutual Insurance Company
175 Berkeley Street
Boston, Massachusetts 02117

Metropolitan Life Insurance Company
School Health Bureau
Health and Welfare Division
One Madison Avenue
New York, New York 10010

National Insurance
Safety Department
246 North High Street
Columbus, Ohio 43215

Prudential Insurance Company of
America
Public Relations and Advertising
Prudential Plaza
Newark, New Jersey 07101

Travelers Insurance Company
Marketing Services
One Tower Square
Hartford, Connecticut 06115

VOLUNTARY HEALTH-RELATED AGENCIES

Alcoholics Anonymous
General Services
P.O. Box 459
Grand Central Station
New York, New York 10017

Allergy Foundation of America
801 Second Avenue
New York, New York 10017

Allied Youth Inc.
1901 Forest Meyer Drive
Arlington, Virginia 22209

American Automobile Association
Pennsylvania Avenue at Seventeenth
Street, N.W.
Washington, D.C. 20006

American Cancer Society
219 East 42d Street
New York, New York 10017

American Diabetes Association
  1 West 48th Street
  New York, New York 10020
American Foundation for the Blind
  15 West 16th Street
  New York, New York 10011
American Health Foundation
  1370 Avenue of the Americas
  New York, New York 10019
American Hearing Society
  919 Eighteenth Street, N.W.
  Washington, D.C. 20006
American Heart Association
  Inquiries Section
  44 East 23d Street
  New York, New York 10010
American Institute of Family Relations
  5287 Sunset Boulevard
  Los Angeles, California 90027
American Lung Association
  1740 Broadway
  New York, New York 10019
American National Red Cross
  Seventeenth and D Streets, N.W.
  Washington, D.C. 20006
American Social Health Association
  1790 Broadway
  New York, New York 10019
Arthritis Foundation
  GPO Box 2525
  New York, New York 10036
Association for Family Living
  Suite 1818
  32 West Randolph Street
  Chicago, Illinois 60601
Association for the Study of Abortion,
Inc.
  120 West 57th Street
  New York, New York 10019
Association for Voluntary
Sterilization
  14 West 40th Street
  New York, New York 10018
Better Vision Institute, Inc.
  230 Park Avenue
  New York, New York 10017
Bicycle Institute of America
  122 East 42d Street
  New York, New York 10017
Center for Science in the Public Interest
  1757 S Street, N.W.
  Washington, D.C. 20009
Child Study Association of America
  Wel-Met, Inc.
  50 Madison Avenue
  New York, New York 10019

Cleveland Health Museum
  8911 Euclid Avenue
  Cleveland, Ohio 44106
Consumers Union of the United
States, Inc.
  256 Washington Street
  Mount Vernon, New York 10550
Council for Exceptional Children
  1920 Association Drive
  Reston, Virginia 22091
E. C. Brown Center for Family
Studies
  1802 Moss Street
  Eugene, Oregon 97463
Educational Foundation for Human
Sexuality
  Montclair State College
  Upper Montclair, New Jersey 07043
Epilepsy Foundation of America
  Information Center
  Suite 406
  1828 L Street, N.W.
  Washington, D.C. 20036
Erickson Educational Foundation
  4047 Hundred Oaks Avenue
  Baton Rouge, Louisiana 70808
Family Planning Program
  Emory University School of Medicine
  80 Butler Street
  Atlanta, Georgia 30303
Family Service Association of America
  44 East 23d Street
  New York, New York 10017
Foundation for Research and Education
in Sickle Cell Disease, Inc.
  423 West 120th Street
  New York, New York 10027
Health Information Foundation
  Public Relations Director
  420 Lexington Avenue
  New York, New York 10017
Hogg Foundation for Mental Health
  P.O. Box 7998
  University of Texas
  Austin, Texas 78712
Institute for Family Research and
Education
  760 Ostrom Avenue
  Syracuse, New York 13210
Institute for Sex Education
  18 South Michigan Avenue
  Chicago, Illinois 60603
Institute for Sex Research, Inc.
  Room 416, Mirrosn Hall
  Indiana University
  Bloomington, Indiana 47401

International Planned Parenthood
Federation
  18-20 Lower Regent Street
  London, S.W. 1, England
Leukemia Society of America, Inc.
  National Headquarters
  211 East 43d Street
  New York, New York 10017
Maternity Center Association
  48 East 92d Street
  New York, New York 10028
Muscular Dystrophy Association of
America, Inc.
  Public Information Department
  810 Seventh Avenue
  New York, New York 10019
National Association for Retarded
Children, Inc.
  386 Park Avenue South
  New York, New York 10000
National Council on Alcoholism, Inc.
  2 East 103d Street
  New York, New York 10000
The National Council on Drug Abuse
  Suite 310
  8 South Michigan Avenue
  Chicago, Illinois 60603
National Council on Family Relations
  1219 University Avenue
  Minneapolis, Minnesota 55414
National Cystic Fibrosis Research
Foundation
  60 East 44th Street
  New York, New York 10017
National Dairy Council
  111 North Canal Street
  Chicago, Illinois 60606
National Easter Seal Society for Crippled
Children and Adults, Inc.
  2023 West Ogden Avenue
  Chicago, Illinois 60612
National Epilepsy League, Inc.
  116 South Michigan Avenue
  Chicago, Illinois 60603
National Foot Health Council, Inc.
  321 Union Street
  Rockland, Massachusetts 02370
National Foundation/March of Dimes
  Box 2000
  1275 Mamaroneck Avenue
  White Plains, New York 10602
National Genetics Foundation
  250 West 57th Street
  New York, New York 10019

National Health Council
  1790 Broadway
  New York, New York 10019
National Hemophilia Foundation
  25 West 39th Street
  New York, New York 10018
National Kidney Foundation
  116 East 27th Street
  New York, New York 10010
National Multiple Sclerosis Society
  257 Park Avenue South
  New York, New York 10010
National Parkinson Foundation, Inc.
  1501 Northwest Ninth Street
  Miami, Florida 33136
National Safety Council
  School and College Department
  425 North Michigan Avenue
  Chicago, Illinois 60611
National Society for the Prevention of
Blindness, Inc.
  79 Madison Avenue
  New York, New York 10016
National Tay-Sachs and Allied Diseases
Association, Inc.
  122 East 42d Street
  New York, New York 10017
National Women's Christian Temperance
Union
  1730 Chicago Avenue
  Evanston, Illinois 60200
Nutrition Foundation, Inc.
  99 Park Avenue
  New York, New York 10016
Planned Parenthood Federation of
America, Inc.
  515 Madison Avenue
  New York, New York 10022
Planned Parenthood-World
Population
  810 Seventh Avenue
  New York, New York 10019
Population Crisis Committee
  1835 K Street, N.W.
  Washington, D.C. 20006
Rutgers University Center of Alcohol
Studies
  Smithers Hall
  Box 554
  New Brunswick, New Jersey 08903
Science Research Associates
  259 East Erie Street
  Chicago, Illinois 60611

Sex Information and Education Council
of the United States
(SIECUS)
  1855 Broadway
  New York, New York 10028

United Cerebral Palsy Association, Inc.
  66 East 34th Street
  New York, New York 10016
Zero Population Growth
  367 State Street
  Los Altos, California 94022

Appendix C

National Health Planning and Resources Development Act of 1974. P.L. 93-641

OVERALL SUMMARY
- Goal
- Previous Legislation
- Needs
- Health Systems Agencies
- State Organization
- Timetable

SUMMARY OF PROVISIONS
- Parts
- Health Service Areas
- Health Systems Agencies
- State Agency
- Financial Assistance

OVERALL SUMMARY OF THE ACT

Goal

"The achievement of equal access to quality health care at reasonable cost."

The Act, signed January 4, 1975 by the President, proposes to achieve the above goal by establishing a nationwide network of health systems agencies with authority to plan, to approve facility expansion in health and mental health, and to establish uniform systems of accounting. This organization supersedes prior planning and review agencies set up since 1946.

Previous legislation

The designers of this Act recognized the following weaknesses in earlier health legislation:

1. the inflationary effect of medicare and medicaid
2. the need for incentives for alternatives to hospital care
3. the unequal availability of health care
4. the need to involve providers in planning the programs
5. the importance of preventive care

Needs

The Act sets forth ten priorities which underscore the following:
- the need for improved health care in rural and depressed areas
- the importance of an integrated system of various levels of care within a geographic area as well as coordination within and among existing provider facilities
- the value of preventive care beginning with studies of causes of diseases as related to nutrition and poor environment; improved public health education; accreditation of group practice, particularly health maintenance organizations
- the importance of improving the quality of patient care including the value of the Professional Standards Review Organizations
- the need for improved health manpower, particularly the training of physician assistants and nurse clinicians

Health systems agencies

Health Systems Agencies must be approved by the Secretary on or before July 4, 1976. They may be nonprofit or public benefit corporations; public planning bodies; or units of local government. The Law requires comments from the Governor on each application prior to the Secretary's approval for a two-year temporary or permanent basis. The composition and staffing and activities of Health Systems Agencies are clearly defined in the Law. Their governing body must include: consumers—minimum 50% plus 1, maximum 60%; providers—minimum 40%, maximum 50% less 1. At least one-third of the providers must be direct providers. Government officials may be either consumers or providers. Once the selected agency is set up, existing CHP—B, RMP, and Hill-Burton agencies are to be phased out by June 30, 1976, or within three months of the designation of the HSA, whichever is later. There will be a period of time when the HSA gradually assumes the following responsibilities:

1. develop a short- and long-term plan for health care delivery
2. implement its plan using local resources giving technical assistance
3. make grants and contracts to public, not-for-profit entities and individuals
4. review and approve or disapprove each proposal for the use of federal funds available from the Community Mental Health Center's Act, Comprehensive Alcohol Abuse and Alcohol Prevention, Treatment and Rehabilitation Act including state funds that come through these Acts
5. review and approve or disapprove request for federal funds from the National Research Institute, Health Research and Teaching Facilities Act, Training of Professional Health Personnel and Nursing Training Act when personnel and services provided under these funds are utilized in the area served by the HSA
6. review and make recommendations for the need for new institutional health services proposed to be offered or developed in the HSA area
7. review within three years of the agency's designation and every five years thereafter all institutional health services and make recommendations to the State Health Planning and Development Agency the appropriateness of such services
8. annually recommend projects for the modernization, construction, and conversion of medical facilities which will help implement the long- and short-range plans and the priorities among such subjects

State organizations

The Act requires the Secretary to designate a State agency chosen by the Governor to be the State health planning and development agency. Designation requires approval of an administrative program for carrying out its work. The State Agency will be advised by a Statewide Health Coordinating Council (SHCC) which must have 60% of its members appointed by the Governor from the boards of directors from the State's HSAs. The Council must also have a consumer majority and one-third must represent "direct providers".

Once functioning, the Council will review and coordinate the HSA plans, with comments to the Secretary; prepare a State health plan incorporating the HSA plans; review for the Secretary HSA budgets and applications for assistance; advise the State Agency on its performance; and review with approval power the State plans and applications for health formula grants to the State.

Timetable

The urgency of the timetable is dictated by the desire to have a nationwide planned system of health care delivery prior to the implementation of national health insurance.

SUMMARY OF PROVISIONS OF THE NATIONAL HEALTH PLANNING AND RESOURCES DEVELOPMENT ACT OF 1974

Parts

The legislation has two principal parts. The first, a new title XV in the PHS (Public Health Service) Act, revises existing health planning programs, all of which expired June 30, 1974. The second, a new title XVI in the PHS Act, revises existing programs for the construction and modernization of health care facilities, which also expired June 30, 1974. Title XVI also provides funds for the health systems agencies for their use in the development of health resources which will implement their plans.

Part A of the new title XV requires the Secretary of the Department of Health, Education and Welfare to issue, by regulation, guidelines concerning national health planning policy within 18 months of enactment. These guidelines are to include a statement of national health planning goals based upon national health priorities specified in the legislation. In issuing the guidelines, the Secretary is to consult with the health systems agencies, the State health planning and development agencies, the Statewide Health Coordinating Councils, the National Council on Health Planning and Development established by this Act, and associations and specialty societies representing medical and other health care providers.

Part B of the new title XV creates a network of health systems agencies responsible for health planning and development throughout the country. In creating such a network, the Governors of the States would be asked to designate throughout the country health service areas for planning and development purposes which meet the requirements specified in the legislation. These requirements are as follows:

1. The area must be a geographic region appropriate for the effective planning and development of health services, determined on the basis of factors including population and the availability of resources to provide all necessary health services for residents of the area.
2. To the extent practicable, the area must include at least one center for the provision of highly specialized health services.
3. Each area must have a population of not less than 500,000 or more than 3 million, except that an area may be less than 500,000 if the area comprises an entire State with a population of less than 500,000 or more than 3 million if

the area includes a standard metropolitan statistical area with a greater population. The legislation also permits the area to be less that 500,000 to a minimum of 200,000 under "unusual circumstances" and below 200,000 in "highly unusual circumstances," both as determined by the Secretary.

4. The area boundaries, to the maximum extent feasible, must be appropriately coordinated with those of Professional Standards Review Organizations, existing regional planning areas, and State planning and administrative areas.

5. The boundaries are also to be established so that, in the planning and development of health services to be offered within the health service area, any economic or geographic barrier to the receipt of such services in nonmetropolitan areas is taken into account. Determination of boundaries must reflect the differences in health planning and health services development needs between nonmetropolitan and metropolitan areas.

6. Each standard metropolitan statistical area (SMSA) must be entirely within the boundaries of a single health service area. This requirement may be waived if a Governor determines, with the approval of the Secretary, that in order to meet the above-mentioned requirements, a health service area may contain only part of the SMSA.

Health service areas

The legislation further provides that the Secretary must designate as health service areas those areas now served by agencies funded under section 314(b) if they meet all the requirements listed above unless the Governor determines that other areas are more appropriate. The Act also provides that no areas need be designated for States which have no county or municipal public health institution or department and which have maintained a health planning system which complies with the purposes of this title. The Secretary may revise the Governor's designations only where they are inconsistent with the above-mentioned requirements. The Secretary is responsible for publishing the health service area boundary designations in the Federal Register within seven months of enactment.

Health systems agencies

In each health service area, the Secretary, after consulting with the Governor of the appropriate State, must then designate either a private nonprofit corporation or a public entity as the health systems agency responsible for health planning and development in that area. A health systems agency may not be or operate an educational institution. The legislation specifies minimum criteria for the legal structure, staff, governing body, and functioning of the health systems agencies. They would be generally responsible for preparing and implementing plans designed to improve the health of the residents of their health service area; to increase the accessibility, acceptability, continuity, and quality of health services in the area; to restrain increases in the cost of providing health services; and to prevent unnecessary duplication of health resources. In performing these responsibilities, the health systems agencies are required to:

- gather and analyze suitable data
- establish health systems plans (goals) and annual implementation plans (objectives and priorities)
- provide either technical and/or limited financial assistance to people seeking to implement provisions of the plans
- coordinate activities with PSROs (Professional Standards Review Organizations) and other appropriate planning and regulatory entities

- review and approve or disapprove applications for Federal funds for health programs within the area
- assist States in the performance of capital expenditures reviews
- assist States in making findings as to the need for new institutional health services proposed to be offered in the area
- assist States in reviewing existing institutional health services offered with respect to the appropriateness of such services
- annually recommend to States projects for the modernization, construction, and conversion of medical facilities in the area

State agency

Part C requires the Secretary to designate an agency of State government chosen by the Governor in each State to serve as the State health planning and development agency (State Agency). In order to be designated, the State Agency must prepare and submit to the Secretary for approval an administrative program for carrying out its functions. The State Agency is to be advised by a Statewide Health Coordinating Council whose composition and responsibilities are specified in the legislation including requirements that the Council:

- have 60% of its members appointed by the Governor from the State's health systems agencies and have a consumer majority
- review annually and coordinate the health systems plans and annual implementation plans of the State's health systems agencies and make comments to the Secretary
- prepare a State health plan made up of the health systems plans of the health systems agencies, taking into account the preliminary plan developed by the State Agency
- review for the Secretary budgets and applications for assistance of health systems agencies
- advise the State Agency on the performance of its functions
- review and approve or disapprove State plans and applications for health-type formula grants to the State

The required functions of the State agency are specified and include:

- conducting the State's health planning activities and implementing the parts of the State health plan and plans of health systems agencies which relate to the government of the State
- preparing a preliminary State plan for approval or disapproval by the Council
- assisting the Council in the review of the State medical facilities plan and in the performance of its functions
- serving as the designated planning agency under Section 1122 of the Social Security Act if the State has made an agreement and administering a State certificate of need program of comparable scope
- reviewing new institutional health services proposed and making findings as to the need for such services
- reviewing existing institutional health services offered with respect to the appropriateness of such services and making public its findings

Any of the functions described above may be performed by another agency of State government upon the request of the Governor under an agreement with the State agency satisfactory to the Secretary.

Part C also provides that the Secretary may make grants for the purpose of demonstrating the effectiveness of rate regulation to a maximum of six States which are regulating, or have indicated their intent to regulate, rates prior to the end of six months after the date of enactment.

Part D contains general provisions applicable to the above programs. These include:

- procedures and criteria for use by the health systems agencies and the State Agencies in performing the reviews required by the Act
- requirements that the Secretary provide technical assistance to health systems agencies and State Agencies and establish a national health planning information center
- a requirement that the Secretary fund at least five centers for the study and development of health planning
- requirements that the Secretary review and approve or disapprove the annual budgets of each health systems agency and State Agency, develop performance standards for health systems agencies and State Agencies and monitor their performance, and review in detail at least every three years the structure, operation, and performance of each health systems agency and State Agency

Parts A, B, C, D, and E of the new title XVI revise the existing medical facilities construction program and relate their activities more closely to the planning programs created by new title XV. Part F provides development funds for each health systems agency to enable the agency to establish and maintain an Area Health Services Development Fund.

Financial assistance

Part A sets forth the general purposes of title XVI which is to provide assistance, through allotments under Part B and loans and loan guarantees and interest subsidies under Part C, for projects for:

1. modernization of medical facilities;
2. construction of new outpatient medical facilities;
3. construction of new inpatient medical facilities in areas which have experienced recent rapid population growth (as defined in regulations of the Secretary); and
4. conversion of existing medical facilities for the provision of new health services.

It is also the purpose to provide grant assistance for construction and modernization projects designed to eliminate or prevent safety hazards or avoid noncompliance with licensure or accreditation standards.

As a condition to the receipt of funds under Parts B and C, a State Agency must have approved by the Secretary a State medical facilities plan. Prior to the Secretary's approval, the plan must be approved by the Statewide Health Coordinating Council in terms of its consistency with the State health plan. The facilities plan is to include a list of the projects for which assistance will be sought and the priorities for the funding of these projects. For each project, an application must be submitted to the Secretary for approval and it must set forth a number of assurances including one that services in assisted facilities will be made available to all persons residing or employed in the areas served by the facilities and that a reasonable volume of services will be available to persons unable to pay.

Part B provides for allotments to the States on the basis of population, financial need, and the need for medical facilities projects. Not more than 20% of a State's allotment may be used for projects for construction of new inpatient facilities in areas which have experienced recent rapid population growth and not less than 25% may be used for projects for outpatient facilities which will serve medically underserved populations, half of which must be expended in rural medically underserved areas. In the case of a project to be assisted under an allotment, the

Federal share may not exceed two-thirds of the costs except that a project in a rural or urban poverty areas may receive 100% Federal funding. This part also directs the Secretary to review compliance with the assurances made under title VI and to those made under the new program. If the Secretary finds that an entity has failed to comply with assurances, he must either withhold payments to the entity or effect compliance by other means authorized by existing law including bringing suit in Federal court. Actions to enforce compliance may be brought by a person other than the Secretary, if the Secretary has either dismissed a complaint made to him by such person or has failed to act on such complaint within six months after the date on which it was filed with him.

Part C authorizes the Secretary to make loans and guarantee loans to non-Federal lenders and the Federal Financing Bank for medical facilities projects. A loan or loan guarantee may not exceed 90% of the costs of a project unless the project is in an urban or rural poverty area, in which case the loan or loan guarantee may cover 100% of the costs.

Part D provides for direct Federal project grants to publicly owned health facilities for construction or modernization projects designed to eliminate or prevent safety hazards or avoid noncompliance with State or voluntary licensure or accreditation standards. The amount of any grant may not exceed 75% of the project costs unless the project is located in an urban or rural poverty area in which case the grant may cover 100% of the costs. Of the funds appropriated for allotment to the States, 22% must be made available for project grants.

Part E contains general provisions pertaining to judicial review, recovery, State control of operations, definitions, financial statements and technical assistance.

Part F relates to the Area Health Services Development Fund and authorizes the Secretary to make development grants to each health systems agency which has a designation agreement in effect, has plans in effect reviewed by the Statewide Health Coordinating Council, and is organized, operated, and performing its functions in a manner satisfactory to the Secretary. A development grant may not exceed $1 per person in the health service area.

Appendix D

School Health Section
Position Paper*
Education for Health in the School
Community Setting

ADOPTED BY
GOVERNING COUNCIL OF THE AMERICAN
PUBLIC HEALTH ASSOCIATION
OCTOBER 23, 1974
NEW ORLEANS, LOUISIANA

The school is a community in which most individuals spend at least twelve years of their lives, and more if they have the advantages of early childhood programs, college education, and continuing education for adults. The health of our school-age youth will determine to a great extent the quality of life each will have during the growing and developing years and on throughout the life cycle. Their capacity to function as health educated adults will in turn help each to realize the fullest potential for self, family, and the various communities of which each individual will be a part.

The American Public Health Association believes that health education should be a continuing process, from conception to death, and that such education must be comprehensive, coordinated, and integrated in *all* community planning for health.

The school, as a social structure, provides an educational setting in which the total health of the child during the impressionable years is of priority concern. No other community setting even approximates the magnitude of the grades K-12 school educational enterprise, with an enrollment in 1973–74 of 45.5 million in nearly 17,000 school districts comprising more than 115,000 schools with some 2.1 million teachers. This is to say nothing of the administrative, supervisory, and service manpower required to maintain these institutions. Additionally, more than 40 percent of children aged three to five are enrolled in early childhood education programs. Thus it seems that the school should be regarded as a social unit providing a focal point to which health planning for all other community settings should relate.

Schools provide an environment conducive to developing skills and competencies which will help the individual confront and examine a complexity of social and cultural forces, persuasive influences, and ever-expanding options, as these affect health behavior. Today's health problems do not lend themselves to yester-

---

* A Position Paper is defined as a major exposition of the Association's viewpoint on broad issues affecting the public's health.

day's solutions. Specificity of cause is multiple rather than singular. The individual must assume increasing responsibility for solutions to major public health problems, and consequently must be educated to do so.

Education for and about health is not synonymous with information. Education is concerned with behavior—a composite of what an individual knows, senses, and values and of what one does and practices. Factual data are but temporary assumptions to be used and cast aside as new information emerges. Health facts unrenewed can become a liability rather than an asset. The health educated citizen is one who possesses resources and abilities that will last throughout a lifetime—such as critical thinking, problem-solving, valuing, self-discipline, and self-direction—and that lead to a sense of responsibility for community and world concerns.

The school curriculum offers an opportunity to view health issues in an integrated context. It is designed to help the learner gain insights about the personal, social, environmental, political, and cultural implications of each issue. Planning for health care delivery, for example, is not simply a matter of providing for manpower, services, and facilities. These things must be considered in concert with housing, employment, transportation, cultural beliefs and values, and the rights and dignity of the persons involved. Nor will nutritional practices be improved substantially by programs based on groupings, labeling, or issuing stamps, because food practices and eating patterns are equally influenced by how, when, where, why, and with whom one eats.

APHA is concerned about the traditional crisis approach to health care. The expense involved in treatment, rehabilitation, recuperation, and restoration to health has sent medical costs soaring. More facilities, more services, and more manpower to staff the facilities and to provide the services appear to be the nation's leading health priorities. The alternative is a redirection of the nation's health goals towards a primary preventive—and constructive—approach to health, through education for every individual.

Because of vested interests, political pressures, mass media sensationalism, and health agency structures with categorical interests, health education programs in schools are compelled to deal with a multitude of separate health issues, with only a few of these given priority at any given time. Too frequently, programs developed to deal with crucial issues are eliminated although the problems remain, because another crisis emerges calling for more new crash programs. A revolving critical issue syndrome has been the result, with the same problems considered crucial a decade or more ago emerging once again. Focusing on selected categorical issues has potential value if time, energy, personnel, and money are available to sustain the emphasis and expand such efforts into an integrated and viable health education framework. A broad concept of healthful living that has consideration for psychosocial dimensions should be the basis for health education.

APHA is encouraged by recent developments in an increasing number of states which attest to recognition of the significance of a comprehensive health education program in grades kindergarten through twelve. Also encouraging are the exemplary programs being established in many school districts, and the expressed intention of the federal overnment to implement an action plan for "Better Health Through Education."
Therefore:

The American Public Health Association supports the concept of a national commitment to a comprehensive, sequential program of health education for all students in the nation's schools, kindergarten through the twelfth grade. The Association will exert leadership through its sections and affiliates to assure for health education:

(1) time in the curriculum commensurate with other subject areas,
(2) professionally qualified teachers and supervisors of health education,
(3) innovative instructional materials and appropriate teaching facilities,

(4) increased financial support at the local, state, and national levels to upgrade the quantity and quality of health education and

(5) a teaching/learning environment in which opportunities for safe and optimal living exist, and one in which a well-organized and complete health service is functioning.

SPECIFIC METHODS TO BE USED FOR IMPLEMENTATION

The American Public Health Association will:

- Publicize and support the concepts expressed in H.R. 2600 (2599 and 2601) and in S. 544 bills of the 94th Congress. First session (Comprehensive School Health Education Act).
- Contact state APHA affiliates and recommend their involvement in offering support and endorsement to the State Commissioner of Education in those states which have within recent years passed K-12 Comprehensive Health Education legislation (e.g., New York, Florida, Illinois); and to offer APHA leadership to other states seeking comprehensive health education legislation for schools.
- Encourage APHA staff members and officers to incorporate in their public messages a statement calling for K-12 comprehensive health education programs in all schools and use the *American Journal of Public Health* and *The Nation's Health* as media for editorials and for reports of legislation.
- Monitor the development and operation of the Bureau of Health Education, CDC, established July 1, 1974, and the proposed National Center for Health Education representing the private sector (both recommended by the President's Committee on Health Education) to assure emphasis on the importance of health education in schools and provision of the adequate funding essential for high quality programs.
- Examine manpower legislation for the health professions to assure that health education professional preparation programs for positions in schools, colleges, and other community settings are specified as eligible for traineeships and other grants.
- Seek grant support to explore and clarify the function of health educators in schools and a variety of other community settings (e.g., colleges, agencies, organizations, hospitals, industry, HMOs, action projects).
- Recommend that each State Department of Education seek budgetary support to add one or more fully qualified health educators to its staff for consultant services to school districts.
- Appoint a task force comprised of appropriate APHA sections and representatives and affiliates to guide the Association's efforts on behalf of health education and designate a staff member to coordinate the activities.

A Partial List of National Organizations and Groups that Support Health Education in Schools
(As Reflected in their Position Statements, Resolutions, Conference Reports, and other Professional Literature)
American Academy of Pediatrics
American Alliance for Health, Physical Education, and Recreation
American Association of School Administrators
American Dental Association
American Medical Association
American Public Health Association
American School Health Association
Council of Chief State School Officers

Department of Health, Education, and Welfare
Department of School Nurses, NEA
International Union for Health Education
Joint Committee on Health Problems in Schools of the National Education
Association and the American Medical Association
National Association of Elementary School Principals
National Association of Secondary School Principals
National Association of State Boards of Education
National Congress of Parents and Teachers
National Education Association
National Health Council
National School Boards Association
School Health Education Study (1961–1972)
Sex Education and Information Council of the United States
Society of Nutrition Education
Society of Public Health Education

Examples of reports from
National Commission on Community Health Services, 1966
President's Commission on National Goals, 1960
President's Committee on Health Education, 1973
Quality of Life Conferences (AMA), 1972, 1973
Schools for the Sixties (NEA Project on Instruction)
Schools for the Seventies (NEA Project on Instruction)
White House Conference on Children and Youth, 1970.

Index

Coalition of National Health Organizations, 10
Coded message, 344. *See also* Information theory
Cognitive development, 25, 54. *See also* Cognitive domain; Intellectual development
Cognitive domain, 50, 92, 149–154, 344
Cognitive learning, 149–154
Cognitive learning theory, 344
Coleman, James C., 132, 133, 134, 140, 165, 183
College proficiency examinations. *See* New York State
Commission on the Reorganization of Secondary Education, 9
Committee. *See* Advisory committees
Communication channel, 344. *See also* Information theory
Communications, 294–295. *See also* Information theory
Community health education, 344
Community health educator. *See* Public health educator
Community health organizations, 49, 237, 344
Community health program, 49, 60, 344
Community health resources. *See* Learning resources
Competency-based teacher education, 199–203
  basic competencies, 200–202
  criteria of, 344
  definition of, 344
Completion items, 326. *See also* Evaluation
Components of the total health program, 345
Comprehensive health program, 25, 57–60. *See also* Health education
  definition of, 345
  primary elements of, 60–64
Comprehensive School Health Education Act, 46, 51–52, 67
Computer-based-resource-units. *See* Computerized learning
Computerized learning, 312, 345
Conant, Richard K., 193, 215
Concept formation, 345. *See also* Health knowledge, and concept development
Conceptual approach. *See* Curriculum development; Curriculum guides; School Health Education Study

Conditioned response, 345. *See also* Conditioning
Conditioned stimulus, 345. *See also* Conditioning
Conditioning
  classical, 144–145, 344
  discrimination in, 145
  and extinction, 144–145
  and generalization of, 145
  operant, 144, 145, 351
  and reinforcement, 144
  and spontaneous recovery, 145
Cone of experiences, 300
Connecticut, 9
Connecticut Citizens Response to Educational Goals, 248–249
Connecticut State Board of Education, 248, 273
Consumer health, 81, 271–272, 276–277
Consummatory response, 175–176, 181. *See also* Motivation
Cooley's anemia. *See* Thalassemia
Coping mechanisms, 79, 345
Coronary thrombosis, 76–77. *See also* Cardiovascular disease
Correlated health experiences, 345. *See also* Health education
Course of study, 345. *See also* Curriculum guides
Creative activities, 345. *See also* Approaches in health education
Creswell, William H. Jr., 8, 18, 241, 245
Criteria, 72–73. *See also* Curriculum development, criteria for; Curriculum guides, criteria; Evaluation, criteria for; Health, criteria for
Critical Health Problems Act, 345. *See also* New York State
Cue function, 179–180, 182, 345. *See also* Motivation
Current methods, 305–310. *See also* Inductive learning; Deductive learning
Curriculum. *See also* Health education; Curriculum development; Curriculum guides
  definition of, 248–250, 345
  design of, 11, 13
  elementary school. *See* Elementary school curriculum
  guides. *See* Curriculum guides
  textbooks as. *See* Curriculum guides; Methodology

Health (*Continued*)

and effectiveness, 124–138. *See also* Human effectiveness

intermediate level of, 34, 35

optimal, 22. *See also* Optimal health

primary level of, 34, 35

relative nature of, 32–33

restoration of, 21, 23

secondary level of, 34, 35

and self-sufficiency, 126–128. *See also* Self-sufficiency

social. *See* Dimensions of health

status. *See* Health status

Health action, 36

Health agencies. *See* Governmental health agencies; Voluntary health agencies

Health attitudes, 49, 73–76, 347. *See also* Attitudinal development

Health behavior, 7, 46, 49, 73–76, 114–115, 179, 347. *See also* Health-directed behavior; Health-related behavior; Psychomotor domain

dynamics of, 158–159

and human energetics, 171

and human plasticity, 171

nonobservable, 75, 158, 350

observable, 75, 158, 350

Health care facilities, 34–45

Health care system, 21, 24, 32, 34, 49, 194, 347

elements of, 36–37

goal of, 36, 40–41

Health content. *See* Health education, content of; Health information

Health curriculum, 347. *See also* Curriculum; Curriculum development; Curriculum guides

Health decisions. *See* Decision-making

Health-directed behavior, 22, 29, 76, 159, 347. *See also* Health-related behavior

Health educated person, 126

Health education, 60, 61, 79, 90–91. *See also* Comprehensive health program; School health program

administrators of, 71. *See also* Health education administrator

of adults. *See* Adult health education

areas of practice, 7

bases for, 68–98

breadth of, 71–72

changes in, 8–10

and community programs, 49

components of, 38–39

comprehensive programs, 25

content of, 76–87. *See also* Informational content

and correlated activities, 50

current, 23–25. *See also* Modern health education

curriculum, 50. *See also* Curriculum development

definition of, 5–6, 40, 45–47, 49, 51, 347

ecological considerations of, 52–55

in elementary schools. *See* Elementary school curriculum

elements of, 17

emphasis of, 27, 38–41

evaluation of, 50–52. *See also* Evaluation

factors affecting, 29

foundational principles of, 50, 74

future of, 16–17

goals of, 13, 17, 24–25, 39, 51, 72–73, 88, 91, 130, 134. *See also* Health goals; Objectives

history of, 7–14

and human effectiveness, 46. *See also* Human effectiveness

incidental experiences, 50

influences of, 53

integrated, 50

and learning, 148–149

and life-styles, 37–39. *See also* Lifestyles

and medical services. *See* Health services

methodology in, 7. *See also* Methodology

modern, 25–26

myths about. *See* Myths

necessity of, 136–137

need for, 70–71

for the 1980's, 15–17

nomenclature of, 48–50

objectives of. *See* Objectives

organization of. *See* Organization and administration

and other academic disciplines, 11

philosophy of. *See* Philosophy

and political action, 5, 223

primitive roots of, 7–8

principles of, 51

and principles of learning, 141–161

process of, 45–46

profession, 6. *See also* Professionalism

program, 38

progress of, 52–53, 90–91

Health restoration, 348
Health science education, 16, 17, 30, 50, 298–299, 348
Health services, 10, 23, 49, 60–61, 298, 348
Health status, 7, 25, 26–28, 29
  defined, 26–27, 40, 348
  factors affecting, 26–28
  and genetic potentials, 111–112
  levels of, 34
Health Systems Agencies, 209, 211
Healthful living, 10, 126–127. See also School environment
Healthful school environment. See School environment
Healthy, becoming, 31–34
Hearing, conservation of, 271
Heart attack, 23, 56. See also Coronary thrombosis
Hebrew Health Code, 8
Heredity, 21, 40. See also Genetics
History of health education. See Health movement; Health education movement
Hochbaum, Godfrey M., 4, 16, 17, 221, 222, 245
Holistic approach to health, 129–132, 166
  definition of, 129
  and internal qualities, 129–130
  uniqueness and, 131–132
Homeostasis, 135, 348. See also Basic needs; Motivation
  and biological level, 166–168
  and health, 166
  and health knowledge, 177
  and interpretive level, 166–168
  and learning, 166–168
  and motivation, 166–168, 180
Horizontal curriculum format. See Curriculum guides
Hoyman, Howard S., 188, 189, 215
Hubbard, William, Jr., 126
Human effectiveness, 25. See also Health, and effectiveness
Human health needs, 101–122. See also Basic needs
Human motivation, 80. See also Motivation
Human needs, 6, 79. See also Basic needs
Human resources. See Learning resources
Human sexuality, 80
Humanity, progress of, 130–131

Huntington's chorea, 56
Huxley, Aldous, 136

Id, 133
Idiographic approach, 131–132, 349. See also Personality development
Ill-health, 115–116
Illich, Ivan, 142
Incentive, 165, 168–169, 170–171, 180, 181, 349. See also Motivation
Incidental health experiences, 349. See also Health education
Independent variable, 323–325, 349. See also Evaluation
Independent study. See Self-directed learning
Individual health, 31–32. See also Health
Individualized learning, 166, 179, 298, 307–308, 349. See also Computerized learning; Current methods; Self-directed learning
Indoctrination, 179
Inductive learning, 179, 305–307, 349. See also Learning; Current methods
Informational approach, 349. See also Curriculum development
Informational content, 13–14, 46, 76. See also Health education, content of
Information theory, 293–296, 349. See also Communications
  and communications, 294–295
  description of, 293–294
  destination of message, 346
  elements of, 293
  encoding, 293, 346
  and feedback. See Psychological feedback
  and noise, 293, 350
Innovative health education, 308–310
Inservice programs, 239–240
Integrated health experiences, 349. See also Health education
Intellectual development, 127–128, 151. See also Cognitive development
Intelligence, 349. See also Intellectual development
Interdepartmental Panel for Health Education of the Public, 212
Internalization, 145, 158, 169, 172–174, 181. See also Learning; Motivation; P-I-S-A

Intervening variables, 334–335. *See also* Evaluation
Ithaca City School District, 308

Jenne, Frank, 8
Joint Committee on Health Education Terminology, 49
Joint Committee on Health Problems in Education, 10, 197, 215
Jordan, Barbara, 218
Jung, Carl, 133

Kendler, Howard H., 155, 156, 161
Kennedy, Edward M., 119, 122
Kennedy, John F., 20
Kilander, H. Frederick, 45, 67
Klausmeur, Herbert, 121
Knowledge. *See* Health knowledge
Knutson, Andie L., 148, 161, 163, 168, 171, 183
Koopman, G. Robert, 249, 290
Korsakoff's psychosis, 117
Krathwohl, David R., 154

Lawlor, John T., 310, 316
Learner-centered curriculum guide, 349. *See also* Curriculum guides
Learner-centered methods, 349. *See also* Methodology
Learner objectives, 25–26, 203. *See also* Objectives
Learner-observational method, 302–303, 349. *See also* Methodology
demonstration method, 302
field trip, 302–303
media resources, 303. *See also* Learner resources
Learners, 46
Learning. *See also* Methodology
active, 25
associationist school of, 144, 145
attitude and. *See* Attitudinal development
cognitive school of, 144–145
concept formation, 151–152. *See also* Health knowledge
definition of, 143–146, 349
and health, 148–149, 178–179
hierarchy of, 148
and internalization. *See* Internalization
and motivation. *See* Motivation, and learning
motivational factors and, 145
needs and. *See* Basic needs
passive, 25

principles of, 146–148. *See also* Health education, and learning
proactive facilitation, 152, 351
proactive inhibition, 152, 351
process of, 25
and public health, 148–149
rate of, 170
and readiness, 169
retroactive facilitation, 152
retroactive inhibition, 152–153
strategies for. *See* Learning strategies
Learning aids. *See* Learning resources
Learning environments, 46, 53–54. *See also* Environment
Learning methods, 295, 349. *See also* Methodology
Learning resources, 46–47, 49, 299–300, 332–333, 349
Learning resources and evaluation committee. *See* Advisory committee
Learning strategies, 295–296, 312–313, 350. *See also* Methodology
Lecture method, 350. *See also* Traditional methods
Lesson plan, 350. *See also* Curriculum guides
Libido, 133
Life expectancy, 29
Life styles, 21, 24, 27, 29, 32, 114, 159, 311. *See also* Health education
Legislation, 9, 11–13. *See also* specific acts

McTernan, Edward J., 195, 215
Mann, Horace, 9
Marriage and family, 82
Maryland Association for Retarded Children, 298
Maslow, Abraham, 105–106, 121, 133, 134, 136. *See also* Basic needs
Massachusetts Institute of Technology, 9
Master plan. *See* Curriculum guides
Matching items, 327. *See also* Evaluation
Material resources. *See* Learning resources
Maturation, 104, 297–298, 350. *See also* Personality development
Mausner, Judith, 81, 98
May, Rollo, 134
Mayshark, Cyrus, 222, 245
Means, Richard K., 8, 90–91, 98
Measurement. *See* Evaluation

Media resources, 350. *See also* Learning resources
Medical care
  cost of, 21, 23
  therapeutic approaches, 28
Medical profession, 24, 49, 195
Medicines, 268–269
Mental health, 59, 264–265
Mental health education, 280
Mental health maintenance, 80
Mental retardation. *See* Down's syndrome
Methodology, 7, 50, 292–316. *See also* Approaches in health education; Current methods; Information theory; Learning methods; Learning strategies; Traditional methods
  and curriculum, 296. *See also* Curriculum; Curriculum development
  definition of, 299, 350
  and learner characteristics, 296–298
  selection of, 296–300
  and teacher characteristics, 298
  and teaching, 295–296
Methods. *See* Methodology; Approaches in health education
Midcentury White House Conference on Children and Youth, 10
Milio, Nancy, 192, 215
Mill, John Stuart, 34–35, 219, 245
Miller, Van, 223, 245
Minnesota, University of, 103
Minnesota Mining and Manufacturing Company, 262
Misconception, 47–48, 114, 350. *See also* Myths; Health misconceptions
Modern health education, 25, 53–55. *See also* Health education
Modern health era, 8
Motivating for health learning, 162–183. *See also* Motivation
Motivation, 23, 25, 164–183. *See also* Basic needs; Incentive; Motives
  applied to health education, 178–180
  and behavior, 164, 179
  extrinsic, 171–172, 181
  factors involved in, 168–172, 173–174
  homeostasis and. *See* Homeostasis
  and intent to learn, 168–169
  intrinsic, 171–172, 181
  and learning, 147, 176–177. *See also* Learning

and needs. *See* Basic needs
  principles of, 164–168
  and punishment, 169–170
  purpose of, 175–176
  and reinforcement, 169
  results of, 177
  rewards and, 169–170
  techniques of, 178–179
Motives. *See also* Basic needs; Homeostasis; Motivation
  and behavior, 174–175, 181
  biogenic, 164–165, 177, 344
  conflicting, 179, 181
  definition of, 164, 180
  sociogenic, 165–166, 177, 353
Multiple-choice items, 326–327. *See also* Evaluation
Myths, 45–52. *See also* Misconceptions

National Association for the Study and Prevention of Tuberculosis, 9
National Center for Health Education, 10
National Clearinghouse for Smoking and Health, 211, 274
National Committee on School Health Policies, 10
National Conference for Cooperation in Health Education, 10
National Conference on Professional Training in Health Education, 10
National Genetics Foundation, 56
National Health Assembly, 211
National Health Council, 211
National Health Planning and Resources Development Act, 10
National Health Test, 70
NEA-AMA Joint Committee on Health Problems in Education, 197
Need, definition of, 350. *See also* Basic needs
Need satisfaction, 108–109. *See also* Basic needs
  counterforces to, 115–119
  and environmental influences, 111–112
  and genetic potentials, 111–112
  and personal behavior, 113–115
Neurotic, 80
New York State
  Boards of Cooperative Educational Services, 226
  Board of Regents, 330–331
  Chapter 787 of Education Laws, 11–13, 345

and college proficiency examinations, 203–204

Commissioner of Education, 13. *See also* Nyquist, Ewald

Education Department, 13, 226, 228, 263, 331

health education regulations, 14

New York University, 226

Noise. *See* Information theory

Nomenclature. *See* Health education, nomenclature of

Nomothetic approach, 131–132. *See also* Personality development

Nonobservable behavior. *See* Health behavior

Nonsense syllables, 350

Nonverbal communications. *See* Communications

Nutrition education, 266, 280

Nyquist, Ewald, 54–55

Oberteuffer, Delbert, 130, 140, 322, 323, 341

Obesity, 27, 32

Objectives. *See also* Behavioral objectives; Goals

defined, 350

domains of, 91–93

enabling, 254

learner, 25–26, 87, 91–93

teacher, 89–91

terminal, 254

Objective test instrument, 350. *See also* Evaluation

Observations. *See* Evaluation, examples of

Official agencies. *See* Governmental health agencies

Operant conditioning. *See* Conditioning

Operant goals, 134. *See also* Health education, goals of

Optimal health, 22, 29, 136. *See also* Health

attainment of, 29–31

chart of, 15

definition of, 26–27, 28–29, 40, 351

and health education, 13–14

role of heredity, 39–40

role of school and community, 30–31

Organic disease, 135–136

Organization and administration, 7, 47, 218–245

activities of, 220

budgetary constraints and, 224

and communications, 224–225, 226–227

factors affecting, 223–224

and inservice programs, 239–240

need for, 220–222

principles of, 219–225

and program effectiveness, 239

purpose of, 219–220

Pap test, 71

Partnership for Health Act, 211

Patient health education, 351. *See also* Patient health educator

Patient health educator, 23, 49, 190, 193–195, 198–199, 321–322. *See also* Health educator

Pavlov, Ivan, 144

Peer approaches. *See* Approaches

Perception, 351

Personal safety, 78. *See also* Safety

Personality development, theories of, 79, 132–134

analytic, 133

existentialism, 134–135

individual, 133.

psychoanalytic, 132–133

self-actualization, 133–134

Persuasion, 155–156

Phenotype, 112, 351

Phenylalanine hydroxilase, 30, 56

Phenylketonuria, 29–30, 56

Philosophy

definition of, 6, 17, 351

of health education, 4, 6, 8, 48–50, 351

historical basis of. *See* Health education, history of

principles of, 6–7, 17

Physical education, 9

Physical health, 5, 58–59, 77–78, 84. *See also* Health

Piaget, J., 127–128, 136

Pigg, R. Morgan Jr., 337

P-I-S-A, 145, 172–174, 181, 351

PKU. *See* Phenylketonuria

Political awareness, 223

Political priorities, 5

Politics and health, 83

Porphyria, 56

Positive health, 178

Positive potentials, 57

Posttest, 351. *See also* Evaluation

Power structure, 238, 351

Predictive posttest, 351. *See also* Evaluation

Premodern Period of Health, 8

Pretest. *See* Evaluation
President's Committee on Health Education, 10, 31–32, 42, 86, 117, 211
Prevention, 27–28
Principles of learning. *See* Learning
Proactive facilitation. *See* Learning
Proactive inhibition. *See* Learning
Problem solving method, 351. *See also* Approaches, learner-centered
Processes, 351. *See also* Methodologies
Professional ethics, 195. *See also* Professionalism
Professionalism, 195–203. *See also* Health education profession
  and certification, 196, 198
  definition of, 195–197, 351
  and political involvement, 196
  role of colleges, 198–199
  standards for, 197–198
Professional preparation, 7
  and certification, 196. *See also* Competency-based teacher education
  and college proficiency examinations. *See* New York State
  and the future, 206–207
  of health education administrator. *See* Health education administrator
  and health education center concept. *See* Health education center concept
  need for change in, 199
  recent innovations, 199–203
  role of colleges. *See* Professionalism
  and secondary school health educator, 203–205
  undergraduate, 198
  universal standards for, 197–198
Proficiency examinations. *See* New York State
Program aim. *See* Aim
Promotion of health, 21–24, 50, 61. *See also* Health
  definition of, 40
  processes for, 34–37
Psychoanalytic theory. *See* Personality development
Psychological feedback, 170, 181, 294, 351. *See also* Evaluation; Feedback
Psychological health, 78–81, 84
Psychological set, 179
Psychomotor domain, 50, 93, 158, 351. *See also* Health behavior
Psychophysiologic disorders, 129. *See also* Psychosomatic health

Psychophysiologic health, 79–80
Psychosis, 80
Psychosocial needs, 165–166, 177. *See also* Basic needs
Psychosocial stages, 107, 108. *See also* Erikson, Erik
Psychosomatic health, 79. *See also* Psychophysiologic disorders
Public health, 279
Public and community health, 81
Public health educator, 49, 189, 190, 192–193, 322. *See also* Health educator
Public relations, 235–237, 351. *See also* Organization and Administration

Question-and-answer method, 351. *See also* Traditional methods
Questionnaire. *See* Evaluation, examples of

Rathbone, Frank, 28, 33, 35, 42
Rathbone, Estelle, 28, 33, 35, 42
Read, Donald A., 151, 161
Recitation method, 352. *See also* Traditional methods
Rehabilitation, 23, 24, 26, 352
Reich, Charles A., 127, 139
Reliability, 352. *See also* Evaluation
Research method, 352. *See also* Approaches, learner-centered
Resource guide, 352. *See also* Curriculum guides
Resources. *See* Learning resources
Retention, 352. *See also* Learning
Retroactive facilitation, 352. *See also* Conditioning
Retroactive inhibition, 352. *See also* Conditioning
Retrospective approach. *See* Evaluation, and learner progress
Retrospective evaluation, 352. *See also* Evaluation
Rogers, Carl, 133, 134, 136, 275, 290
Roman health promotion, 8
Ross, Helen S., 16, 18
Ruch, Floyd, 115, 122, 134
Russell, Robert D., 296, 315, 318

Safety, 82–83, 267–268, 280–281
Samuel Bronfman Foundation, 262
Sanitary Commission of Massachusetts, 9
San Ramon Unified School District, 274

Strategies. *See* Learning strategies; Methodology
Strategy, defined, 353
Subjective test, 353. *See also* Evaluation
Subliminal, 353
Sulkin, Sidney, 247, 290
Sumption, Merle, 234, 236, 245
Superego, 133
Surveys. *See* Evaluation, examples of

Tanner, Daniel, 149–150, 161
Tay-Sacks disease, 55
Teacher, 46
Teacher-centered approaches. *See* Methodolgy
Teacher-centered curriculum guide, 353. *See also* Curriculum guide
Teacher-centered methods, 353. *See also* Approaches in health education
Teacher competencies, 89, 298. *See also* Professional preparation
Teacher-learner relations, 275
Teacher-made tests, 336. *See also* Evaluation
Teacher objectives. *See* Objectives
Teacher training, 13. *See also* Professional preparation
Teaching, 25. *See also* Approaches in health education; Methodology
Teaching/learning teams, 353. *See also* Advisory committees
Teaching methods, 353. *See also* Approaches in health education; Methodology
Teaching resources, 49. *See also* Learning resources
Teaching strategies, 353. *See also* Strategies
Techniques, 353. *See also* Methodology
Terminal goal, 72, 353. *See also* Goal; Objectives
Textbook method, 353. *See also* Curriculum guides; Methodology
Thalassemia, 55–56
Therapeutic approaches. *See* Medical care
Tillich, Paul, 134
Tinkelman, Sherman E., 325, 341
Tosteson, Daniel, 67
Trabasso, Thomas R., 127
Traditional health education, 25, 53–55. *See also* Traditional methods

Traditional methods, 300–304. *See also* Methodology
Transfer of learning, 353. *See also* Learning
Transmitter of message, 353. *See also* Information theory
Treatment, 26–28. *See also* Disease
Tresnowscki, Bernard R., 69
Triad of health education, 262
True-false items, 326. *See also* Evaluation
Turner, C. E., 10
Typhoid fever, 113–114

Unconditioned response, 353. *See also* Conditioning
Unconditioned stimulus, 353. *See also* Conditioning
U.S. Department of Health, Education and Welfare, 42, 65, 211
United States Public Health Service, 211

Validity. *See* Evaluation; Face validity
Values clarification, 79, 134, 166, 311–312, 353. *See also* Approaches in health education, experimental
Venereal diseases, 85–86
Verbal communication. *See* Communications
Vertical curriculum format. *See* Curriculum guides
Vision, conservation of, 271
Voluntary health agencies, 50, 354. *See also specific agencies*

Walker, Rosabelle, 51, 67, 118, 122
Ward, Barbara, 44
Warga, Richard G., 128, 140
White House Conference on Child Health and Protection, 9, 10
Whitman, Walt, 113
Wilhelm, Fred T., 250, 290
Willgoose, Carl, 45, 67, 263, 290
Wilner, Daniel, 51, 67, 118, 122
Women's Christian Temperance Union, 9
Woodward, Kenneth, 215
World health, 281–282
World Health Organization, 26–27, 33

York College, 200

Zimmering, Stanley, 195, 215
Zimmerli, William H., 229